(Fibromyalgia

**THE DOCTOR'S COMPLETE GUIDE TO
VITAMINS AND MINERALS**
BRINGS YOU HEALTH-ENHANCING,
LIFESAVING BENEFITS OF
VITAMINS, MINERALS, AND ESSENTIAL NUTRIENTS.

DR. MARY DAN EADES'S
INNOVATIVE **A-TO-Z LISTING OF AILMENTS AND
CONDITIONS**
REVEALS THE LATEST MEDICAL KNOWLEDGE ABOUT

- NIACIN TO INCREASE MOBILITY AND DECREASE
  PAIN OF **ARTHRITIS**

- TRYPTOPHAN TO CURB **BINGE EATING**

- AVOIDING RED MEAT AND EGG YOLKS TO FIGHT
  THE COMMON COLD

- MACRONUTIENT DIETS TO BOOST **ENERGY** AND
  END **FATIGUE**

- FOLIC ACID MOUTH RINSE TO REDUCE **GINGIVITIS**

- ESSENTIAL FATTY ACIDS TO DECREASE FREQUENCY
  OF **HEADACHES**

- VITAMIN C AND BIOFLAVONOIDS TO HELP RELIEVE
  FLUID RETENTION AND HOT FLASHES THAT
  ACCOMPANY **MENOPAUSE**

- CALCIUM AND IRON FOR **BRITTLE NAILS**

- MAGNESIUM TO RELIEVE SYMPTOMS RELATED
  TO **PMS**

- CHELATED ZINC TO REDUCE **PROSTATE GLAND
  ENLARGEMENT**

- VITAMIN E TO PROTECT AGAINST **SKIN CANCER**

- PANTOTHENIC ACID TO RELIEVE **STRESS**

- GLA AND EPA FISH OIL TO STOP **YEAST INFECTIONS**

AND MORE . . .

THE DOCTOR'S COMPLETE GUIDE TO VITAMINS AND MINERALS

Revised Edition

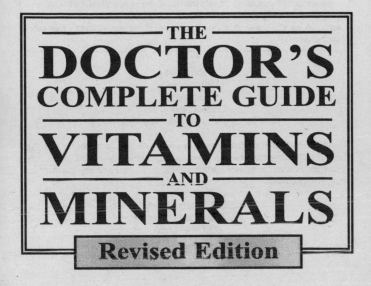

MARY DAN EADES, M.D.

Produced by
The Philip Lief Group, Inc.

A DELL BOOK

Published by
Dell Publishing
a division of
Random House, Inc.
1540 Broadway, New York, New York 10036

Published by arrangement with
The Philip Lief Group, Inc.
130 Wall Street
Princeton, NJ 08850

Dell books may be purchased for business or promotional use or for special sales. For information please write to: Special Markets Department, Random House, Inc., 1540 Broadway, New York, NY 10036.

ISBN: 0-440-23645-2

Printed in the United States of America

Published simultaneously in Canada

July 2000

10 9 8 7 6 5 4 3 2 1

OPM

For my sons,
Ted, Dan, and Scott

with love

CONTENTS

Section Two: Diseases, Disorders, and Conditions from A to Z

ACKNOWLEDGMENTS

I wish to thank Gary Sunshine, Lee Ann Chearneyi, and Philip Lief of The Philip Lief Group for their help and encouragement and for once more giving me the chance to work with them. The lion's share of my gratitude, however, I will have to reserve for my family (my husband Mike, and my boys, Ted, Dan, and Scott) for putting up with me during the writing—a task that is never easy and even less fun. Many thanks, as well, to my faithful clinic staff—to Valerie, Linda, and Rita—who helped to juggle my patient schedule and for the most part left me alone to write when I could.

INTRODUCTION

This book is the natural outgrowth of an interest in nutrition and good health that first began at a very personal level for me and my husband in the late 1970s. He had completed medical school training and I was finishing mine when we met, fell in love, subsequently married, and declared our mutual intention to stay young, fit, and healthy forever. We were not alone—both of us being card-carrying members of the Baby Boomer Generation—in our quest to fend off the ravages of age, but the downside risk of not doing so weighed more heavily on me. As a teenager, I had seen my very strong, active, intelligent, "can-do" father succumb to the ravages of cardiovascular disease (his first heart attack came at 40) and of virulent rheumatoid arthritis. During his 40s, I watched as he underwent a metamorphosis from a 6'4" hearty man who could do anything to a cardiac and arthritic cripple in constant pain. My mother, who I believe became determined to precede my father from this world, smoked her way into an aggressive lung cancer and died at 55. My father died of intractable congestive heart failure three years later at 58. And I, before I was 30, was left bereft of my parents and vowing, as Scarlett O'Hara had, with God as my witness, not to suffer the same fate.

And so my husband (who is also a physician, my partner, and my mentor in the world of nutritional metabolic medicine) and I set about trying to make ourselves knowledgeable in nutrition. The idea of two doctors trying to "make themselves knowledgeable" in nutrition may seem odd to you, but believe me when I say that the amount of general nutrition offered at most medical schools is appallingly meager (and ours was no exception). Certainly, our medical training paid lip service to the fact that "good nutrition" (whatever *that* is) is important in keeping patients healthy. I know most medical schools teach the rudiments of nutrition on that basis, but it's *generally* slim pickings in nutritional education. In some medical courses, physicians learn about vitamins and minerals and how they work from a biochemical standpoint, but nowhere in our training did anyone ever make clear what a potent weapon against disease food, vitamins, and minerals can be. And how much more cost-effective by comparison to virtually any prescription medication. And so the task of understanding this field fell to us to do ourselves.

My husband qualifies as one of the world's most voracious readers, certainly the most broadly read of any person I have ever known. And that made our job easier. We set about reading and studying on our own to try to chart a course of common sense that we hoped would provide us with healthy, long, productive lives. We undertook this educational quest in our spare time, while building and running a chain of general practice outpatient clinics in Little Rock, Arkansas, where we live.

We became involved in national and international specialty societies in areas related to nutritional health, weight control, and longevity, subscribed to their journals, attended their symposia and meetings, and tried to incorporate the principles of nutrition and vitamin and mineral therapy we had learned into our daily practice to as great an extent as possible. After nearly a dozen years in general medical practice, we were able to sell our clinics, retaining the portion of the practice that intrigued us most—weight control and nutritional metabolic rehabilitation—and now devote our full time to it. We currently operate the Arkansas Center for Health and Weight Control, where our guiding premise is to provide nutritional strategies for improving the lives of our patients (as well as our own). And although I cannot personally be your nutritional specialist, through the use of this book, I hope to give you the information you need to develop a nutritional strategy to improve your own life as well. Soon, I'll tell you how you can get the most from this book, but first let me digress to share with you a bit of my own philosophy about vitamins, minerals, herbs, and supplements as medicines.

In the fall of 1992, my husband and I attended a conference in Tulsa, Oklahoma, on the use of nutrition as an accompaniment to improve the conventional treatment of cancers. Although the main thrust of our clinical practice is the nutritional management of obesity and the metabolic health disorders related to it, such as high blood pressure, heart disease, cholesterol problems, and diabetes, and not cancer treatment per se, we were still quite interested to see what was new on the frontiers of therapeutic nutrition from experts around the world. The credentials of all the faculty assembled for this seminar were impressive, but the highlight of the event was the participation of Dr. Linus Pauling. Dr. Pauling—as most people interested in nutrition and vitamin supplementation already know—spent the last 30 or so years of his long and illustrious career researching ascorbic acid and attempting to plumb the depths of its many clinical benefits. But what you may not necessarily recall is that Dr. Pauling, who ranks alongside Albert Einstein as one of the premier scientific minds of the twentieth century, had the singular distinction of having been awarded two—count them, *two*—unshared Nobel Prizes. The first in 1954, a science prize in chemistry for his monumental contribution to that field in elucidating the nature of the chemical bond, and the second, in 1962, a Nobel Peace Prize, received for his fearlessly speaking out against atmospheric testing of the atomic bomb and bringing to light the serious danger it represented to humankind in terms of birth defects and miscarriages. We all owe Dr. Pauling an enormous debt of gratitude for standing up (armed with a head of knowledge and an understanding of atomic chemistry) against the combined voices of the superpowers who shamelessly downplayed the dangers of such open atomic testing. Here was a man of gigantic stature in both the scientific community and the world, and you can imagine how delighted we were to discover that he was to speak to the group assembled there in Tulsa.

Dr. Pauling developed an interest in ascorbic acid about 30 years or so ago almost by serendipity. Apparently, he had given an address to a group in New York and, in it, remarked that he wished he could live another 25 years (he was then in his mid-60s) to see some of the principles he had puzzled out come to fruition. And he had hope that he might, he had said, because his health was reasonably good, he was rarely ill, suffering only from an occasional cold. That admission garnered a note from Irwin Stone, who commented that if he really wanted to avoid those occasional colds and live longer, he would be well advised to take several grams of vitamin C each day.

Being scientifically curious, Dr. Pauling delved more deeply into what basis there might be for such a claim and came away with a firm belief that it was not bunk. There appeared to him to be enough validity to the idea to justify doing some experimentation of his own. When he published his own thoughts on the subject in a book called *Vitamin C and the Common Cold,* touting the value in health of taking doses ranging from 4 to 5 grams up to even 12 to 15 grams of vitamin C each day and claiming that doing so would prevent and cure a cold, his views were roundly and soundly dismissed by much of the traditional medical establishment. Here was a man whose keenly curious mind had revolutionized chemistry, who had been the one voice willing to expose the dangers of open-atmosphere atomic testing, now sharing with the world a hypothesis that something as simple as vitamin C might prove to be a potent nutritional weapon against viral and other illnesses. That would have seemed to be news worth hearing, at least worthy of real scientific inquiry. After all, it wouldn't be the first time in history that a humble vitamin proved to be the miracle cure of serious disease, nor would it have been the first time in history that Linus Pauling was right and others were wrong. But without an honest trial of the hypothesis, the traditional medical establishment pooh-poohed him. Lesser lights of the scientific world scoffed at him, smirked and whispered "poor old Linus has gone round the bend, gone off the deep end with this vitamin C stuff." But as it had done before, time would prove him out.

Dr. Pauling passed away in 1994 at the age of 93, but the research he so diligently began into the potential beneficial effects of ascorbic acid on heart disease, cancer, and viral illness is still being actively pursued by his followers at the Pauling Institute of Science and Medicine in Palo Alto, California. Until the end of his life, he was still in the pursuit of the key to longevity and good health through proper nutrition; he was still flying around the country lecturing to groups like ours. The lecture he presented to us was cogent, witty, humorous, and scientifically informative. I can say without reservation that I was amazed at his ability, and pleased. After all, how many 92-year-olds do you know who have it together enough to give a detailed lecture on a complex subject? I can take that even a step further: How many 92-year-olds do you know? We felt privileged to have been there. Afterward, my husband and I stood, applauding, along with an entire auditorium of international experts in the field of nutrition to pay tribute to this man and his contributions to nutritional science.

Even a momentary discrediting of a person of Linus Pauling's scientific stature, when he proposed a theory that strayed outside the mainstream of traditional establishment medicine, should shame us. That is not to say that clinicians—or laypeople, either, for that matter—should blindly believe anything that someone of scientific note speaks, but neither should we become so narrow and so sure in our thinking that we fail to give a fair and open hearing to novel ideas, even if they seem a bit far-fetched. Openness to unconventional thought freed us from smallpox and protected our children from polio. The courage to stand up as a single voice stating a position running counter to the conventional thinking of the many brought Columbus safely to the New World, instead of off the edge of a flat earth. That same courage, embodied in Dr. Pauling, saved us all from an atmosphere polluted with atomic fallout that our own government would have had us think harmless.

It is in that spirit of questioning investigation that I began to write this vitamin and mineral encyclopedia, which I hope gives you insight into the truths about vitamin and mineral nutrition. I have tried to bring to light what scientific evidence I could uncover to validate "old wives' tales" of putative benefits for specific nutrients or to debunk those myths and tell you why they seem to be false. Where there appears to be benefit, but no hard science backs up the claim, I have made every effort to so state. Where there could be harm from supplementation of a nutrient, I have pointed it out, so that I may follow every physician's principal guiding dictum to "Do No Harm." But throughout the research and the writing of this book, I have attempted to keep an open mind to every possible benefit that may have medical validity, even including those claims that at least appear to have some merit, so long as they cannot cause damage. After all, the goal of vitamin and mineral supplementation is to optimize health, not to damage it. With that in mind, I invite you to join me now in exploring the nutritional facts that fill this work. So that you'll get the most benefit from it, let me take just a moment to tell you how to find what you want to know.

How to Use This Book

The book is divided into two main sections. In the first section, I have provided you with a bit of vitamin history, detailing the circumstances of their discovery and describing for you the classic vitamin deficiency disorders of beriberi, scurvy, pellagra, and rickets. Then I have included a discussion about what vitamins and minerals are and how they generally work in the body. I have tried to keep the science and chemistry of it to a minimum, which may bore the chemistry buffs to tears, but should be enough to give readers of a less chemically scientific bent a clearer understanding of what's going on. Sections on nutraceuticals, antioxidants, free radicals, eicosonoids, and the importance of macronutrients on the effect of the micronutrients should bring you up to speed on the hotbeds of current research areas. In my discussion of the DRI (or Dietary Reference Intake) for the vitamins and minerals, you will learn how these recommendation numbers came about. After that, we'll delve into the idea of whether supplementation is necessary, including a section about the dangers of getting too much of a good thing.

Section I includes an A-to-Z listing of virtually every vitamin, mineral, and nutrient, with some key facts about each one: how it works, its functions in the body, the foods that provide it, the recommended dosages and forms, its interactions with other nutrients or with drugs, and the symptoms of deficiency or of toxicity associated with it. If, for example, you wanted to find out what vitamin D could do for you, or whether taking it could cause problems, or how best to get it from foods, you should look here. New to this revised edition is the Herbal Encyclopedia, which list 37 herbs—from alfalfa to wild yam—with the same key facts for each as provided in the vitamin and mineral section. With herbs like St. John's wort and echinacea now household words, it is important to familiarize yourself with the major herbs, just as you would the major vitamins and minerals. Research has revealed—or, should I say, confirmed, since many of the treatments have been used in some cultures for centuries—the amazing benefits of herbs to prevent, manage, or treat dozens of conditions and diseases, with virtually none of the side effects of conventional medicine.

In Section II, you will find the real heart of the book. Here I have compiled, again in A-to-Z fashion, a comprehensive listing of diseases, disorders, and conditions, along with information on which vitamin(s), mineral(s), and herbs may be important to alleviating that problem. I have tried to make the listings as "reader friendly" as possible, with the disorders entered in layman's terms to make it easier for you to find what you're after. For example, you could look here by symptom or disorder to find out what vitamins or minerals might help dry skin, bleeding gums, painful joints, or the risk for prostate cancer. And if there is more than one commonly used name for an ailment, I have listed each name and directed you to the "mother listing." For example, there may be listings for dry skin, dermatitis, seborrhea, and scaly skin and scalp, but a discussion found only under dermatitis, with the other listings cross-referenced as "see Dermatitis." When the information is the same or very, very similar, I have chosen to combine the entries in this fashion, so that I will be able to give a fuller discussion in one place without being repetitive. For each disorder or condition, I have discussed both conventional and traditional medical wisdom as well as the most up-to-date information I could find.

My goal in writing this book is to provide you with an easy-to-use, up-to-the-minute reference, laid out in a manner that will let you go right to the issue that concerns you at the moment. If you wonder, for example, whether there is a vitamin that you can take to improve the luster of your hair, or help relieve painful menstrual periods, or strengthen your immune system when you have a major virus, you should be able to pick up this book and turn to what interests you and easily find out what you want to know. I hope I have accomplished that goal, that you will enjoy the reading, and that you will benefit in health and longevity from the information I have provided.

One word of caution, however: I do urge you to remember that since I can't see you, take your history, or examine you personally, I would recommend you consult your personal physician about any medical condition beforehand. This book is not intended as a substitute for advice of the appropriate medical professional. Always consult your doctor or appropriate medical professional before making any major dietary changes or taking any vitamin supplementation. And certainly, I would ask you

never to stop or change a treatment your physician has prescribed in favor of vitamin or mineral treatments without first
consulting him or her—doing so can sometimes be very dangerous. Instead, I hope you will use this book as an addition to your
physician's instructions. If you have or can find a physician who
also believes in the power of nutrition, so much the better
for you.

SECTION I
Understanding Vitamins

VITAMINS: A HISTORICAL PERSPECTIVE

Nutrition, or the lack of it, has shaped the world. The pages of history record human suffering, disease, and the disability occasioned by malnourishment through the millennia. From the first description of beriberi in ancient Chinese writings (2500 B.C.) to the blight of scurvy that crippled or destroyed armies and navies from the time of Hippocrates to the Crusades, nutritional deficiency played a role. And it didn't end then. Human suffering from malnutrition followed us straight into the early twentieth century, when physicians filled mental institutions of the post–Civil War American South to overflowing with the hopelessly insane and disabled, many of whom suffered only from lack of the B vitamin niacin. How different a history humankind might have recorded were it not for the diseases occasioned by epidemic vitamin and mineral malnourishment.

Although throughout history medical investigators struggled to discover the link between illness and certain food habits, the concept of dietary deficiency causing disease did not become widely accepted until the late nineteenth century. Prior to that time, the prevailing scientific wisdom held that the diseases called scurvy, beriberi, pellagra, and rickets—which modern nutritional and medical science now accept without question as being caused solely by vitamin deficiencies—were caused by an unknown infectious agent or a toxin or poison in the food. At the turn of the twentieth century, several researchers began to believe that perhaps certain foods contained an "accessory food factor" that prevented disease. Based on early investigations, researchers believed that the critical "accessory food factor" belonged to a group of organic nitrogen-containing compounds called amines. They named their discovery "vital amines" (from the Latin *vita* for life, and the chemical class of *amines*) or vitamines. Continued study would ultimately prove that the compounds were not amines at all, but the name for the food factors stuck. In deference to accuracy or to avoid confusion, the pioneers of nutritional research decided to drop the final "e," creating the name by which we call them today: *vitamins*.[1]

Each disorder and the vitamin deficiency that causes it has a unique and interesting place in medical history, replete with the missed clues, false trails, and serendipity with which the advancement of medical knowledge often stumbles and bumbles forward. I ask you to thumb through the pages of nutritional history with me now as we examine the Big Four dietary deficiency disorders in turn.

The Classic Vitamin Deficiency Diseases

Beriberi: Thiamine (Vitamin B₁) Deficiency

Over 4000 years ago, the ancient Chinese first described the disorder we recognize today as thiamine deficiency. This disorder, with the unusual name *beriberi,* strikes a wide assortment of body systems. Impairment of the nervous system and muscles from insufficient thiamine in the diet causes symptoms ranging from pain and weakness to paralysis and wasting; in the gastrointestinal tract, lack of thiamine may cause nausea, vomiting, bowel sluggishness, and constipation; and mental aberrations from mild irritability to frank depression, dementia, and paranoia can occur as well. Carried to its extreme, thiamine deficiency proves fatal.

It is not surprising that the ancient Chinese, in their voluminous writings on medicine, would have identified and first recorded the symptoms of this vitamin deficiency disease, since thiamine is found in the husks or bran of rice, a main staple in the Orient. Once the rice has been milled to remove the bran, however, most of the thiamine is lost. And so, with the advent of milling processes, the incidence of beriberi among the Chinese increased. Modern food manufacturers add thiamine back into milled rice products—a process called enriching the rice. But even today, beriberi occurs in third world countries where populations rely on milled, unenriched, white rice as a main dietary staple.

In the nineteenth century, a Japanese naval scientist named Kanehiro Takaki observed that some crews on long voyages at sea fell victim to an alarming number of cases of a deadly form of nerve inflammation, while the crews of other ships did not. In examining the dietary differences between ships, Takaki noted that the crews that escaped serious health problems carried less polished rice and more meat, fish, vegetables, wheat, and milk than the stricken crews. The addition of these foods (which all are rich in thiamine) to the sailors' diets prevented nerve problems and deaths from beriberi, which prevailing medical wisdom of the day held to be infectious—an opinion mainstream medical scientists continued to hold even after Takaki published his observations in a prestigious medical journal. The idea that disease could be caused by lack of some substance in the diet simply hadn't taken root in medical thought at that time. It was not, in fact, until 1890 that a Dutch physician named Christiaan Eijkman observed the causative connection between beriberi and diets high in polished rice. Ten years later, his colleague, Gerrit Grijns, proved that the disease could be prevented by adding the polishings back into the diet. One small mental step for Drs. Eijkman and Grijns, one giant leap for the nutritional good of humankind.[2, 3]

Pellagra: Niacin (Vitamin B$_3$) Deficiency

Medical historians credit an eighteenth-century Spaniard named Gaspar Casal for the first Western description (c. 1735) of pellagra, as well as for his observation of its frequent occurrence among people relying on maize (corn) as a staple. Although the disease did occur commonly in Spain, it also claimed victims in southern France, Italy (its name is, in fact, from the Italian *pelle agra,* meaning rough skin),[4] and the Balkan states in Europe.

In the Americas, pellagra occurred widely in the midwestern and southeastern portions of the United States and swept with a vengeance through the rural South following the Civil War, where impoverished populations subsisted on milled cornmeal, white flour, sweet potatoes, rice, and sugar: all foods with little usable niacin (or other B vitamins, for that matter). Although whole corn does contain niacin, humans cannot absorb the vitamin from corn.

It occurs in a "bound" form—called niacytin—in which the niacin is attached to another large fibrous substance that the human gastrointestinal tract cannot readily absorb. However, treatment of the cornmeal with an alkaline solution, such as lime—a culinary practice common for centuries in Mexico and the southwestern United States to make it suitable for tortilla preparation—releases the vitamin from its nyacytin bound form, freeing the niacin in the corn for absorption by the intestine. Reliance on the lowly tortilla spared the Mexican and southwestern Indian populations from the ravages of pellagra even though corn is a dietary staple in these areas, too.

Deficiency of niacin causes the development of not only an inflamed scaly skin eruption, swollen red tongue, and irritation of the intestinal lining with diarrhea, but severe mental disturbance, as well. In fact, as recently as the 1920s, medical specialists condemned huge numbers of unfortunate people to the grisly confines of mental institutions for intractable mental derangement that could have been cured by adequate niacin in their diets.

Niacin insufficiency still occurs in Asia and southern Africa, where maize constitutes a significant portion of the diet.

Scurvy: Ascorbic Acid (Vitamin C) Deficiency

Although it was not until 1932 that Hungarian scientist Albert Szent-Gyorgyi discovered vitamin C (and subsequently received the Nobel Prize for his efforts), the disease resulting from insufficient dietary intake of this vitamin has existed in medical writings since 1500 B.C. *Scurvy,* as the deficiency is called, likely holds the honor of most famous (or infamous) of all the classic deficiency diseases. Rare would be the American schoolchild whose history or science education did not include lessons about the ravages of scurvy among the sailors in the British navy. In fact, some historians credit the discovery by British naval physician James Lind in 1753 that lemons, limes, and fresh green produce would prevent scurvy on long sea voyages and the implementing of a policy taking these foods on board British ships with the subsequent era of dominance of the British navy at sea.[5] The reliance of the British navy on this means of nutritional supplementation led eighteenth-century Americans to coin the nickname "Limeys" to refer to British sailors.

Even though this method of scurvy prevention had been used for over a century and a half, we often fail to heed the lessons of history, to overlook them, or to discount them at any rate. And so scurvy did not disappear after the publication of Dr. Lind's findings in the mid–eighteenth century. As incredible as it seems, there are Americans living today who were children way back in 1912 when Captain Robert Scott headed his ill-fated expedition to the South Pole. Without a supply of foods containing vitamin C, every person on the expedition died of scurvy.

What, then, is scurvy? The symptoms of the disorder usually begin insidiously with lassitude, fatigue, and irritability, followed by bleeding and inflammation of the gums, loosening of the teeth, bruising, then finally hemorrhaging, which can prove fatal. The problem arises because of the key role that vitamin C plays in the production of strong, well-formed collagen, the chief protein component of fibrous tissue, without which the body would literally fall apart. When the body has insufficient vitamin C, the collagen manufactured to build and maintain the fibrous tissue framework becomes weaker. This weaker, flimsier tissue tears and breaks more easily, as evidenced most visibly by the fragility of the walls of the blood vessels, which rupture and bleed.

The other equally if not more important function of vitamin C—namely, its role as a potent antioxidant—also figures into the development of scurvy. I'll explain what an antioxidant is and together we'll take a look how antioxidants protect us from aging and disease shortly, but for the moment, let's move on to the last of the classic deficiency diseases: rickets.

Rickets: Vitamin D (Cholecalciferol) Deficiency

Since antiquity, developing children have succumbed to rickets the disease that results in bowed, bent, or otherwise misshapen bones. Rickets develops from two specific deficiencies: a diet deficient in vitamin D (cholecalciferol) and an environment without sufficient sunshine, which acts on substances in the skin to make vitamin D work. Dietary deficiency might occur as the result of famine, extreme poverty, or cultural dietary restraints. But how could a child grow up deficient in sunshine? Living, for example, in arctic regions where the "dark" season limits hours of sunlight and heavy clothing against the cold limits what little light there is from reaching the skin could make a child susceptible to the disorder. Lack of sunlight could occur if the air were fouled by pollutants that block out the sunlight—perhaps from volcanic eruption in antiquity, or from industrial smokestacks in the eighteenth century, or from severe smog in modern times. (Let me add here that just a few intermittent days of smoggy haze is not enough to cause deficiency in vitamin D.) Even cultural mores can influence the development of rickets from insufficient sunlight. In India, for example, the incidence of rickets in rich, well-fed Muslims under 20 years of age is an astounding 70%, whereas rickets occurs in only 20% of the well-fed upper-class Hindus and almost not at all among the lower-class Hindus eating very poor diets. The remarkable difference here is a cultural custom: the Muslims remain primarily indoors and keep the young children continually indoors, the well-off Hindu families spend less time indoors, and the poor may literally live outside.[6]

Although the skeletal record of humankind records the presence of rickets throughout human history, it was not until 1650 that an English physician, Francis Glisson, gave medical history its first concise description of the disease. (Daniel Whistler, another English physician, had written a thesis describing rickets in 1645; however, many historians believe that he relied heavily on the work of Glisson for his information.)[7]

Rickets reached epidemic proportions during the industrial revolution in England when young, still-developing children marched off before dawn to work until night in the factories and mines. Rarely seeing the sun because of spending long hours indoors or subterraneously, living on diets composed primarily of gruel, bread, and other starchy vegetables, with little meat or milk, the young children of eighteenth-century industrialized English cities could not help but fall victim to deficiency of vitamin D. Rural children on diets of eggs, butter, meat, and plenty of sunshine exposure escaped the fate of their city cousins.

Vitamin D occurs naturally only in foods of animal origin: liver, butter, egg yolk, and fatty-fleshed fish—such as mackerel, herring, salmon, cod, or oils extracted from fish liver. (Note: Milk in its natural state does not contain much vitamin D, but for many years, manufacturers have fortified milk products sold in the United States with vitamin D. We Americans, therefore, have become accustomed to thinking of milk as a good source of vitamin D and calcium for strong bones, which nowadays in its fortified state, it is.)

By the middle of the eighteenth century, medical practitioners clearly understood that rickets could be prevented or cured by adding cod liver oil to the diet; however, the connection became muddled a bit because they also quite clearly recognized that sunlight exposure prevented or cured rickets, Medical research did not dispel the confusion surrounding the biochemical basis of why both of these regimens worked until years later. And so, the practice of dosing the family with cod liver oil for nearly any ailment gained a broad popularity base, much to the chagrin of the children. The taste is potent to say the least, and thanks to fortification of dairy products with vitamin D_2 and plenty of sunshine (actually, the ultraviolet light converts a skin chemical to cholecalciferol or vitamin D_3), America's infants and young children can escape the regular doses of cod liver oil that plagued their forebears.

You're now acquainted with the role that vitamins have played in history, and it should be readily apparent to you that they are critically important to our good health and survival. But why? What are they, anyway? What do they do? How do they work their invisible magic in the human machine?

What Are Vitamins?

The term *vitamin* applies only to a specific group of organic compounds—those composed of chains of carbon, hydrogen, and oxygen in various arrangements, augmented sometimes with nitrogen, sulfur, phosphorus, and occasional other chemical elements—that medical science has shown are necessary to life. For us to say that a substance is a vitamin, it has to be something your body requires for good health and normal functioning—in other words, you've got to take it into your diet regularly in some amount, however small, or you will become ill. *Its absence from your diet must result in your developing an identifiable and reproducible disease or disorder.* I emphasize the last statement to make clear the difference between those substances that truly function as vitamins and other compounds, termed "false vitamins," that you may derive some benefit from, that may make you feel somewhat better when you take them, but that do not result in a specific deficiency disease if you don't. That doesn't mean you should not take it; it simply means that technically we can't call it a "true" vitamin. We can, however, call it a *nutrient*, which is nothing more than a component of food that nourishes our body. A nutrient can be essential to life or nonessential. A vitamin, on the other hand, can only be essential.

To complicate matters further, even a "true" vitamin is not

always a vitamin. For example, most mammals produce their own vitamin C (ascorbic acid) and therefore do not require addition of it in their diets for good health. For these species, ascorbic acid is not a vitamin, even though it is precisely that same compound carrying out the same functions as what we refer to as vitamin C. We humans, you and I, along with certain primates, the guinea pig, and the fruit-eating bat—all species that have lost the ability to produce our own vitamin C—must regularly eat a diet that provides us with an adequate amount of vitamin C or else suffer disease and disability and finally die from the lack. For us, the apes, the guinea pig, and those bats, ascorbic acid is indeed a vitamin, meeting the two basic criteria: (1) we cannot make it ourselves and therefore must eat foods containing it; and (2) it is absolutely necessary for our lives and health, and we will develop specific, identifiable symptoms every time we are without it.

Alphabet Soup

The Nonsense of Vitamin Names

Medical scientists first began to try to identify the "accessory food factor" by searching for a single substance in rice polishings that prevented beriberi. By 1906, however, Frederick Gowland Hopkins published work demonstrating that a different sort of food factor also occurred in milk, and then further experiments by other workers turned up yet another food factor in the water extract of yeast. The appearance of several of these "food factors" demanded some sort of naming system by which they could be differentiated. Because one factor appeared to be a substance dissolved in the butterfat of milk and another factor dissolved in the water from a yeast solution, the terms *fat soluble* and *water soluble* arose. The two factors were initially dubbed "fat-soluble A" and "water-soluble B," and then by the logical progression of that system, vitamin C for a third substance in fruit that prevented scurvy. It is from these humble and reasonably logical origins that we get what has become a very confusing nomenclature of vitamins.

After these orderly beginnings, a little further down the discovery road, research teams discovered a whole series of factors within both the fat-soluble A and the water-soluble B groups. The first new fat-soluble component, one that influenced growth and development, became—you guessed it—vitamin D, since that was the next available letter in the alphabetical scheme. Then further research demonstrated multiple components of the water-soluble Bs, each one of which has specific disease-preventing capabilities, and each of which was given a B-vitamin subnumber. And so, this scheme ultimately gave us vitamins A, B_1, B_2, B_3, B_6, B_{12}, C, D, E, and K. We don't have a B_4, B_7, B_8, B_9, B_{10}, or B_{11} because these "vitamins" that were discovered by various researchers subsequently turned out in truth to be some minor variant of vitamins B_1, B_2, B_3, B_6, or B_{12}.[8]

In recent years, medical and nutritional researchers have tried to supplant the alphabet soup nomenclature with the actual chemical names of the vitamin compounds, but old habits die hard. Throughout both the lay and professional literature, cobalamin will still more often be called B_{12}, but thiamine has replaced B_1 and niacin has replaced B_3, ascorbic acid and vitamin C both appear often, but more people recognize vitamin D than its chemical name cholecalciferol, and so on. I will try throughout to call the substances by their commonest names, whether that's of the ABC system or otherwise; bear with me if I slip up.

How Do Vitamins Work?

What a piece of work is man!
How noble in reason!
How infinite in faculties!
In form and moving how express and admirable!
In action how like an angel!
In apprehension how like a god!
The beauty of the world, the paragon of animals!
—*Hamlet* II.ii.203
William Shakespeare

Hamlet ended his observations on man in Act 2, Scene 2 by calling him a quintessence of dust. Perhaps a quintessence of chemicals might have been closer to the truth. The energy required to blink the eyelid, to move a finger, to take a breath; the nerve signals that make the heart beat, that sense and respond to the need to breathe, to eat, to sleep—perchance to dream, as Shakespeare's tortured prince would have said—depends on an intricately choreographed interplay of chemistry. What a piece of work, indeed; a miraculous, complex, convoluted work of art.

But enough of literature, back to chemistry. Each of those finely tuned chemical reactions that makes us a piece of work depends on helper substances called enzymes to speed up (or catalyze) the reaction. And each of those enzymes requires some kind of helper of its own (called a cofactor) to be whole and active. And those cofactors—or coenzymes, as they are sometimes also called—are very often vitamins or minerals or both. So distilled to the essence—or quintessence—we're a big bag of chemistry that couldn't happen without vitamins and minerals.

The chemical reactions that the enzymes and their vitamin and mineral cofactors speed up usually involve moving around (or transferring) different chemical structures, transforming one kind of molecule to another, or the addition or removal of hydrogen atoms between molecules (oxidation/reduction reactions). The main vitamins that act as coenzymes in these kinds of reactions are biotin, vitamin B_{12}, folic acid, niacin, pantothenic acid, vitamin B_6, riboflavin, and thiamine.[9] The oxidation reactions, especially, are important to us because of their role in the aging process. Let's take a moment to look a little deeper into this particular chemical reaction: oxidation.

Oxidation and Reduction

Broken down to our simplest subunits, we are merely a nearly infinite collection of atoms and molecules. Every organ, every tissue, every protein, enzyme, or cell shares this trait as a lowest common denominator of life. The atoms that make us what we are exist in a state of electrical neutrality or balance, with all their electrons happily paired. The electrons are negatively charged particles that orbit in pairs around the atom's nucleus or center of positively charged and neutrally uncharged particles. Normally, the number of positives in the center matches the number of negatives whirling about it, leaving the atom electrically balanced. However, if everything stayed electrically neutral, we couldn't survive. Our bodies depend upon the generation of energy through the shuffling of these electrons from one kind of molecule to another in a controlled fashion. This activity is called a redox reaction and occurs in each cell, primarily in structures within the cell called the mitochondria. Think of these mitochondria as little energy factories.

The name *redox* derives from the two phases of this kind of energy-transferring activity: reduction, a process by which a molecule gains (or accepts) an electron from another substance, and oxidation, the reverse process in which a molecule loses (or donates) an electron to another molecule. In the donating process, the electron given or lost breaks up a matched pair of electrons that were happily in orbit around the nucleus, converting the molecule into what biochemists term a *free radical*. Once formed, the free radical becomes intensely reactive, by which I mean it becomes very desirous of mating up its lonely single or free electron with one from another molecule. The formation of a free radical sets in motion a sort of biochemical equivalent of robbing Peter to pay Paul: atom A takes B's electron, B takes C's, C takes D's, and so on. As long as the cascading process stays controlled, all is well.

Free Radical Chic

The formation of free radicals, however, does not always occur to our benefit. Damaging effects of chemicals, sunlight, ozone, cigarette smoke, food additives, and oxygen contribute to the formation of free radicals that lead to aging and disease development. Day by day, the evidence suggesting that free radical damage to human tissue is the driving force behind conditions ranging from arthritis to cataracts to heart disease to cancer grows stronger. But the free radical theory, so *en vogue* today, is not new. Dr. Denham Harman, professor emeritus at the University of Nebraska, originated the idea in 1954 and has spent much of the last 40 years defending the notion against the unified forces of establishment medicine, which tended to downplay its importance and to pooh-pooh its validity. Dr. Denham, now in his mid-70s, must feel an enormous sense of vindication these days, with researchers the world over jumping on his bandwagon. Let me take a few moments to tell you about the theory of the radicals and touch on just some of the current work under way that points the accusing finger at these subcellular kamikazes.

As I mentioned in the preceding section, free radicals form when molecules oxidize. Once stripped of one of its happy pair of electrons, the molecule (now a radical) becomes intensely reactive, and in its mindless quest to restore its own electrical balance, will rob an electron from some other molecule. That process may (and usually in these instances does) damage the victim molecule: damage it, alter it, or age it. The innocent molecule in question could be a subunit of any cell of any tissue in the body. Often the free radicals do their dirty work to the DNA (deoxyribonucleic acid) that makes up the genetic material in the nucleus of every cell and that houses all the information that makes us work. Severe damage to the genetic material will at best render the cell useless and at worst turn it into a rogue cell, uncontrolled and wild, that can become the seed of cancerous change. So free radicals are bad news. Or are they?

As is so often the case in life, there are two sides to this coin. Free radicals are, on one hand, unequivocally biologically damaging, and on the other, unequivocally necessary for health. The proper functioning of a healthy immune system depends on a burst of free radicals being released from the white blood cells in their defensive assault on viruses and bacteria. Without free radicals as weapons, the killing power of these immune fighters would be nil, and we would be rendered defenseless against infection. It's that old dichotomy: one man's meat is another man's poison, I believe it goes.

So what can we do to protect ourselves from—or at least minimize—the unfavorable kind of free radical attack? You guessed it: vitamins and minerals of the right kind and in sufficient doses will fend off the damage. Since the damage is primarily oxidative, the group of vitamins and minerals receiving the greatest research attention in containing free radical damage fall into a category called, naturally enough, the *antioxidants*. Let's take a look at the research (some of it quite new) into several specific members of this important group: the vitamins A, C, and E, beta-carotene (a nutrient related to vitamin A), the minerals selenium and zinc, and the peptide glutathione. Although disagreement among experts still exists about whether you should consider higher doses of these nutrients and vitamins as preventives and therapies for disease, the case *for* such a role is quite strong.

Take vitamin E (tocopherol), for instance. In the early days after its discovery, nutritionists and alternative practitioners touted roles for this vitamin for everything from dandruff to wrinkles, but without a surfeit of medical evidence, the "fad" of taking vitamin E faded. The medical establishment decried these claims as quackery and snake oil. Now, after much more intensive medical examination, Dr. Meir Stampfer, at the American Heart Association's annual meeting in November 1992, stated that taking a supplemental dose of 100 IU of vitamin E per day cut the risk of heart disease by 46% in a recent Harvard Health Study involving quite a large group of nurses (87,000). Another Harvard study, the Physicians' Health Study, showed a 50% reduction in expected heart attacks in 333 males (known to have heart disease) who took 30 mg beta-carotene every other day. Quite a swing in perspective.

On the immune system front, a study conducted by the Human Nutrition Research Center on Aging showed that 800 IU of vitamin E could boost immune response in the elderly. And yet another study, this one by the Memorial University of Newfoundland, corroborates that role, suggesting that the addition of supplemental doses of vitamin E and beta-carotene taken along with the standard U.S. Department of Agriculture recommended dietary allowance (or RDA) for all other vitamins and minerals reduced infection-related illness by 50% in 96 healthy elderly volunteers.[10] And going beyond infection fighting, beta-carotene (the vitamin A relative found in plants) at a dose of 30 mg daily caused precancerous lesions of the lining of the mouth (called leukoplakiae, meaning white patches) to shrink or disappear in 70% of the participants in an Arizona Cancer Center research study.

Along that same line, a 12-year-long Swiss study conducted on 3000 men recently found that low blood levels of beta-carotene and retinol (vitamin A) correlated highly with increased risk for lung cancer and with death from cancer of all kinds. Researchers project corroborating work, currently under way in the United States, to be finished this year. This series of tests, dubbed CARET, for Carotene and Retinol Efficacy Trials, looks at this connection between the carotenoids and the retinols and cancer prevention. The hypothesis hinges on the knowledge that beta-carotene acts as a protective antioxidant, preventing cellular damage, and retinol acts to normalize cell growth and intercellular communication. In concert, the researchers hope the pair of vitamins will reduce the occurrence of lung cancer.

Work, presented at a symposium on Adjuvant Nutrition in Cancer Treatment by Mark Levine, M.D., of the National Institute of Health/Johns Hopkins University, shows that vitamin C may be a critical antioxidant protector to immune cells. These particular defense cells kill foreign invaders (bacteria, fungi, cancerous cells) by what amounts to dumping oxidizing free radicals onto them. To be able to do that, however, means the immune defender cells have to storehouse and convey their free radical toxins. Vitamin C may allow these defenders to do so without risk to themselves. At that same symposium, Dr. Linus Pauling spoke about the role vitamin C—or rather the lack of sufficient amounts of it—appears to play in the development of atherosclerotic heart and blood vessel disease, based on new work coming from the Linus Pauling Institute of Science and Medicine. This new information dovetails nicely with the already proven effect that vitamin C can lower serum cholesterol.

Another study, also presented at the above-mentioned symposium, was conducted to determine whether supplemental vitamin C would improve the strength and integrity of blood vessels in the feet and hands, kidneys, and retinas of diabetic patients. It concluded that 1 gram of the vitamin daily indeed improved the strength of capillaries. Although that statement may seem pretty tame, it's really quite remarkable in the light that the overwhelming majority of health complications that befall the diabetic person are a direct consequence of disease of small blood vessels and capillaries. So, clearly a scientifically conducted clinical study proving that you could correct these terrible diabetic problems by something as simple and direct as vitamin C supplementation would be nothing short of a monumental breakthrough.[11]

Information presented at the American Academy of Ophthalmology meeting in the late fall of 1992 by Dr. David Newsome of Tulane University showed improvement in at least one-third of people with macular degeneration placed on antioxidant vitamins and zinc. Macular degeneration is a condition in which the most acutely seeing portion of the retina, called the macula, begins to fall apart, ultimately leading to severe visual impairment or blindness. A Finnish study on accumulated data from patients dating from 1966 to 1972 found the correlation of low blood levels of alpha-tocopherol (vitamin E) and beta-carotene with a doubling of risk for the subsequent development of cataracts.[12]

Daily, the information mounts clarifying the protective, preventive, and therapeutic roles for the antioxidant vitamins in human disease. And more and more it appears that once again Dr. Pauling sounded the call to arms in the war on aging and disease when he began to advocate vitamin C. Perhaps there's a connection between the fact that he began to protect himself with 18,000 grams of ascorbic acid and 800 IU per day of alpha-tocopherol in his 60s and the fact that he lived to celebrate his 94th birthday. Whatever the role that vitamin and mineral supplementation played for Dr. Pauling, and whatever role it may play in your war on aging and disease, vitamins and minerals alone cannot save you from an overall unhealthy lifestyle. I think Dr. Jeffrey Blumberg said it best: "Vitamins are like seat belts. Wearing a seat belt doesn't give you a license to drive recklessly, it just protects you in case of an accident. Vitamin supplements work in the same way: they don't give you a license to eat poorly and otherwise abuse your health, but provide an added cushion of protection."[13]

Turn with me now and let's look at the bigger picture—the basic diet you eat—and the role it will play in your response to vitamin and mineral supplementation.

Leveling the Playing Field: Macronutrient Effects

What, you may be asking yourself, is a macronutrient? And what, pray, does it have to do with playing fields, level or otherwise? Fair question. The macronutrients are the major dietary fuels, that is the proteins, carbohydrates (starches and sugars), and fats that make up the foods we eat. Everything from bagels to bananas to T-bone steaks is composed of varying amounts of protein, carbohydrate, or fat—the *macro*nutrients that create the field upon which the actions of the vitamin and mineral *micro*nutrients takes place.[14] If, as Dr. Blumberg so glibly put it, vitamins are like seat belts, then the basic foods we eat are the whole bloomin' car. And without a safe, well-built car, what good are the seat belts? The moral of which is: before you spend your valuable time and hard-earned dollars seeking out and taking micronutrient supplements, I would recommend that you start by building a level playing field. By that I mean that if you begin with sound general dietary composition, you will reap far greater and more predictable benefit from the vitamins and minerals you add to that basic framework. Let me illustrate for you.

Say, for example, a group of nutritional researchers turns out a beautiful scientific study on the beneficial role of a particular vitamin—it could be any vitamin—on a certain medical condition. And no sooner has the ink dried on their paper than some other research team—studying the same vitamin effect—turns out an equally beautiful and scientific study that shows the vitamin to be of no benefit in that condition. What could possibly explain such totally conflicting data? Is one group of researchers inept? Unscrupulous? Poorly trained? Although I suppose anything's possible, the truth is that both groups probably reported exactly what they found as accurately as they could. In one instance, the vitamin appeared to benefit the condition, in another it did not. Simple, but *why?*

The why of it may arise from the two studies being fought out on "unlevel" playing fields. Study participants in one group may have eaten a diet that provided a basic background of protein, carbohydrate, and fat that created a favorable chemical environment for the vitamin to act—and they benefited from the supplementation. And the other group, perhaps, did not.

Vitamin and mineral research abounds with such conflicting data, but very often, the studies ignore the macronutrient composition of the diet and focus only on the dosage and effect (if any) of the micronutrient in question. Let me forge ahead with this concept to illustrate for you how the composition of the diet you eat will play a major role in how well you respond to vitamin and mineral supplementation.

—— The Yin and Yang of Human Health ——

The Chinese concept of yin and yang—the universe existing in a delicate balance of opposing forces such as good and evil, light and dark, happiness and despair—serves as an appropriate metaphor for the workings of the human body. For virtually every body chemical that exerts a "good" influence, there exists its "evil twin," a body chemical that does the opposite. (I say "evil" twin, but in reality, that's too simple. I would better serve the truth to say *opposite twin,* because oftentimes, the opposite force in body chemistry to "good" is not "bad." It's just "opposite.") For example, one body chemical might relax blood vessels and thereby reduce blood pressure; its opposing chemical then would constrict blood vessels and increase blood pressure. Yin and yang. To keep our bodies humming along like well-oiled human machines, we would naturally like the "good" influences to carry the day. And here is where the role of macronutrients—the food we consume—comes into the picture. I will lay out for you an optimal macronutrient strategy in just a moment, but first let me digress one step further to explain why this strategy is so important.

The Eicosinoid Messengers

Among the key players in promoting the "good" side of the yin and yang of health—of critical importance in getting that playing field level—are a group of body chemicals called the *eicosinoids* (pronounced: eye-kah'-sin-oyds), which influence and regulate a wide range of body functions, including blood pressure, the immune system, blood clotting, inflammation, and pain control. We can maintain a supply of these eicosinoids by eating certain kinds of polyunsaturated fats, the primary one being linoleic acid. Our bodies can take this basic kind of fat and alter it in stepwise fashion to make the various members of the eicosinoid gang.

The action of the eicosinoids, as chemical messengers, typifies the yin and yang of health, because there are very clearly "good" ones and "bad" ones. The "good" group promotes such healthy occurrences as lowered blood pressure, thinner blood to prevent abnormal clotting that can lead to heart attacks, reduced inflammation and the pain that occurs in such diseases as arthritis, and a stronger immune system especially against attack by viruses. And the "bad" group? Well, they do precisely the reverse. But here's the kicker. Our bodies make both the good and the bad kinds of these chemical messengers starting with *the same dietary fat: linoleic acid.* Whether the linoleic acid in the foods you eat becomes an eicosinoid beneficial to you or one of the group detrimental to you depends largely on the overall composition of your diet.

Recent research into what basic dietary framework would favor the production of mainly the "good" messengers indicates that a diet that controls the output of insulin (a metabolic hormone that increases when we overeat starches and sugars) benefits most people. What would the macronutrient composition of such a diet look like?

According to the National Research Council, you should get 35% of your daily calories from complex carbohydrates, which are found in grains, breads, and starchy vegetables. Fifteen percent of your calories should be obtained from simple carbohydrates, those high-sugar foods such as sweets and fruits. The Mayo Health Clinic recommends similar amounts, suggesting that 60% of your daily calories come from carbohydrates.

You should get another 15 to 20% of your daily calories from protein sources such as lean meats, nonfat dairy products, soy products, and beans. The number of calories you eat from these protein foods must be enough to provide you with at least one-half gram of protein for each pound of lean body weight. Your lean body weight (LBW) is your weight with all the water and fat tissue removed: the muscles, organs, bones, skin. You can calculate it by various means:

1) You can figure it yourself; the details of such methods are readily found in either of two good books noted below.[15]

2) There are computerized machines that will calculate body

composition for you. You may find such machines by checking with your physician, a diet specialist in your area, or a fitness center.

3) You can use the rough guestimate method outlined below. This method won't be totally accurate, but it will at least get you into the ballpark easily and with little arithmetic.

Gender	Build	Approximate LBW
Female	slender	75–80% of weight
Female	moderately overweight	65% of weight
Female	obese	55–60% of weight
Male	slender	80–85% of weight
Male	moderately overweight	70% of weight
Male	obese	60–65% of weight

Once you locate the category that most nearly describes you, take your weight in pounds and multiply it by the percent (to the right of the description) as a decimal. The answer will be your approximate lean body weight. (Example: A woman, describing herself as moderately overweight, weighing 165 pounds would calculate her lean body weight as follows: $165 \times .65 = 107.25$ pounds. If for each of those 107 pounds, she must eat $\frac{1}{2}$ gram of lean protein each day, her daily intake of protein would be 107/2 or 53.5 grams *as a minimum* to preserve lean tissue.)

I would encourage you to purchase a complete book of food values (there are dozens of them at almost any bookstore) that details for you the protein, fat, carbohydrate, and calorie level of most foods. Some of these reference sources even include the values of typical fast foods, prepackaged foods, and junk foods, as well as the fiber content and major vitamin and mineral content. Roam through the pages of your book of food counts and get a feel for the nutritional content of the foods you eat, the ones you like, and even the ones you avoid. Only by becoming well versed in the macronutrients in the diet you currently eat can you know what changes you could make that would improve it.

The remaining portion of your daily caloric intake (30%) should come from beneficial fats: cold-pressed olive oil, canola oil, marine lipid (the beneficial oils found in the flesh of cold-water fish, such as herring, salmon, mackerel, and tuna), and a little animal fat (about 10%).

Okay. I promised earlier that I would make it clear to you why dietary composition and its effect on insulin control is so all-fired important. The answer for that takes us back to the eicosinoids. Remember I said that the kicker was that the body could make either the "good" kind or the "bad" kind from the same dietary fat? Well, to a large degree, the level of insulin we produce is what determines which way the wind blows in eicosinoid production. In the stepwise alteration of linoleic acid to make eicosinoids, there are two major steps controlled by enzymes. The first critical step is controlled by an enzyme I'll call D6D (which, for anyone interested, stands for delta 6 desaturase) and the second, by another enzyme I'll call D5D (standing for, you guessed it, delta 5 desaturase). Insulin acts *against* D6D in the first step to slow it down. The result is that the production of the raw material that our body could turn into either kind of eicosinoid falls off. Insulin further acts to *improve* the action of D5D in the second step, to speed up its action, which might at first blush sound beneficial, but which in truth steps up the production of the bad kind of eicosinoid. So under the influence of insulin, your body makes fewer total eicosinoids, and what you do make will be mostly of the "bad" variety. This situation damages your overall state of health and makes it much more difficult for even large amounts of vitamin and mineral nutrients to have much of an impact.

On the other hand, if you begin with an excellent diet that favors the production of these "good" eicosinoid messengers, you've leveled the playing field and given the micronutrients a fighting chance to do their good works. Begin today to put your macronutrient house in order, designing a diet for yourself along the lines of Dr. Sears's, perhaps the country's foremost researcher in essential fats. This will not only improve your health and vitality, but will enhance your response to the vitamin and mineral therapies I am going to describe.

Minerals and Good Health

We've examined, now, the proper kind of diet to encourage your body to make the "good" series of eicosinoid messengers that will put you in the best and most receptive position to get the most benefit from the vitamins you will need to achieve optimal health and combat specific illnesses, but what about the minerals? What role do they play in human health and why do you need them?

Minerals, like vitamins, often act as cofactors that help speed up the billions of chemical reactions going on in your body all the time. But minerals also have other duties. Calcium, for example, gives strength and hardness to your bones and teeth and stimulates the contraction of muscle fibers throughout your body; phosphorus, like calcium, provides strength to bones and teeth and is necessary for you to properly metabolize protein, fat, and carbohydrate. It also acts as a cofactor for many enzyme systems (chemical reactions) and regulates the use of B vitamins. If you became deficient in critical minerals, you could become seriously ill. Profound deficiencies could even cause death. You must be certain your diet contains all the necessary minerals. Here's an easy device to help you remember at least the major elements (minerals) deemed necessary for human health by the USFDA, although it's not quite complete. There are additional minerals—zinc, chromium, selenium, molybdenum, and others—that the human body requires to function optimally, but here are the biggies: "C HOPKINS Café: Mighty Good Food plus Salt."

Translation:	C	carbon
	H	hydrogen
	O	oxygen
	P	phosphorus
	K	potassium (*kalium,* see below)
	I	iodine
	N	nitrogen
	S	sulfur
	Ca	calcium
	Fe	iron (*ferrous,* see below)
Mighty good		magnesium (OK, that's a reach)
Food		fluoride
plus salt		sodium and chloride ("table salt")

All letter names follow actual elemental abbreviations except: K stands for kalium, the elemental name for potassium (which is a common name derived from potash, a source of the element); Fe is the chemical symbol for iron, derived from the Latin *ferrous;* "mighty good" loosely stands for Mg, the chemical symbol for magnesium, but at least it sort of makes sense in the phrase; and finally plus salt brings in sodium and chloride, the two elements that combine to form table salt. Now perhaps you're set for your next round of Trivial Pursuit, a guest appearance on *Jeopardy,* or a quiz in a Health and Nutrition class. Or at least you know which mineral elements you need for good health, but how best to get them? In foods rich in them? From supplements?

Certainly, eating a varied diet that provides plenty of these minerals—calcium from dairy products, potassium from broccoli, iron from red meat—would be ideal; however, that nutritional utopia is often not possible. Perhaps you need calcium but can't tolerate dairy products, for example. Or perhaps you need a larger amount of a certain mineral to combat a specific illness or disease; for example, magnesium in higher doses than you can get from foods to alleviate such symptoms as dizziness, ringing in your ears, or leg cramps. Then you must obviously rely on supplements.

Before you begin to supplement minerals, however, you need some basic information on how your body absorbs them, because these nutrients jealously guard their own positions in your body and vigorously compete with each other for entry. Taking a large amount of some minerals can create deficiencies in others. Let me illustrate how this works.

The Single Ion Channel Theory

Minerals often occur, especially in supplemental form, as combination salts (such as the iron salt ferrous sulfate, chemical symbol $Fe_2(SO_4)_3$ or table salt, sodium chloride, chemical symbol NaCl) that must be broken apart before your body can absorb it. When a mineral salt breaks apart, each part becomes what is called an *ion,* a particle of the element that has an electrical chemical charge. In the examples above, breaking apart the ferrous sulfate would yield two iron ions with positive charges and three sulfate molecules with negative charges. The lining surface of your intestine has a protein mucous coating that is slightly negatively charged. This coating attracts the positively charged mineral ions (like iron above), and like the two poles of a magnet, the positive and negative attract and stick. In the individual lining cells themselves, nature has provided an entry port, called the *single ion channel,* that permits safe passage of one ion at a time. You can envision this channel like a funnel tube.

Imagine the mineral ions in your stomach as tiny balls. Each mineral is a different color: iron is red; zinc is blue; phosphorus, green; copper, yellow; and so on. For the sake of illustration, assume that there are 100 balls of each color in the belly of the funnel with an opening large enough for only one ball at a time to pass through the spout. Since there are equal numbers of balls of each color, the law of averages tells us that about the same number of balls of each color will pass through the funnel in a given space of time: red, blue, green, yellow, all the colored balls with an equal chance of passing through the spout. But imagine that someone suddenly dumps 1000 yellow balls into the belly of the funnel. Now there are over ten times more yellow balls competing with the other colors to enter the spout. Naturally, since there are so many more of them, more yellow balls will get through, and since only one ball can pass at a time, that means passage of the other colors will of necessity be reduced.

By this same means, the single ion channel permits only one ion of certain minerals to enter the cell at a time. Dumping a huge extra load of an ionic mineral into the system (your body) can create deficiencies in other minerals through unfair competition for absorption, just as happened with the yellow balls. So what can you do? How can you supplement with extra minerals without creating deficiencies? You've got to fool Mother Nature. Let me show you how it's done.

The Magic of Chelation

(Or: sometimes it *is* nice to fool Mother Nature)

I've said that minerals in their broken-down, ionic forms must pass through the ion channel in single file, and that's true. But what if we could disguise them somehow, put a mask over their charges? What would happen then? Would the cells take them in? The answer is yes, and the disguise is effected by a process called *chelation*. Let's examine this process.

If our goal is to get complete or near-complete absorption of a mineral, perhaps we can smuggle it in attached to something that the body not only absorbs well, but actively seeks to absorb. Amino acids, the building blocks of protein essential to human life, fill that bill. The intestinal lining has systems in place to actively absorb these protein subunits, and the structure of the amino acids themselves provides the means for disguise. Recall from our earlier discussion that the mineral ions have a positive electrical charge. Certain critical spots along the amino acid structure have negative charges, and as with magnets, opposite charges attract and stick. When we put in the right amount of certain amino acids (glycine or aspartic acid, for example), the negative points on the amino acid bind or stick to the positive points of the mineral ion, clustering around it much like iron filings cluster around the negative pole of a magnet, forming what we call an amino acid/mineral *chelate*. With the mineral hidden in the middle of the cluster, all the lining of the intestine "sees" is the amino acids that surround the ion. The lining cells actively snatch up and absorb the amino acids, and voilà! The mineral is smuggled in and absorbed without ever darkening the door of the ion channel.

Chelation of ionic minerals allows for better absorption without the risk of competition causing deficiencies in other minerals and better tolerance, because the negative amino acid charges balance out the positive charges on the mineral ion. What does that mean to you? That you will have less stomach upset from taking a chelated mineral than from an ionic one. If you've ever taken large doses of ferrous sulfate to correct iron deficiency anemia (as I once had to do), you will appreciate not having to put up with the feeling that while you weren't looking, someone took a Brillo pad to the lining of your stomach. The less obvious benefit of chelation is that you absorb what you spent your hard-earned dollars to buy and, therefore, get the health benefit you seek from taking less of it. Chelation is truly "living better through chemistry"! We should all be thankful someone thought of it.

DRIs: Faux Improvement?

In 1941, the United States Food and Nutrition Board came up with a set of figures called the *Recommended Daily Allowances*. Each vitamin and mineral was assigned a number representative of the amount these experts deemed necessary for maintaining good health. The RDAs were our nutritional guidelines for over 50 years, until experts realized that the figures from the 1940s no longer applied to today's population due to changes in environment, lifestyle, and basic needs. Truth be told, the RDAs never really *were* effective for maintaining health; they were barely sufficient to stave off malnutrition and disease. In January 1997, the new and improved RDAs were unveiled, now called the *Dietary Reference Intakes*. The figures for most nutrients are higher than the RDAs, but the old problem remains: These numbers don't aim for optimal health; many physicians and nutritionists feel they're merely slightly changed numbers from the RDAs. Indeed, though most DRIs are higher than their predecessors, some are mysteriously lower. Most physicians and nutritionists have the same concerns with the DRIs that they had with the RDAs. Let's take a look at those concerns individually.

DRIs
"Nutritional" Analyses

The term *Dietary Reference Intake* (DRI) is new. It replaces the *Recommended Daily Allowance* (RDA) published in 1941 by the National Academy of Sciences.

What does the DRI figure take into consideration?

Each DRI includes the Estimated Average Requirement (EAR), the RDA, the Adequate Intake (AI), and the Tolerable Upper Intake Level (UL).

• The EAR is the daily intake value that is estimated to meet the requirement, as defined by the specified indicator of adequacy, in half of the individuals in a life-stage or gender group.

• The RDA is the average daily dietary intake level that is sufficient to meet the nutrient requirement of 97 to 98% of healthy individuals in a particular life-stage and gender group.

• The AI is a reference intake used instead of an RDA. If sufficient scientific evidence is not available to calculate an EAR, then the AI comes into play. The AI is a value based on experimentally derived intake levels of observed mean nutrient intakes by a group of healthy people.

• The UL is the highest level of nutrient intake that is likely to pose no risks of adverse health effects to almost all individuals in the general population.

Food Myths and the American Lifestyle

The DRIs are intended to be met solely through diet, not through supplementation. But how realistic is this expectation? Most people simply don't eat a well-balanced diet; I know of very few people who intentionally count their intake of complex carbohydrates or protein in an effort to meet the recommendations of the National Research Council. It just doesn't happen. And the DRIs fail to take into consideration the fact that at any given time, as much as one-third of the American population is dieting and so is getting a daily intake of less than the normal 2000 to 3000 calories which the DRIs are based on. Add to that the fact that these new figures don't consider individual lifestyles, habits, nutrient bioavailability, or the loss of nutrients that happens during storage, processing, and cooking, and you have numbers that, well, don't mean a whole lot to a whole lot of people.

One Size Fits All?

The DRIs are meant for the general population, based on a set of criteria determined by the panel. But what is the "average, healthy person"? That search leads you down the same path as the one that tries to find the "normal American family." The fact is, the average person does not exist any more than the average family does. The DRIs don't consider individual needs. Everything we encounter throughout our lives—environmental pollution, stress, disease—affects each of us differently. Not one person is the same as he was ten years ago, five years ago, even three months ago. We are ever-changing, and our nutritional needs change with us. The DRIs don't change; they're engraved in stone, and the recommendations are for everyone from age four and older.

What of Optimum Health?

Like the RDAs, the DRIs are designed only to prevent overt deficiency symptoms. But is that enough? Are we willing to settle for not being deficient, when we can just as easily achieve optimum health, whatever that may be for each individual? Your answer to these questions, I hope, is a definitive no. And this is the attitude of many physicians and nutritionists, including the panel of experts who designed the DRIs. Even these people recognize the limitations of the new figures.

———— **Where Do We Go from Here?** ————

Experts everywhere in the fields of healing and nutrition argue that we need to determine figures that are more useful, more beneficial than the DRIs. It is generally agreed upon that these figures wouldn't be in the form of one figure per nutrient, but rather a *range of figures,* according to various individual factors. At this point, no panel has been formed to deal with this issue. What the experts need to realize is that maintaining proper nutritional balances is like healing; it is a process, not a one-time event. Everyone's journey is made at a different pace, in a different place.

And so I urge you to use the DRIs I've included in this book as a mere starting point; don't hedge your bets on them. Take into consideration your own needs and habits. Equally important is consulting a nutritionist or physician you unequivocally trust. This is your life we're talking about. If you value it enough to read this book, surely it's worth going the distance.

Notes

1. John Yudkin, *The Penguin Encyclopedia of Nutrition* (Middlesex, England: Penguin Books, Ltd., 1986), 374.

2. Eleanor R. Williams, *Nutritional Principles, Issues, and Applications* (New York: McGraw-Hill, Inc., 1984), 277–278.

3. Herbert L. Newbold, *Meganutrients: A Prescription for Total Health* (Los Angeles: The Body Press, 1987), 146–147.

4. Yudkin, 281.

5. Yudkin, 219.

6. Newbold, 280.

7. Yudkin, 178, 316.

8. Yudkin, 375.

9. Donald and Judith Voet, *Biochemistry* (New York: John Wiley & Sons, 1990), 322.

10. P. J. Skerrett, "Mighty Vitamins," *Medical World News* (January 1993): 28.

11. E. Cheraskin, "Vitamin C . . . Who Needs It?" *Health & Nutrition Update,* no. 4 (Winter 1992): 6.

12. Skerrett, 26.

13. Skerrett, 32.

14. The prefixes of these terms take their root from the Latin words for large (macro) and small (micro).

15. Michael R. Eades, *Thin So Fast* (New York: Warner Books, 1989), and Garth Fisher, et al., *How to Lower Your Fat Thermostat* (Provo: Vitality House Intl., Inc., 1983).

16. Shari Lieberman, and Nancy Bruning, *The Real Vitamin and Mineral Book* (New York: Avery Publishing Group, 1997), 18–28.

VITAMINS, MINERALS, AND NUTRIENTS FROM A TO Z

In this section, I have provided you with an extensive listing of the vitamins, minerals, and nutrients important to human health. Each entry contains several subheadings: *Important Facts* gives the kind of nutrient and a brief history about the nutrient. *Food Sources* tells which foods are richest in the nutrient. You should always try first to increase your intake of a nutrient by eating more of the foods that contain it and then move on to supplementation. *Functions in the Body* tells you how the nutrient benefits your health, its mode of action. *Interactions* provides you with a listing of how the nutrient interacts with other nutrients, medications, foods, and so on. Do they compete with each other? Help each other? *Recommended Usage* gives you the DRI listings and my own suggestions for adequate intake. Here you will also find any information about the preferred way (or best form) to supplement that nutrient. *Symptoms of Deficiency* catalogs all the possible signs and symptoms you might experience if your diet is deficient in the nutrient. *Symptoms of Toxicity* gives you the same kind of guidelines to know if you're taking too much of the nutrient. *Safety Information* provides you with a listing of facts pertinent to the safe use of the nutrient, such as unsafe forms of the nutrient or dangers of supplementation with the nutrient.

Refer to this section to check all these listings, especially the last three listings, before you supplement with any nutrient in an effort to remedy a specific condition.

——————— **A (Retinol)** ———————

Important Facts—Antioxidant, fat-soluble vitamin.

This vitamin holds the distinction that, in 1920, it was the first vitamin discovered and named—hence the compound called retinol got the designation as *vitamin A* under the alphabetical nomenclature system. It is fat soluble, therefore stored by the liver, and because of that storage capability, substantially toxic if taken for sustained periods in high doses. Fat solubility also means that vitamin A does not dissolve in water; however, a little of the vitamin (about 15% to 35%) is still lost during the boiling, steaming, and canning of vegetables. The vitamin also withstands the heat of cooking, but can be destroyed by air through the process of oxidation.

Food Sources—Liver, sweet potatoes, asparagus, cantaloupe, carrots, spinach, broccoli, winter squash, raw apricots, fortified fluid milk.

Functions in the Body—The most widely known function of vitamin A must surely be prevention of night blindness. Everyone, it seems, has heard that "old wives' tale" (which is perfectly sound medically) about eating carrots (rich in precursors of the vitamin) to help you see in the dark. Even Egyptian papyri as far back as 1500 B.C. document night blindness, a condition for which the physicians of that time prescribed the eating of ox liver. Once again, empiric treatment proves correct, since liver (whether of beef, ox, water buffalo, codfish, or any other kind) contains very high amounts of vitamin A.

Aside from vision, vitamin A also functions in the integrity and maintenance of the epithelial cells that make up your skin, the membranes lining your mouth, the length of your intestines, and your respiratory and reproductive passages. These cells also require vitamin A to normally produce the mucus that protects and lubricates them.

In your reproductive tract, vitamin A is a necessary cofactor (or helper) in sperm production and ovum (egg) development. And in the skeletal system, you need the vitamin for normal bone growth and development.

A recently reported Swiss study of vitamin A and its precursor (a forerunner that the body turns into active vitamin) beta-carotene and the development of lung cancer in an "at-risk" population of smokers and workers exposed to asbestos (both of which correlate strongly with lung cancer) reported a reduction of over 50% in lung cancer development among the group taking the vitamin compared to the control group. Current clinical trials in prevention of cervical cancer and breast cancer are using beta-carotene. It may also be helpful in the prevention of colon cancer and melanoma. It appears to help prevent cancer by neutralizing those nasty free radicals.

Interactions—

• Vitamin E (tocopherol) protects vitamin A from oxidation in the gut as well as in the tissues. (See the discussion of oxidation and free radicals on pages 18–19 for more information.) Consequently, if you're deficient in vitamin E, you may not be able to absorb enough vitamin A, and for this reason, the two should be supplemented together.

• Zinc deficiency can impair the metabolism of vitamin A to its active forms. Because your body can't make vitamin A binding protein—the carrier molecule that fairways vitamin A through the intestinal wall and releases it into the blood—without enough zinc, deficiency of zinc can create problems with the release of vitamin A to the tissues. The two are interdependent such that vitamin A enhances zinc absorption and zinc returns the favor.

• Mineral oil, which you might sometimes take by mouth as a laxative, can dissolve fat-soluble substances (such as vitamin A and beta-carotene). These vitamins then pass worthlessly on through your intestine, since they are bound up by the mineral oil, which your body cannot absorb. Chronic use of mineral oil, therefore, can render a person deficient in vitamin A.

• On the other side of the fat-soluble interaction story, however, proper absorption of vitamin A requires some fat and protein in the diet. The difference between dietary fat and mineral oil is that your body *can* absorb dietary fat along with the vitamin A dissolved in it; not so for mineral oil.

• Absorption of vitamin A also requires adequate daily protein intake for the production of sufficient amounts of vitamin A binding protein (see discussion of zinc above).

Recommended Usage—The RDI for vitamin A is 5000 IU for adults and 8000 IU for pregnant and lactating women. Children's dosages vary according to weight and age. A child weighing between 70 and 100 pounds should be given ¾ the adult dose; a child weighing under 70 pounds (and over the age of six) should be given half the adult dose. For children under the age of six, consult your physician. In the case of a potentially toxic vitamin, such as vitamin A, additional supplementation should only be undertaken under the supervision of a qualified physician able to examine you regularly.

The carotenoids, such as beta-carotene, which your body converts to active vitamin A, but which are derived from vegetable and fruit sources, do not carry the toxicity risk of vitamin A that comes from animal sources. You can take higher amounts of beta-carotene in supplemental form, on the order of 10 to 15 mg or 15,000 IU to 25,000 IU per day, without risk. It is important to take only natural beta-carotene, however, if you have hypothyroidism.

Symptoms of Deficiency—Acne, dry dull hair, dry skin, fatigue, poor growth, insomnia, thickened scaly skin on the palms and soles of the feet, frequent infections, night blindness, weight loss, dry eyes (progressing to ulceration of the cornea if untreated), and dry mouth.

Symptoms of Toxicity—Probably no vitamin toxicity syndrome has received more study than hypervitaminosis A. Symptoms include: pain in abdomen, bones, and joints; fatigue; malaise and lethargy; night sweats; headache with nausea and vomiting, which may occur because of increased pressure inside the skull; hair loss; menstrual irregularities or cessation; enlargement of the liver and spleen; other gastrointestinal disturbances; cracking of the corners of the mouth; irritability; generalized itching; brittle nails; and finally, once again, dry itching skin (I'm certain you must be saying, "Strange that the same symptom can occur with too much or too little vitamin A," but such is indeed the case).

Safety Information—Toxicity varies widely, with doses of 1 million IU taken daily for 5 years posing no threat to health in some people and doses of as little as 25,000 IU causing symptoms of hypervitaminosis A. You must be careful and acquaint yourself thoroughly with the signs of toxicity given in this listing when you supplement vitamin A for specific purposes.

Very high doses of vitamin A have produced birth defects in laboratory animals and have been linked to birth defects such as cleft palate, hearing defects, and other congenital defects in the babies of women who have taken high doses. Foods high in vitamin A may also cause these problems. The maximum daily intake of vitamin A for pregnant women is 8000 IU.

─────────── **B₁ (see Thiamine)** ───────────

─────────── **B₂ (see Riboflavin)** ───────────

─────────── **B₃ (see Niacin)** ───────────

─────────── **B₅ (Pantothenic Acid)** ───────────

Important Facts—Water-soluble vitamin.

As its name (derived from the Greek *panthos,* meaning everywhere) suggests, this vitamin is widely distributed in nature. It is destroyed by dry heat, such as baking and grilling, by acid and alkali solutions used in canning or freezing, and by processing of foods (such as wheat flour, refined sugar, and heat-treated commercial fats and oils). Unlike riboflavin, niacin, and thiamine, this member of the B-complex group is not added as an enricher into white flour.

Food Sources—Occurs widely, but sources with highest content are meat, nuts, liver, peanuts, whole wheat, wheat germ, brewer's yeast, bran, egg yolk, chicken, and green vegetables, including broccoli.

Functions in the Body—Pantothenic acid forms one part of a vital substance called *coenzyme A,* which is necessary for energy production and the metabolism of carbohydrate and fatty acids. It is necessary for the normal synthesis of red blood cells, brain chemicals, cholesterol, and native corticosteroids, critical to our withstanding physical (and emotional) stress. In the immune system, pantothenic acid helps to stimulate antibody production. It is also needed for normal functioning of the gastrointestinal tract and may be helpful in treating depression and anxiety.

Interactions—Adequate amounts of pantothenic acid are necessary for the proper absorption and metabolism of folic acid, so there is a positive interaction there. Otherwise, this vitamin does not appear to adversely affect other vitamins, nutrients, or medications.

Recommended Usage—Need for this vitamin (as is true for all the B group and C) increases dramatically under physical or emotional stress or with illness. Orthomolecular physicians (those who subscribe to the use of high doses of vitamins and minerals to treat diseases) routinely prescribe doses in the 200 to 400 mg per day range during such times when native steroid (stress hormone) production is high.[1] However, the DRI is 10 mg.

Symptoms of Deficiency—Because the vitamin is ubiquitous in foods, deficiency rarely occurs in humans unless specifically created for study purposes. During these special circumstances, volunteers kept deficient for 9 to 10 weeks developed symptoms associated with deficiency that included: abdominal pains, hair loss, loss of appetite, nerve function impairments such as burning foot pain and loss of coordination, emotional symptoms of depression, irritability and nervousness, muscle spasms, weakness, fatigue, nausea and vomiting, rapid heartbeat, low blood pressure, eczema, and insomnia. In animal models, deficiency results in a broad range of problems that involve abnormal growth of young; spontaneous abortion of young; infertility; abnormalities of hair, skin, and pigment; malfunction of the gastrointestinal system and neurologic system; and sudden death. The graying of fur in rats made deficient in pantothenic acid and the subsequent reversal of the color loss upon resupplementation led researchers to postulate that additional dosage of the vitamin in humans might prevent or reverse graying of human hair. Certainly, this is an intriguing hypothesis to those of us hitting that phase of life when the "salt" has begun to overtake the "pepper" in our hair; however, clinical trials of oral and topical supplementation for this purpose have proven disappointing to date.

Symptoms of Toxicity—Very nontoxic. Some orthomolecular physicians describe using doses of up to 10,000 mg without adverse effect.

Safety Information—Safe and nontoxic.

B₆ (Pyridoxine)

Important Facts—Water-soluble vitamin.

Processing of foods can result in considerable loss of vitamin B_6: from as little as 15% to as much as 70% is lost in freezing of fruits and vegetables, 50% to 70% from processing meats, 50% to as high as 90% from milling grains.

Food Sources—Although this vitamin is found in all foods, brewer's yeast, carrots, chicken, eggs, fish, meat, peas, spinach, sunflower seeds, walnuts, and wheat germ contain the highest amounts. Other sources include liver, soybeans, bananas, poultry, beef, tuna, pork, veal, kidney, salmon, lima beans, peanuts, and avocados. Also, whole grains, unmilled, contain the vitamin in somewhat smaller amounts.

Functions in the Body—Your body needs vitamin B_6 for proper protein metabolism and essential fatty acids, to use stored "muscle starch" (glycogen), and to produce brain chemicals and the hemoglobin portion of red blood cells. Your body takes pyridoxal—one form of the vitamin that occurs in three forms—and makes a helper molecule (coenzyme) called PLP (pyridoxal phosphate), which more than 60 different enzyme systems depend on to function properly. One such system involves turning dietary tryptophan (an important amino acid or protein building block) into niacin (see Niacin, Vitamin B_3).

In medical research on female rats found to have low blood levels of vitamin B_6 because of deficient intake during pregnancy, doses of as much as 70 times the RDA have failed to restore the levels to normal. This finding could be interpreted in two very different ways: the deficiency was not real (i.e., the rats excreted the excess intake), or during the stress of the pregnant state the demand for the vitamin rose so sharply that even massive supplementation could not keep up with the demand. The interesting note that this vitamin has proven useful in combating morning sickness in pregnant women certainly seems to indicate that there may be an increased need for the vitamin in this condition.

This vitamin plays a role in cancer immunity and aids in the prevention of arteriosclerosis. It inhibits the formation of a toxic chemical called homocysteine, which attacks the heart muscle and allows the buildup of cholesterol around the heart muscle. It is also helpful in the treatment of asthma, arthritis, and allergies.

Interactions—
• Alcohol intake increases your need for additional dietary vitamin B_6 because alcohol increases the rate of breakdown of PLP, lowering body stores of this critical coenzyme.

• Isoniazid, a drug used in the treatment of tuberculosis, binds to the vitamin and inactivates it.

• Antidepressants, estrogen therapy, diuretics, and cortisone drugs deplete the body's supply of B_6.

• Penicillamine, a drug marketed under the trade name Cuprimine for the treatment of rheumatoid arthritis, also binds and inactivates this vitamin. (Note that this is not the antibiotic penicillin, but penicill*amine*.)

• Smoking lowers your body's vitamin B_6 stores.

• Some studies show that women on oral contraceptive agents have lower levels of this vitamin and that supplemental vitamin B_6 in doses of 25 to 50 mg per day alleviated disorders in users of the "pill," including: abnormal glucose tolerance, increased blood triglyceride levels, premenstrual swelling, and depression.[2]

• Drugs for Parkinson's disease can be inactivated by vitamin B_6. Therefore if you suffer from this disease you should not take increased amounts of this vitamin, because you could alter the effective blood levels of drugs critical to therapy of your disease.

Recommended Usage—To promote good health, I would recommend most adults take at least 50 mg per day. The DRI is 2 mg for men and women, 2.5 mg for pregnant and lactating women.

However, a woman's B_6 needs increase during pregnancy and lactation, and to ensure your baby does not become deficient in this vitamin, I would recommend at least 50 mg per day, which healthy adults also do well on.

Orthomolecular physicians (practitioners who subscribe to the use of high doses of vitamins and minerals to treat diseases) prescribe daily doses of 600 mg without incident; however, I would not recommend that you use doses exceeding 50 mg per day except under the direct supervision of a physician who is able to examine you regularly and who knows your history thoroughly.[4] (See Safety Information.)

Symptoms of Deficiency—Acne, spotty hair loss, anemia, loss of appetite, nausea, cracking of the corners of the mouth, painful tongue, mouth ulcers, conjunctivitis (irritation of the filmy covering over the eyes), depression, nervousness, irritability, dizziness, numbness, pins and needles or electric shock sensations, sleepiness, fatigue, weakness, poor wound healing, joint pains, flaky skin, a sore tongue, hearing problems, and growth retardation.

Symptoms of Toxicity—Numerous verified reports state that doses of as little as 200 mg to as much as 2000 to 5000 mg may cause numbness and tingling of the nerves supplying the hands and feet, as well as actual loss of sensation in these areas. Women involved in one study of this vitamin at an average dose of 117 mg per day for 2.9 years to combat premenstrual syndrome described the usual numbness and tingling, but also reported sensitive/painful skin sensations, bone pain, muscle weakness, and muscle twitches. Another study reports an associated decreased ability to memorize on doses of vitamin B_6 of 100 mg per day.

Safety Information—The *New England Journal of Medicine* reported cases of severe nerve damage in patients taking 2000 mg of vitamin B_6 per day. Similar symptoms have occurred on far smaller doses (in the 200 to 300 mg per day range). For safety's sake, I would caution you not to supplement vitamin B_6 at greater than a 50 mg per day dose without careful experienced medical follow-up. (Even at this dose, should you experience tingling in fingers, hands, toes, or feet, you should discontinue excess supplementation.)

—————— **B_{12} (Cobalamin)** ——————

Important Facts—Water-soluble vitamin.

Although it is water soluble, vitamin B_{12} is stored to some degree in the liver, kidney, lungs, and spleen. This minor degree of storage will not lead to your building up toxic levels of the vitamin, as can happen with fat-soluble vitamins. The vitamin is relatively stable in heat and light, and normal cooking temperatures do not destroy significant quantities of it. However, temperatures sufficient to sterilize and not merely pasteurize milk products may deplete milk of up to 70% of its vitamin B_{12}. Therefore, the practice of sterilizing milk for baby's consumption by boiling bottles of it at 119 degrees C for 13 minutes (versus using commercially prepared, enriched formulas and gently warming before feedings) could result in vitamin B_{12} deficiency if that overprocessed milk were the sole (or a major) nutritional source of the baby's diet.

Food Sources—Vitamin B_{12} occurs naturally mostly in foods from animal sources, with the highest levels found in organ meats (liver, kidney, and heart) and in bivalve mollusks (clams and oysters). Lesser, but still high, amounts occur in nonfat dry milk, other seafood sources (crab, salmon, sardines), and egg yolks. Moderate amounts come from muscle meats (beef, chicken, pork, fish), yet other seafood sources (tuna, haddock, swordfish, lobster, scallops, flounder), and Camembert and Limburger cheeses. Fluid milk and cheddar and cottage cheeses contain the lowest amounts. Sea vegetables such as dulse, kelp, kombu, and nori also contain this vitamin, as do soybeans and soy products.

Functions in the Body—Vitamin B_{12} functions in the body in cellular division, an activity carried on by every living cell. So, from that statement alone, you can easily gauge the importance of this vitamin to good health. Those tissues that divide most rapidly depend most heavily on adequate levels of vitamin B_{12}: the blood cells, immune cells, skin cells, and cells that line your intestine. Although we don't understand exactly how it works, vitamin B_{12} also plays a crucial role in the production of the covering of nerves (called the myelin sheath, because the protein material itself is called myelin), and chronic deficiency of it will lead to severe and irreversible nerve damage.

Interactions—Vitamin C in large amounts may interfere with your ability to absorb vitamin B_{12} from your food. If you supplement vitamin C to this degree (1000 mg or more with each meal), you should periodically ask your physician to check the level of vitamin B_{12} in your blood. If your blood levels decline, you may need to take vitamin B_{12} in shot form periodically, maybe 3 or 4 times a year.

Recommended Usage—Vitamin B_{12} is such a potent vitamin that the amounts necessary to provide protection from deficiency are measured in *micro*grams, not milligrams. (One microgram is 1/1000th of a milligram.) The DRI for this vitamin is 6 *micro*grams for adult men and women and 8 *micro*grams for pregnant and lactating women.

Some people do not absorb vitamin B_{12} well from the gastrointestinal tract for a variety of reasons: intestinal tract diseases, such as Crohn's disease or ulcerative colitis, sprue and other severe food sensitivities that cause intestinal inflammation, and chronic diarrhea. But the poor absorption may also be because they lack a special protein produced by the stomach lining—called intrinsic factor—which stimulates the intestinal lining to absorb the vitamin. Finally, some people fail to absorb much B_{12} because there isn't much there, as would occur with a person following a strict vegetarian diet (one without the addition of eggs or milk products).

Strict vegetarians can take vitamin B_{12} preparations orally, because there is nothing wrong with their ability to absorb the vitamin in the intestine. However, for a person who cannot absorb vitamin B_{12} when taken by mouth, injection is the only available route. The injectable vitamin B_{12} comes in two forms: as cyanocobalamin or hydroxocobalamin. Both are depot (sustained or long-lasting release) forms with a standard dose of 1000 *micro*grams per milliliter. Let me hasten to add, for the needle-phobics in the group, that injectable vitamin B_{12} is painless to take. Even with my own morbid aversion to needles—ones pointed in *my* direction, anyway—that was honed to a razor's edge during a childhood bout with scarlet fever requiring numerous penicillin injections, a shot of vitamin B_{12} is so innocuous that even I will take one. Should your physician suggest your taking this vitamin by injection, rest assured, you have zero to fear in the taking and much to gain.

The single-milliliter dose, commonly used in clinical practice as often as weekly to combat deficiency states, is many times greater than the DRI. But, because the vitamin is water soluble and quite nontoxic, this amount of vitamin is safe, with any excess excreted in the urine. Both the cyano- and hydroxo- forms break down to yield the vitamin B_{12} molecule; however, there are some minor differences. The most widely used (and cheaper) form, cyanocobalamin, may cause flushing or other mild allergic reactions in a few people, although this kind of reaction is rare. If allergic flushing does occur when you take the cyano- form, switching to the hydroxocobalamin form of the vitamin will usually solve the allergic problem.

Symptoms of Deficiency—Anemia; gastrointestinal problems such as constipation or cramping; fatigue; moodiness; depression; dizziness; a smooth, red inflamed tongue; headaches; irritability; numbness and other nerve problems; heart rhythm abnormalities; and finally nerve and spinal cord damage.

Symptoms of Toxicity—There are reports that supplementation with vitamin B_{12} may induce an acnelike eruption on the skin or worsening of acne if present.[5] Otherwise, I know of no documented adverse symptoms.

Safety Information—Vitamin B_{12} orally or by injection is safe and nontoxic.

Bioflavonoids

Important Facts—Pseudovitamin (vitamin-like). Antioxidant.

When Szenty-Gyorgyi first identified vitamin C, he extracted a compound from Hungarian peppers that contained high amounts of vitamin C along with another substance that he called vitamin P (for "paprika" and "permeability"). He felt that this vitamin P when added to vitamin C improved C's action on strengthening fragile capillaries. We now call these vitamin P compounds *flavonoids* or *bioflavonoids,* because in the strictest sense they are not vitamins. Recall that for a substance to be a vitamin, it must be absolutely necessary for life and consistently produce an identifiable deficiency disorder when absent from the diet.

The bioflavonoids, though not vitamins, are important in their action as "vitamin helpers." They are used extensively in the treatment of athletic injuries because they relieve pain, bumps, and bruises. They also lessen symptoms associated with prolonged bleeding and low serum calcium. Bioflavonoids have an antibacterial effect and promote circulation, stimulate bile production, lower cholesterol levels, and treat cataracts. Quercetin is a bioflavonoid that is used to treat and prevent asthma symptoms. The flavonoids occur widely in plants, both edible portions and flowers, giving them their colors: the flavonoid citron gives the yellow color to lemon peel, for example.

Food Sources—The compounds concentrate in the peelings or skin of most fruits and vegetables, and beverages such as tea, coffee, wine, and beer contain significant amounts. Other sources include apricots, cherries, grapefruit, grapes, lemons, oranges, prunes, and rose hips.

Functions in the Body—The bioflavonoids probably act as chelators of metals and as antioxidants, although their role is not clear. For more information about antioxidants see page 20 and chelation see pages 30–31.

Interactions—The bioflavonoids enhance the action of vitamin C.

Recommended Usage—Because these compounds occur so widely in fruits, vegetables, and common beverages, the typical American diet provides about 1 gram of these substances per day, which in most cases should be sufficient. In the event of supplementation of excess vitamin C, you can increase your intake of the flavonoids by choosing a supplement that contains them. Except for specific conditions as listed in this text, you need not take extra amounts of bioflavonoid.

Symptoms of Deficiency—None. The substance is not essential.

Symptoms of Toxicity—None specified in the medical literature.

Biotin

Important Facts—Water-soluble vitamin.

You can store some of this sulfur-containing vitamin of the B-complex group in your liver, even though the vitamin is technically water soluble.

Food Sources—The highest concentrations of biotin come from liver (100 to 200 *micro*grams per 100 grams of liver), kidney and pancreas, followed by soy flour (60 to 70 *micro*grams per 100 grams), egg yolk (16 *micro*grams per 100 grams), cereal (3 to 30 *micro*grams per 100 grams), and yeast (100 to 200 *micro*grams per 100 grams).

Functions in the Body—We need biotin for proper energy metabolism and for growth; for the production of fatty acids, antibodies, digestive enzymes; and in niacin metabolism. The vitamin also has insulinlike activity in lowering blood sugar. Researchers have discovered nine enzyme systems in the body that require biotin to work.

As is also the case for vitamin K, friendly resident bacteria in your intestinal tract produce biotin; however, the amount of the vitamin you actually absorb from this source is a point of debate: some research suggests you can absorb enough to meet your body's needs without the addition of any food or additional supplementation under *normal* conditions. However, if you must take prolonged courses of antibiotics—and this is true for both children and adults—you could sharply reduce the production of biotin by wiping out the friendly intestinal bacterial population, making supplementation necessary.

Interactions—
• Raw egg white contains a substance called avidin—a biotin antivitamin—that binds to biotin and prevents its absorption into your blood. Heating denatures (irrevocably alters the structure of) the avidin in egg white, and therefore cooked eggs pose no problem in preventing you from absorbing the biotin from foods you eat.
• Alcohol impairs your ability to absorb biotin and, therefore, chronic abuse of alcohol can make you deficient in biotin.
• Conversion of biotin to its active form requires magnesium, so if you are deficient in magnesium, you can also become deficient in biotin.
• Antibiotics increase your need for biotin by killing the intestinal bacteria that produce it for you.

*Recommended Usage—*Natural d-biotin is the only form (of eight possibilities) known to be fully active. (Other forms are not fully active vitamins. Oxybiotin has reduced activity and desthiobiotin retains no activity whatsoever.) It's rare under normal circumstances that you would become deficient in biotin, and except as a remedy for specific medical conditions, little reason to supplement exists. The DRI listing for biotin is 300 *micro*grams.

Also, if you indulge in the "athlete's breakfast" of large numbers of *raw* eggs (the risk of contracting Salmonella aside) you will need to take biotin supplements (at least 500 *micro*grams per day) on an empty stomach or risk deficiency of biotin because of the antivitamin avidin (see Interactions) found in raw egg white.

*Symptoms of Deficiency—*Spotty loss of hair, anemia, loss of appetite and nausea, depression, fatigue, high blood cholesterol, elevated blood sugar, sleeplessness, pain and weakness of the muscles, dry skin, grayish cast to the skin, pale smooth tongue.

*Symptoms of Toxicity—*No reports of toxic effect have occurred with daily intakes as high as 10 mg per day.

*Safety Information—*Biotin is safe and nontoxic.

────────────── **Boron** ──────────────

Important Facts—Ultratrace mineral.

Discovered in 1910, boron has been considered an essential element for plants since 1923. But not until fairly recently (1985) has evidence accumulated to suggest that this trace element might also be essential to good health in people.

Food Sources—Fruits, vegetables, nuts, wine, cider, and beer.

Functions in the Body—You need boron to build and maintain healthy bones, to maintain healthy cell membranes (absolutely critical for normal cell function and therefore for life), and even possibly as a helper for certain enzyme (chemical) reactions that your body carries out. Boron also promotes the metabolism of calcium, phosphorus, and magnesium. In addition, it enhances brain function and increases alertness.

Interactions—A boron deficiency accentuates a vitamin D deficiency. Elderly people can benefit from taking a supplement of 2 to 3 mg daily to enhance their calcium absorption.

Health Benefits—Because of its ability to enhance calcium absorption, this trace mineral is useful in treating and preventing any bone disorders, including osteoporosis and arthritis.

Recommended Usage—No specific recommendations for requirements in people are yet available, but recent work suggests a daily intake of 3 mg per day. I would not recommend going over this amount.

Symptoms of Deficiency—No deficiency symptoms have been identified.

Symptoms of Toxicity—Nausea, vomiting, diarrhea, skin rashes, and lethargy.

Safety Information—At doses of over 150 mg per liter in drinking water, boron can cause toxic symptoms. No symptoms have been determined in dosages ranging from 3 to 6 mg.

────────────── **C (Ascorbic Acid)** ──────────────

Important Facts—Water-soluble vitamin. Antioxidant.

Vitamin C is a powerful antioxidant and a cofactor for many enzymes. Your body cannot store the vitamin, so you must supplement it regularly. Because it is both water soluble and heat labile, cooking destroys it.

Food Sources—Highest levels are found in berries, sweet peppers, broccoli, citrus fruits, strawberries, melons, tomatoes, raw cabbage, and leafy greens such as spinach, turnip, and mustard greens. Among animal foods, only liver contains vitamin C.

Functions in the Body—In your body, vitamin C functions primarily in the formation of collagen, the chief protein substance of your body's framework. Vitamin C also participates in the activation or production of vital body chemicals—such as norepinephrine, needed for the "fight or flight" response: the unconscious raising of your pulse rate, blood flow to your muscles, blood pressure elevation, and heightened sense of readiness that you experience when danger threatens. Two other important roles for vitamin C are as a *detoxifier,* helping to cleanse your body of toxins ranging from cigarette smoke to carbon monoxide to snake venom[6] and as an *antioxidant* (see discussion of antioxidants on page 20). In this capacity, it functions as a molecule designed to protect your body, its essential fats, and the fat-soluble vitamins (especially A and E) from the damaging effects of oxygen. In fact, recent evidence indicates that vitamin C works synergistically with vitamin E. While vitamin E scavenges for free radicals in cell membranes, vitamin C attacks free radicals in biologic fluids. By working together, these vitamins extend each other's antioxidant activity. The antioxidant property of ascorbic acid in citrus juices (such as lemon juice) prevents browning of the cut surfaces of susceptible fruits and vegetables, such as apples, peaches, and avocados. All this antioxidant activity makes vitamin C a mighty soldier in the war on aging.

This nutrient is a major component in the health of the immune system. There is a growing body of evidence that it helps enhance resistance to diseases ranging from infections to cancer. Vitamin C has also helped reduce the symptoms of allergies and asthma.

Although research on vitamin C as an anticancer agent has yielded conflicting results, even the National Cancer Institute and the American Cancer Society feel the evidence is strong enough to warrant a diet high in vitamin C as a possible preventive measure.

Vitamin C helps prevent high blood pressure and atherosclerosis, which makes it a valuable treatment against cardiovascular disease.

Studies have linked increased levels of vitamin C with a reduction of serum cholesterol. Vitamin C also helps repair damaged arterial walls, which prevents cholesterol deposits from forming. In one clinical trial, patients with atherosclerosis given 1000 mg of vitamin C daily could walk farther without pain or breathlessness than could unsupplemented patients.

And finally, vitamin C enhances the absorption of iron from the intestinal tract by chelating it (see the discussion on chelation of minerals on pages 30–31).

Interactions—

• The citrus biovflavinoids (vitamin-like molecules naturally present in the peeling of citrus fruits) improve your ability to absorb and hold vitamin C by about 35%.[7] But does that mean you should eat the peeling of your grapefruits and oranges? Not unless you particularly like to do that. You can purchase vitamin C supplements that contain bioflavinoids or you can purchase the bioflavinoiods separately.

• Birth control pills and aspirin. Some research suggests that oral contraceptive agents (birth control pills) may reduce your blood levels of vitamin C. Large doses of aspirin (such as that which might be used to treat arthritis) may cause you to flush more vitamin C through your kidneys and waste it in urine, which could in time make you deficient in it.[8]

• Alcohol, analgesics, antidepressants, anticoagulants, and steroids may have the same results as aspirin and oral contraceptives.

• Smoking seriously depletes your stores of vitamin C.

• Vitamin C makes your intestine absorb aluminum better, and since aluminum can be toxic to you, you should not take supplemental ascorbic acid at the same time as any medication that contains aluminum (such as some antacid liquids, like Alternagel).[9]

• Large doses of this vitamin can alter the results of lab tests, including Pap smears. Diabetics should be aware that testing the urine for sugar could be inaccurate if they're taking a lot of vitamin C.

• Some diabetes medications may not be as effective when taken with vitamin C.

• Early studies suggested that large doses of vitamin C (1 gram or more taken with meals) can interfere with your ability to absorb vitamin B_{12} from food or supplements you take. Subsequent research has shown that vitamin C does not have this effect.

Recommended Usage—The DRI for vitamin C is 60 mg daily for men and women. However, in the face of an abundance of research, even the government is beginning to question the adequacy of this recommendation. Dr. Mark Levine and colleagues at the National Institutes of Health conducted research and concluded that the current recommendation of 60 mg should be increased to 200 mg per day. Some data recommend daily intake as high as 1000 mg!

To derive the maximum benefits from vitamin C, take your supplement in divided doses throughout the day. Estrified vitamin C (Ester-C) is a truly effective form of the vitamin, especially for those living with chronic illnesses such as AIDS and cancer. This particular form enters the bloodstream and tissues four times faster than standard vitamin C, moves into the blood cells more efficiently, and stays in the body tissues longer. Just as important is the fact that only one-third as much is lost through excretion. Dr. Linus Pauling, who studied the vitamin and its uses extensively beginning in the 1960s, based his recommendation for intake on careful scientific study of the levels of the vitamin in animals that produce their own vitamin C.[11] From that perspective, Dr. Pauling believed that the weight of the healthy human animal would require an ascorbic acid intake of 3000 to 4000 mg (3 to 4 grams) per day at a minimum up to 18 to 20 grams for larger individuals.

Disease, stress, fever, and toxic exposures (such as cigarette smoke) increase your demand for vitamin C. Some orthomolecular physicians (practitioners who subscribe to the use of large doses of vitamins and minerals to treat diseases) prescribe doses of 200 grams (that's 200,000 mg) per day (which may have to be administered by vein instead of mouth at this level) to treat major chronic viral illnesses such as mononucleosis and as adjuvant therapy in cases of terminal cancers.[12] Their data show very promising and intriguing responses to these megadose levels with few toxic side effects. Work concerning ascorbic acid's effects in cancer treatment is currently being done at the Pauling Institute (in Palo Alto, California) and in Canada and Scotland.

Symptoms of Deficiency—Bleeding gums, loosening of the teeth, easy bruising, poor wound healing, hair loss, dry skin, irritability, joint pains, fatigue, loss of the sense of well-being, and depression.

Symptoms of Toxicity—Very well tolerated even in high doses. The only consistently documented symptom of taking too much vitamin C is diarrhea. The intake level that exceeds bowel tolerance for ascorbic acid—that is, the amount taken daily that will cause loose stools—is quite variable person to person. And even in a single person, bowel tolerance varies situationally, since your gastrointestinal tract will tolerate more vitamin C in states of stress or disease as your body's demand for the vitamin increases.[13]

Safety Information—
• Some concern about the development of kidney stones as a result of increased vitamin C intake arose several years back because ascorbic acid breaks down to form oxalic acid, a major player in the formation of one type of kidney stones (calcium oxalate stones). In practice, however, even in patients taking extremely high doses of 15,000 to 30,000 mg or more per day for extended periods, no significant increase in kidney stone formation has occurred.
• Large doses (above the RDA) could cause hemolysis (red blood cell rupture) in people who suffer from a lack of a specific enzyme called glucose-6-phosphate dehydrogenase. Therefore, people with this inherited disorder should take increased amounts of vitamin C only under careful physician supervision.
• Do not take more than 5000 mg of vitamin C daily if you are pregnant. Infants may become dependent on this supplement and develop scurvy when deprived of the accustomed megadoses after birth.

——————————— **Calcium** ———————————

Important Facts—Mineral.
Calcium is among the most abundant elements (minerals) in the human body, comprising a total of 1000 to 1200 grams in the adult human. It is helpful in treating and preventing colon cancer, high blood pressure, high cholesterol, kidney stones, migraine headaches, dysmenorrhea, osteoporosis, PMS, gingivitis, and rickets.

Food Sources—Dairy products provide the major source for calcium intake, making up 55% of the intake in the United States.

Vegetable sources include green leafy vegetables, such as broccoli, kale, spinach, collard and turnip greens (see Oxalate Interactions), cabbage, cauliflower, asparagus, lime-processed tortillas, egg yolks, beans, lentils, nuts, figs, calcium-precipitated tofu, and calcium-fortified foods. Another good source of dietary calcium not often considered comes from the soft bones of salmon and sardines, which we eat when we consume these foods.

Functions in the Body—The major role of calcium is in maintaining integrity of the skeletal system, which, in fact, houses 99% of the body's calcium. The giant reservoir of calcium contained here remains in a constant state of flux with the pool of calcium in the bloodstream, and serves as a buffer to keep the levels in circulation remarkably stable. The other 1% plays a crucial role in the coagulation of blood, in the generation and transmission of nerve impulses, in the contraction of muscle fibers, and in the activation of certain enzyme systems and the release of some hormones.

And the skeleton itself is not a permanent depot site for calcium, but quite dynamic, with new calcium crystals forming as others break down. The rate of this tearing down and building anew—called the turnover rate—varies markedly with age: youngsters may turn over 100% of the calcium in their bone mass in the first year of life, older children may turn over 10% per year, and adults may only turn over 2% to 3% annually. Peak bone mass may not occur until about age 25. And by age 40 to 50, the resorption or tearing down may exceed the deposition or building up and total bone mass may gradually decline. The increase in loss of bone begins earlier and with graver consequences in women than men, in whites than blacks, in shorter people than taller ones, so that in general, the short white woman is most at risk for the medical consequence of bone loss, called osteoporosis. (Let me hasten to add that there is a significant heredity component to the development of this condition, as well.) However, this predilection accounts for the preponderance of hip fractures in bones weakened by calcium loss in this particular subgroup of women.

There is evidence that calcium helps prevent colon cancer. Several studies show that people who eat a typical high-fat diet may be protected from this form of cancer by supplementing 1200 to 1500 mg of calcium daily. Within two to three months after supplementation had begun, the subjects' colon linings showed that the number of fast-growing cells associated with cancer had significantly decreased. A Dutch study of over 2500 people supported this conclusion.

Interactions—

• Vitamin D is required for you to adequately absorb calcium from the gastrointestinal tract.

• Stress and immobilization can reduce your ability to absorb calcium from the gastrointestinal tract.

• Spinach, which contains oxalates, will combine with calcium forming the unabsorbable compound, calcium oxalate. It is worth noting, however, that one study suggests that while the oxalate contained in green leafy vegetables, like spinach, does inhibit the absorption of the calcium from the spinach itself, it may not impair absorption of calcium from other foods eaten at the same time.[14]

• Phytic acid in the bran of whole grains also combines with calcium, forming calcium phytilate, which, too, is not absorbable by the human gastrointestinal tract.

• Other foods that interfere with the absorption of calcium are cocoa, soybeans, and foods with a high phosphate content—which may include carbonated cola beverages.

• Gastric acid must be present in the stomach for the proper absorption of some forms of calcium, in particular the calcium carbonate form. A lack of sufficient stomach hydrochloric acid could occur in a number of medical conditions; most notably, there may be a marked reduction of stomach acid in people taking large doses of antacid medications or taking acid-inhibiting drugs for ulcers. Such drugs would include Tagamet (cimetidine), Zantac (ranitidine), and Pepcid (famotidine). However, this association is not true across the board, according to a study done by T. A. Knox and associates in 1989, which showed that the citrate form of calcium absorbs 10 times as well in the face of decreased stomach acid.

• Protein in the diet influences calcium absorption, as well. On diets high in protein, about 15% of the calcium taken in by mouth absorbs, while a person on a low-protein diet absorbs only about 5%.[15] The other side of that coin is that the body's needs for calcium increase on a higher-fat/higher-protein diet, so perhaps it is fitting that the body absorbs calcium better in a situation in which it will need more of it.

• A light meal enhances calcium absorption better than taking it on an empty stomach.

• Caffeine increases the loss of calcium through the kidneys.

• Magnesium may reduce calcium absorption from the intestinal tract. However, severe magnesium deficiency can also cause hypocalcemia (or low blood calcium).

• Taking iron with calcium reduces the effect of both minerals.

• Too much calcium can interfere with zinc absorption, and excess zinc can interfere with calcium absorption. A hair analysis can determine the levels of these minerals.

• Increased calcium intake without adequate phosphorus (a ratio of 2 calcium to 1 phosphorus or more) may inhibit the synthesis or absorption of vitamin K, which in theory could cause a decrease in normal blood clotting.

• Some antibiotics, such as penicillin and neomycin, may enhance the intestinal absorption of calcium.

• Drugs such as cortisol (cortisone and its relatives), anticonvulsant medications, and thyroid hormone may decrease the intestinal absorption of calcium.

Recommended Usage—The American Medical Association and many scientists recommend at least 1500 mg for postmenopausal women. The DRI for calcium is somewhat lower than that, at 1000 mg for everyone over the age of 4. Pregnant or lactating women should get a daily intake of 1300 mg. High calcium intake during pregnancy has been shown to prevent hypertension and premature birth.

Remember that the carbonate form of the mineral does not absorb well in a non-acid stomach and that the citrate form absorbs up to 10 times as well in these conditions.

Symptoms of Deficiency—Agitation, hyperactivity, nervousness and irritability, brittle fingernails, eczema, insomnia, high blood pressure, localized numbness and tingling sensations or numbness of an arm or leg, muscle cramps or even tetany (grabbing or locking spasms), clouded or confused thinking, delusions, depression, heart palpitations, stunted growth, disease of the gums and tooth support structures, and tooth decay.

Symptoms of Toxicity—Loss of appetite, muscle weakness, a fleeting inability to speak, difficulty with balance in walking, depression of the knee jerk reflex (and others), and mental and emotional symptoms ranging from the development of psychoses (major personality breaks with loss of touch with reality) to memory impairment to depression and irritability. (This is another time where the symptoms of too much are the same as those of too little. Like Goldilocks with her porridge, with regard to depression and irritability, your body wants the calcium level to be "just right.")

Safety Information—Taking daily doses of calcium above 2 grams (2000 mg) can cause hyperparathyroidism. The parathyroid glands (embedded in the thyroid gland in the front of your neck) produce and release a hormone called, naturally enough, parathyroid hormone. The release of this hormone occurs when the blood level of calcium falls, causing an increase in bone resorption (tearing down) to provide more calcium in the blood pool.

When you take calcium in great excess of its fellow elemental members in bone building (magnesium and phosphorus) in a ratio of calcium to phosphorus of more than 2 to 1, an actual reduction of bone strength can result. These minerals need to stay in the proper balance in your diet.

Carnitine

Important Facts—Vitamin-like molecule.

Carnitine first entered the nutritional picture in 1952 when researchers discovered it to be an essential nutrient to the mealworm. By extension, scientists began to wonder about an essential role in people. It took another 11 years for medical research to uncover a specific role for this nutrient. Although carnitine is actually related to the B vitamins, it has a chemical structure similar to that of amino acids and is usually considered together with them.

Your body can make carnitine by remodeling the amino acids (protein building blocks) lysine and methionine, and as long as your diet provides plenty of these amino acids, you will not become deficient.

Food Sources—Milk products and meats.

Functions in the Body—The clearest role for carnitine in your body is in burning fat for energy. In order to burn fat (or fatty acids, really) for fuel in muscle, heart, and liver tissues, the fatty acids must get into the mitochondria, little powerhouses of chemical activity inside the cells. Carnitine works to carry these molecules of fat into the mitochondria to be burned there. Without sufficient carnitine, the fat molecules are denied entry into the mitochondrial furnace and return to the blood, causing an increase in triglycerides. Because the oxidation or burning of fatty acids is a major source of energy for the heart muscle, scientists have hypothesized that carnitine deficiency might damage the heart. Indeed, research shows carnitine supplementation benefits the heart in many ways. It improves exercise tolerance and heartbeat regularity in patients with angina pectoris, decreases the incidence of heart failure and reduces the need for pacemaker transplants in patients with heart disorders, reduces the number of deaths due to inflammation of heart muscle tissue, and has been used to successfully increase levels of high-density lipoproteins, which are associated with a reduced risk of heart disease. Other studies have shown that carnitine can reduce the level of damage to the heart from cardiac surgery. It is also believed that carnitine deficiency may contribute to certain types of muscular dystrophy.

Interactions—
• No adverse interactions are known.
• Vitamin B_6 is necessary to convert the amino acids lysine and methionine into carnitine.

Recommended Usage—Nutritionists recommend 500 mg daily if you choose to supplement with this amino acid. As long as you make certain to eat the amount of complete protein required by your lean body mass for good health, you should have plenty of carnitine itself and its amino acid forerunners. You will find specific recommendations on calculating protein needs in the discussion on macronutrients on page 23.

Symptoms of Deficiency—All studies to date have involved animal and not human information, but based on those studies, deficiency might cause fatigue, weariness, and poor liver, heart, and kidney function.

Vegetarians need to supplement carnitine because it is found only in animal proteins.

Symptoms of Toxicity—None, from the carnitine found in food sources (natural carnitine or l-carnitine).

Safety Information—Nutritional scientists comment that the mirror-image molecule, d-carnitine, could cause problems.* Unfortunately, the literature did not specify the exact kind of problems that could develop, only that the d-form or mixtures of the d- and l-forms probably should not be given to people.

—— Cholecalciferol (see Vitamin D) ——

—————————— Choline ——————————

Important Facts—Vitamin-like molecule.

Choline functions as a true vitamin in certain mammals (the dog, cat, rat, and guinea pig, for example) but not in humans. A healthy, normally functioning human body can produce choline, and therefore, if your diet lacks the substance, you will not develop an identifiable deficiency disease. Choline falls into a category that nutritional science dubs "false vitamins." (Some nutritionists group choline and its near relative inositol as "minor" B vitamins; however, that name is not strictly correct for the reasons stated above.)

Your body uses choline to produce certain brain chemicals, to mobilize fat (especially removing it from the liver), and for the normal transmission of nerve impulses, but your body can normally concoct enough of it from other nutrients to do the job in the face of dietary lack. Such lack would occur only under extreme privation, because choline is present in so many foods. It is found in a broad variety of plant foods as free choline, in animal sources, and in soy as a part of the lecithin molecule.

Food Sources—Egg yolks, legumes, liver, soybeans, oatmeal, cauliflower, kale and cabbage, and peanuts. It is a component of lecithin, which is available in most drug and health food stores carrying nutritional supplements.

_____

*"D" and "l" refer to the direction that a chemical molecule is oriented in space: to the right is "dextro" rotated, or "d," and to the left is "levo" rotated, or "l." Changing the orientation of the molecule often changes its chemical properties. For example, codeine is a potent pain medication, cough suppressant, and potentially addictive narcotic; dextromethorphan is the "d" mirror image of codeine that retains the cough-suppressing properties (it's the DM of over-the-counter remedies), but none of the pain-relieving or addicting properties.

Functions in the Body—

Choline alone has no role; however, it forms parts of a critically important brain chemical (acetylcholine) and is also required for the synthesis of the major fatty components of the membrane of every cell in the body.

Because choline is used to make acetylcholine, an adequate supply of choline is critical for nerve function. A deficit of this nutrient may play a role in the development of certain disorders, including Parkinson's disease and Alzheimer's disease. In doses of 500 to 3000 mg daily, choline has resulted in a significant improvement in children who were seriously developmentally delayed.

Studies by M. T. Childs and his colleagues in 1981[16] and supported by the work of other researchers, as well, demonstrated that dietary choline (in the form of lecithin) increased your high-density, "good," cholesterol and reduced the low-density, "bad," sort. Such a change would normalize your blood lipid values and reduce your risk of heart disease.

Other work suggests that choline plays some role in the brain processes involved in learning and memory that decline with age, perhaps through its role in brain chemical production. Memory enhancement occurred in study participants taking choline and cholinelike medications.

Some studies suggest that choline deficiency may contribute to the development of cirrhosis of the liver in alcoholics. In lab animals, numerous studies document the fact that choline-deficient diets result in a fatty infiltration of the liver much like that seen in alcoholic damage. The infiltration of fat into the liver reverses with the addition of adequate choline in the diet.

Interactions—

• On choline-deficient diets, the level of carnitine—a body chemical critically important for you to be able to burn fatty acids as fuel for energy production—in the heart, liver, and skeletal muscle declines.

• Phenobarbital, a medication used to prevent seizures, may interfere with your ability to absorb choline.

• Methotrexate, used to treat cancers and rheumatoid arthritis, may also interfere with your ability to absorb choline from your intestinal tract.

Recommended Usage—There is no established DRI for this nutrient. However, some nutritionists recommend a daily intake of 100 mg, and I agree with this figure.

Symptoms of Deficiency—Fat intolerance (diarrhea and bloating from eating fat), hypertension, growth impairment, stomach ulcers, heart rhythm changes, and poor liver and kidney function.

Symptoms of Toxicity—None described. Doses of 3 to 12 grams per day, used to treat alcoholic cirrhosis of the liver for months, have caused no ill effects. Even doses over 100 grams daily for over four months may cause no problems in some people, but cause a fishy body odor, vomiting, salivation, dizziness, depression, sweating, and intestinal distress in others.

Safety Information—Some reports of allergic reactions occurring to choline chloride. Also, free choline supplementation may cause a fishy odor when the body degrades it. Supplementing choline by taking lecithin does not cause this odor.

Chromium

Important Facts—Mineral.

In the late 1950s, two researchers, named Schwarz and Mertz, reported that rats fed a diet deficient in chromium developed sugar intolerance and that replacing the chromium in the diets of these "diabetic-like" rats restored them to normal. This marked the first recognition that animals required chromium for normal life. Since that time, researchers have recognized a similar role for chromium in human health.

Food Sources—Brewer's yeast, brown rice, wheat germ, liver, meat, cheese, legumes, beans, peas, whole grains, black pepper, and molasses.

Functions in the Body—The primary role of chromium in your body is in blood sugar regulation as a "glucose tolerance factor," or GTF. Chromium works with insulin to drive sugar from your blood into the tissues of your body for use or storage. This mineral is so important in sugar tolerance that severe deficiencies of it cause a diabetes-like illness to develop. Chromium levels fall low during and after childbearing, in childhood diabetes, and in coronary artery disease (hardening of the arteries to the heart). Deficiency of chromium during pregnancy may explain the diabetes that develops during pregnancy (gestational diabetes), and through its interaction with insulin may also contribute to the rapid weight gain, fluid retention, and rise in blood pressure some women experience during pregnancy and afterward.

More recently, chromium (in the form of chromium picolinate) is being studied for its potential role in altering body composition. In preliminary animal and human studies, it has been shown to increase fat loss and lean muscle tissue gain. For this reason, and for the fact that it reduces sugar cravings by stabilizing the metabolism of sugars, chromium is valuable in the treatment and prevention of obesity.

Interactions—
• Calcium carbonate (a form of calcium often used in over-the-counter calcium supplements) can impair your ability to absorb chromium and could ultimately cause you to become deficient.
• Sugar increases your need for chromium and at the same time may increase your loss of chromium in urine.
• Do not take supplemental chromium if you have diabetes. Chromium can affect insulin requirements.

Recommended Usage—Use only the chromium picolinate form to take the DRI dosage of 120 *micro*grams daily. Picolinate enables chromium to enter the body's cells more effectively. Chromium polynicotinate is an effective form of this mineral also.

Symptoms of Deficiency—Anxiety, fatigue, sugar intolerance (borderline diabetes), stunted growth, high cholesterol.

Symptoms of Toxicity—Symptoms that could develop, but are rare, include: skin rashes, stomach ulcers, and poor kidney and liver function.

Safety Information—Even in very high doses in experimental animals, chromium seems to cause no ill effects.

Copper

Important Facts—Mineral.
Humankind has recognized the importance of copper as a metal since the Bronze Age (bronze being a copper-tin alloy) when we fashioned it into tools and weapons. But as a nutrient essential to

human health, its history is much shorter. Not until 1966 did scientists first document a recognized deficiency disease for copper.

Food Sources—Organ meats such as liver, seafood, nuts and seeds, whole-grain cereals, raisins, cherries, cocoa.

Functions in the Body—Although it sometimes occurs in people with severe protein malnourishment (severe anorexia or starvation), in sprue (discussed in Section II), and in other rare conditions that cause the kidney to waste protein, copper deficiency rarely occurs if you are able to eat.

Copper works in concert with iron in making red blood cells, and it is a major component of the outer coating of nerve fibers, collagen, the chief structural protein of your body, and in the production of skin pigments. It is involved in the healing process and is needed for healthy nerves and joints.

Interactions—
• Alcohol may worsen deficiency of copper.
• Egg yolk can bind with copper in your intestine and prevent its absorption.
• A diet high in fructose (a component of both fruit sugar and table sugar) can contribute to copper deficiency.
• Iron may reduce your ability to absorb copper from your intestinal tract.
• Molybdenum increases your loss of copper in urine.
• Phytates (binders in green leafy vegetables and grains) can reduce your ability to absorb copper from foods.
• Supplementing vitamin C in high doses can decrease your absorption of copper from food if you take your vitamin C with meals. Your best bet is to take your vitamin C by itself.
• Zinc in its ionic form can compete with copper to be absorbed through the ion channel in your cells. If you supplement minerals in chelated form, deficiencies caused by competition for entry into the body will not occur. Refer to the discussion in Section I on chelation of minerals (pages 30–31) for more information about how this happens.

Recommended Usage—In most instances, if you eat a diet rich in foods that contain copper, you will adequately meet your copper needs. In specific cases when you need extra copper, take a chelated copper supplement in a dose of 2 to 5 mg per day.

Symptoms of Deficiency—Spotty hair loss, anemia, rashes, emphysema, fatigue, high cholesterol, frequent infections, low white blood count, depression, heart muscle damage, osteoporosis (thin, weak bones).

Symptoms of Toxicity—Muscle and joint pain, irritability, and depression (again, a symptom that occurs with too much as well as too little copper).

Safety Information—Except in certain rare diseases that cause you to store copper (Wilson's disease, for example), toxicity from dietary intake of copper is extremely rare.

D (Cholecalciferol)

Important Facts—Fat-soluble vitamin.

Because this vitamin is fat soluble and stored to some degree by the body, it could build up to a potentially toxic level if you take large amounts of it. Even with little coming into your diet, however, you would rarely become deficient in vitamin D as long as you have exposure to plenty of sunlight. Your skin contains an inactive precursor of the vitamin (a forerunner that your body turns into the active vitamin) that the ultraviolet light in sunshine acts upon. The amount of vitamin D formed by your skin from the action of sunlight on it depends, among other things, upon the length of sunlight exposure, your skin pigmentation (with dark-skinned people activating less of the precursor and so more susceptible to deficiency), and level of pollutants in the atmosphere where you live.[18] We call the vitamin D formed in this manner "natural" vitamin D, or vitamin D_3. This is also the form of vitamin D that occurs in the foods of animal origin.

A "synthetic" vitamin D forms by the action of ultraviolet light on certain yeast fungi; called vitamin D_2, this is the form of the vitamin used in fortifying foods, such as milk products.

Your liver must then act on either the vitamin D_3 your skin makes or the vitamin D_2 you get from fortified foods to make them functional.

Food Sources—Fish liver oil (cod liver oil), fatty-fleshed fish, sweet potatoes, egg yolks, vegetable oils, butter, and (in America) vitamin D–fortified milk products.

Functions in the Body—Cholecalciferol acts primarily to maintain bone integrity through enhanced absorption of the minerals required to build and maintain the skeletal structure. While this is vitamin D's main function, studies have revealed other possible roles. When combined with calcium, vitamin D has been found to possess anticancer properties. In some people, low levels of the vitamin may increase blood pressure. Vitamin D also plays a role in the treatment of some immunological disorders such as multiple sclerosis and psoriasis. It may also improve muscle strength.

Interactions—
• Vitamin D stimulates your intestine to absorb calcium, and because calcium and iron will compete with each other for absorption, vigorous supplementation of vitamin D can lead to iron deficiency.
• Vitamin D also stimulates your intestine to increase absorption of magnesium, one of calcium's bone-building partners.
• It causes your kidney not to waste phosphate in the urine, again to provide your body with the other of calcium's bone-building partners.
• Deficiency of vitamin E impairs proper metabolism of vitamin D in the liver (where the precursor forms are activated).
• Sunlight, although not usually thought of as a nutrient, is important to stimulate the body to produce the vitamin. The elderly, especially, are vulnerable to deficiency of vitamin D: they may spend little time outdoors in the sun and they may eat very deficient diets. And because with aging they are able to convert only about half as much of the precursor molecule in their skin to vitamin D as they could when they were young, older people may become deficient enough in vitamin D during the late fall and winter months to develop obvious symptoms of deficiency.[19]

Recommended Usage—The DRI for vitamin D is 400 IU or 10 *micro*grams (a *micro*gram is one 1/100th of a *milli*gram) per day for normal, healthy adults. Unless you are using the vitamin as a specific remedy (as specified by your physician or in this text) for illness, this amount of vitamin should be enough. Adequate exposure to full-spectrum sunlight will usually provide enough vitamin D to prevent deficiency, although the latitude, time of year, and custom of dress can influence conversion. Fortification of milk products will provide sufficient vitamin D to those people not intolerant of milk products.

Symptoms of Deficiency—Burning of the mouth and throat, nervousness, sweating of the scalp, diarrhea, insomnia, mineral weakness of the bones, and nearsightedness. The classic deficiency syndrome is called *rickets*.

Symptoms of Toxicity—Irritability, weakness, nausea, vomiting, diarrhea, thirst, headache, loss of appetite.

Safety Information—
• Hypercalcemia, or high serum calcium, can occur from overuse (more than 1000 IU daily) of vitamin D in the diet. Symptoms can range from irritability to muscle spasm to actual seizure activity. Longer-term effects include calcification (or deposits of calcium) in the tissues (kidneys, lungs, arteries).

• In babies, excess vitamin D can cause a syndrome physicians refer to as "failure to thrive," which includes poor growth and development, poor weight gain, irritability, and poor feeding.

• This kind of hypervitaminosis occurred widely in England after World War II, when manufacturers of baby foods and formula powders there began to fortify their products with what proved to be an excess of vitamin D. Babies whose total intake came from these commercial sources consumed too much of the vitamin. Because it is a stored vitamin and can build up to toxic levels, the excess caused failure to thrive, absorption of excess calcium, and from that, irritability, seizures, coma, and even death when the cause went unrecognized. (Such a syndrome did not occur in America during those years to my knowledge, nor should it occur with the commercially prepared baby foods used nowadays, which do not contain an excess of the vitamin.)

• Although some sources put 158,000 IU as the "toxic" dose, studies report that daily doses of as little as 10 times the RDA (or about 4000 IU) of vitamin D may cause loss of appetite, nausea, thirst, diarrhea, muscular weakness, and joint pains.[20] You should rarely have to take a dose of vitamin D greater than 800 to 1200 IU per day for any condition specified in this text.

E (Tocopherol)

Important Facts—Fat-soluble vitamin. Antioxidant.

This vitamin was discovered in 1922—number five in serial order under the alphabetical classification and, hence, dubbed vitamin E—as the deficiency in the diets of lab rats that was responsible for fetal death in pregnant females and for testicular atrophy in male rats. From these humble and less than illustrious beginnings has sprung forth a wealth of information on this vitamin, destined to become one of our most potent allies in defense of our bodies from free radical damage. It is one of America's most popular vitamin supplements, second only to vitamin C. Some experts estimate that if we all took adequate vitamin E supplements, we could reduce our health-care costs by $8 billion!

Research scientists chose the name tocopherol for vitamin E from the Greek—*tos* (childbirth) and *phero* (to bring forth) and *ol* (the chemical designation for an alcohol, which it technically is)—to reflect its original role in restoring reproductive function to lab rats.

The vitamin exists in at least eight different configurations, all of which have activity similar to the "original" molecule (alpha-tocopherol), the most abundant and active form. It remains the standard against which we compare the activity of the others; their potency, we express in tocopherol equivalents.

Food Sources—Richest sources are wheat germ oil, sunflower oil, cottonseed oil, safflower oil, corn oil, margarine, sunflower seeds, almonds, and peanuts.

Functions in the Body—In its antioxidant capacity, tocopherol becomes incorporated in the cell membrane to scavenge free radicals that would weaken this most basic cellular defensive line. In immune cells, it strengthens and protects the membranes surrounding the lysosomes as well. These lysosomes are tiny bags of potent chemicals with free radical potential that the immune cells storehouse, ready for transport to the site of attack by viruses, bacteria, and any other "foreign" invader. Here, much like the armies of old poured cauldrons of boiling oil onto their enemy below, the immune cells dump destructive chemicals on the body's enemies to kill them. Unfortunately, just as would have been the case in times of old, if the boiling oil inadvertently lands on your own men, it kills them, too. Release of these toxic defenders into our own healthy tissues could destroy them as well. Tocopherol serves to sop up these free radicals at the site before they can do us harm. Recent studies seem to suggest that this critical function may protect us from arteriosclerosis and resultant heart disease, from the formation of cataracts, and from rapid aging of all our tissues. What this means, in short, is a slowing-down of the aging process.

More than 50 human studies have been conducted on the role of vitamins in the prevention of cancer. These studies tell us that vitamin E protects us from lung, esophageal, and colorectal cancer, and possibly from cancer of the cervix and breast as well. If animal studies are any indication of human physiology, then vitamin E also reduces the incidence of cancer of the skin, mouth, colon, and breast. Applied topically, vitamin E protects the skin of animals against free radical damage caused by ultraviolet light.

This miracle vitamin is also useful in treating existing cancers. In human studies, vitamin E was given to cancer patients, and the supplement appeared to protect normal cells from the damaging effects of chemotherapy drugs without protecting the cancer cells. So the side effects were relieved, but the drugs' effectiveness was uninhibited.

This vitamin has been studied for its effects on circulation, but results have been conflicting and inconclusive in some cases. However, some of the results are quite hopeful. Vitamin E does improve blood flow to the extremities. Some practitioners have reported success when using vitamin E to treat angina, arteriosclerosis, and thrombophlebitis.

Several studies suggest that vitamin E plays a vital role in the metabolism of fats in the arterial wall and lowers cholesterol levels in the blood.

Although earlier studies linking vitamin E with heart disease prevention were "iffy," 1993 brought two large-scale Harvard studies that changed all that. The Nurses' Health Study followed 87,000 nurses for eight years, during which the women regularly filled out questionnaires about their lifestyles and diets. After making adjustments for varying factors such as age and use of other vitamins, researchers found that women who had the highest intake of vitamin E had a 36 percent lower risk of major coronary disease than did those with the lowest intake.

Another study followed 22,000 male physicians for 4 years. Men who consumed at least 100 IU of vitamin E for at least 2 years had a 40 percent reduction in risk of heart disease.

These studies, along with other recent research, have strengthened the conviction of physicians who believe there is evidence supporting the use of vitamin E in the prevention of heart disease.

Studies have linked vitamin E with the reduction of scar formation and decreased healing time for wounds.

Vitamin E seems to enhance resistance to disease, as shown by animal and human studies. It may also positively affect the nervous system. Symptoms of neuromuscular disease in children improved after vitamin E supplementation.

Vitamin E alleviates symptoms associated with PMS and helps reduce the incidence of hot flashes in menopausal women.

Scientists are still conducting tests on vitamin E and coming up with new functions for it all the time. Two studies have shown that supplementation of the vitamin reduces the need for insulin in diabetics by improving insulin function. Vitamin E, in combination with vitamin C and beta-carotene, is being used in the prevention and treatment of cataracts.

Interactions—

• Dietary polyunsaturated fats (PUFA) and oils increase the requirement for tocopherol, with the need to prevent deficiency varying from 5 mg to as much as 20 mg per day. The rough ratio for intake to prevent deficiency of tocopherols as intake of PUFA increases is 0.4 mg tocopherol for each gram of PUFA.[21]

• A deficiency of tocopherol can lower tissue magnesium levels.

• Selenium and tocopherol interact so closely that supplementation to correct deficiency (or improve optimal health) using one demands proportionate supplementation of the other.

• When taken with tocopherol, inorganic (or ferric) iron will oxidize the tocopherol and render it inactive in the intestine.

• The ferrous form of iron (more commonly used in oral iron supplements) does not cause this oxidation.

• Deficiency of zinc may worsen symptoms of tocopherol deficiency.

• Insulin requirements may decrease during supplementation of vitamin E succinate. Diabetics must monitor blood sugar closely to regulate their insulin dose according to a planned reduction schedule according to their physician's recommendation.

• Two preliminary studies (in 1978 and 1979) suggesting a decrease in thyroid hormone levels on megadoses of vitamin E appeared to be disproved by controlled double-blinding methods in a study conducted by M. F. Brin in 1989 and published in the *Annals of the New York Academy of Science*.

Recommended Usage—
• Recently published work suggests that the succinate form of vitamin E may be more effective at scavenging free radicals than the acetate form of vitamin E.[22]

• The International Unit (IU) dosages are based on a conversion of 1 mg activity of alpha-tocopherol = 1 IU.

• Orthomolecular physicians (practitioners who subscribe to the use of large doses of vitamins and minerals in treating diseases) sometimes recommend doses of 1200 IU to 3000 IU and more. Except in the treatment of specific disease conditions, I generally agree with the DRI of 30 IU as adequate antioxidant protection for adults. (See Safety Information regarding the possible blood pressure elevation that can occur in some people at doses of over 100 IU.)

Symptoms of Deficiency—Nerve and muscle problems, such as decreased reflexes, difficulty walking, weakened eye movement muscles, decreased ability to feel vibration. Deficiency also causes shortening of the life of the red blood cells. Work based on animal studies (calf, rat, hamster, mouse, guinea pig, dog, and monkey) raises the question that the heart muscle and reproductive tract may also suffer in vitamin E deficiency.

Symptoms of Toxicity—Relatively nontoxic.

A review of over 10,000 cases of supplementation using doses ranging from 200 to 3000 IU per day for as much as 11 years produced no significant side effects.[23] You can develop transient nausea, flatulence, or diarrhea at high doses, and some people will develop an elevation of blood pressure.

Safety Information—
• Supplementation using the oily form of tocopherol (versus the water-soluble form) may cause an increase in your blood pressure and serum triglycerides, and may reduce your insulin requirement if you are an insulin-dependent diabetic. In the latter instance, it is important that you check blood sugar regularly if you begin to take vitamin E, because you may need to reduce your usual insulin doses. It is also important that when you supplement with this vitamin, you begin slowly, with 100 IU or less. Take that dose for one week, then get an average blood pressure reading (the average of 4 or 5 blood pressure readings taken over the space of several days). If your blood pressure does not exceed an average of 140/90, you may continue to

increase your intake of vitamin E to whatever level treatment of a specific condition demands, in increments of 200 IU, taking blood pressures after each increase. Do not continue to increase your dose of vitamin E if your average blood pressure rises above 140/90.

• Exceedingly high doses *might* cause birth defects. Doses on the order of 40,000 IU, taken during pregnancy, have caused birth defects according to correspondence from researchers Martinez-Frias and Salvador in the British medical publication *Lancet* (1 [1988]: 236). However, another bit of British research, published in the *British Medical Journal,* exonerated doses under 10,000 IU in this regard. (That means any dose I would recommend in this reading will be safe for you, if your blood pressure tolerates it, and has never caused birth defects.)

Fluoride

Important Facts—Mineral.

The role of this mineral in preventing dental cavities first came to light 50 years ago, although there is still disagreement in the dental/medical community about exactly how it does this. Aside from this role in dental health, experts question whether there is a clear benefit for fluoride as a mineral essential to human health. Many communities add fluoride to the city water supply. The U.S. Government Food and Nutrition Board (the RDI folks) recommends that communities add fluoride to the water supply if the natural fluoride level is below 0.7 mg per liter. Check with your local water company if you are uncertain whether your community's water contains added fluoride.

Food Sources—Tea, marine fish eaten with their bones (such as sardines, kippers, herring, mackerel, and salmon), and any foods prepared in water from a fluoridated supply. If you get your water from a well or a nonfluoridated water system, you may want to inquire at your local health department about checking the mineral content of your water. If it's low in fluoride, you want to be certain to eat more of foods rich in fluoride and to use fluoride toothpaste and fluoride dental rinse to protect your (and especially your children's) teeth.

Functions in the Body—Fluoride works with calcium and phosphorus in providing hardness and strength to bones and teeth.

Interactions—Aluminum, both in cookware surfaces and in antacid medications containing aluminum (Alternagel, for example), can bind the fluoride in food and reduce the amount of fluoride available in the food. Teflon cooking utensils do not bind fluoride.

Recommended Usage—There is no DRI for fluoride. The National Academy of Sciences–National Research Council recommends 1.5 to 4 mg daily, which is what most people get from their fluoridated drinking water. Except as indicated for treating specific medical conditions as outlined in this text, this amount of fluoride should be sufficient.

Symptoms of Deficiency—Weak brittle bones and teeth, cavities in teeth.

Symptoms of Toxicity—Poor bone health, poor kidney function, nerve and muscle problems, and brown mottling of tooth enamel in children (on doses of 2 to 8 mg per kilogram of body weight, which would mean 20 to 80 mg per day for a 22-pound child, 40 to 120 mg per day for a 44-pound child—certainly not small doses).

Safety Information—At the doses recommended in this text, fluoride is safe and nontoxic.

—————————— **Folic Acid** —————— —

Important Facts—Water-soluble vitamin.

Folic acid takes its name from the Latin word for leaf, *folium,* because it was first made in the laboratory from spinach leaves. The vitamin is easily destroyed by cooking and is susceptible to loss through processing and canning of vegetables and refining of grains.

Food Sources—Brewer's yeast, liver, green leafy vegetables such as asparagus and broccoli, cheese, mushrooms, oranges, whole wheat, root vegetables, and legumes.

Functions in the Body—Folic acid and a group of related compounds, collectively referred to as folacin, serve as coenzymes or helpers for chemical reactions involved in your body's ability to make protein and are required for normal red blood cell production and cellular division, the splitting of two cells into one—an activity that every living cell must be able to do in order to survive. And so you can easily see that this vitamin is critically important for your body to produce new cells: skin cells, hair cells, immune-fighting white blood cells, red blood cells—to name but a few. But folic acid also acts in the processes of removing fat stored in your liver and of converting one amino acid to another to rebuild and maintain body proteins—the amino acids being the building blocks of protein. It also strengthens immunity by aiding in the proper formation and functioning of white blood cells.

Folic acid is crucial during pregnancy. It is vital for normal fetal development, and studies have shown that a daily intake of 800 *micro*grams of folic acid in early pregnancy may prevent the vast majority of neural tube defects such as spina bifida and anencephaly. It also helps prevent premature birth. The trick here is to supplement *before* conception and continue for at least the first trimester. If a woman waits until she knows she is pregnant, it may be too late because fetal development begins during the first six weeks of pregnancy. For this reason, experts recommend that every woman of childbearing age take a folic acid supplement daily.

Interactions—

• B-complex vitamins. Because your body requires folic acid to be able to absorb the other members of the B-complex group (especially vitamin B_5), deficiency of folic acid can create deficiencies of others in the complex.

• Alcohol. If you abuse alcohol, you need extra folic acid, because alcohol in the intestine decreases intestinal absorption of this vitamin and a liver damaged by alcohol can't metabolize and use the vitamin as well.

• Taking oral contraceptive agents (birth control pills) also increases your body's demand for folic acid and allows you to become deficient in the vitamin over time. Correcting that deficiency could be lifesaving.

Adding extra folate to the diet of young women who take the birth control pill may decrease their risk of developing cervical cancer. Also, since many women stop taking the birth control pill in order to become pregnant, deficiency of folic acid caused by prolonged "pill" use may be important in other ways. (See discussion above.)

• Vitamin B_{12}. Deficiency of either B_{12} or folic acid causes the same kind of anemia, and replacing either one in your diet will correct the anemia. This kind of anemia—one that produces large pale red blood cells—is the most easily identified symptom of vitamin B_{12} deficiency (also called pernicious anemia). The problem is that anemia is the least severe symptom in pernicious anemia; severe wasting and nerve damage will follow if your body doesn't get some B_{12}. By correcting the anemia with folic acid, you could mask the first recognizable sign of B_{12} deficiency long enough to cause permanent nerve damage. Therefore, if you take a dose of folic acid greater than 1 to 2 mg per day, you must be certain that you do not have a deficiency in vitamin B_{12} by having your physician check its level in your blood or by supplementing with B_{12}, preferably in shot form to preclude any chance of your not absorbing it.

• Phenytoin (Dilantin), used for seizure control, competes with folic acid for absorption into the body. Each tries to prevent your intestine from properly absorbing the other. The two substances also engage in this competition to get into brain cells, which could alter the amount of Dilantin that makes it to the site of its action. In very large doses, folic acid (100 or more times the RDA) may cause seizures in such people.[24]

Recommended Usage—The DRI dosages for folic acid are from 400 (for adult men and women) to 800 *micrograms*. Women who are pregnant or lactating should be sure to get the upper-end dosage.

Women who supplement with folic acid and currently take or recently took oral contraceptives are at risk for lower zinc concentrations. A zinc supplement would be a good idea in this case.

Symptoms of Deficiency—Anemia, fatigue, weakness, headache, faintness, pallor, red sore tongue, diarrhea, weight loss, irritability, poor memory, hostility, and paranoia.

Symptoms of Toxicity—There are no *certain* symptoms of toxicity documented for folic acid, even at dosages of several hundred times the RDA (except as noted above in patients on seizure medication). However, 60% of the participants in one study (involving 14 normal subjects) receiving folic acid at a dose of 15 mg per day developed abdominal distention, flatulence, nausea, and anorexia, sleep disturbances with vivid dreams, malaise, and irritability after one month that researchers thought *might* have been caused by this large dose of folic acid.[26]

On the other side of the coin, Kurt A. Oster, M.D., reports using folic acid to combat arteriosclerotic (hardening of the arteries) disease in doses of as much as 80 mg per day without toxic effects.

Safety Information—The FDA (Food and Drug Administration) decreed in 1960 that over-the-counter vitamin supplements could not contain more than 400 *micro*grams of folic acid. This limit was established not because folic acid is itself toxic but to prevent people's taking doses of folic acid large enough to mask the visible blood profile symptoms of pernicious anemia (caused by B_{12} deficiency, see discussion on page 75). Pernicious anemia is easily treatable, but if it goes undetected can cause irreversible nerve damage. Today you can find supplements containing up to 800 *micro*grams of folic acid. However, if you take more folic acid than the recommended dose, you should have your B_{12} level checked periodically to be certain you are not deficient.

Inositol

Important Facts—Vitamin-like molecule.

A researcher named Wooley first described a dietary deficiency of inositol in mice, and since that time, nutritional scientists have debated whether it might be essential to good human health as well. It has been found to be vital for hair growth. In addition, inositol is involved in the synthesis of phospholipids, which are essential to the digestion and absorption of fats, facilitate the uptake of fatty acids by the cells, and regulate the transport of material in and out of the cells.

Food Sources—Brewer's yeast, lecithin, dark green leafy vegetables—such as spinach, turnip, and mustard greens—lentils, butter beans.

Functions in the Body—Because of the abilities mentioned above, inositol helps prevent hardening of the arteries, metabolizes fat and cholesterol, removes fats from the liver, and is important in the formation of lecithin.

Interactions—Inositol, as found in the dark green leafy vegetables and other vegetables containing high amounts of phytic acid (inositol hexaphosphate), will bind to calcium, zinc, and iron in the intestine and prevent you from absorbing these minerals normally. Caffeine may increase your need for inositol.

Recommended Usage—The typical American diet reportedly contains about 1 gram of inositol, and except in diabetics who may require supplementation of 1 to 2 grams per day, that is probably more than sufficient. In addition to foods containing inositol, you can supplement it by taking lecithin granules: two tablespoons twice daily.

Symptoms of Deficiency—Spotty hair loss, constipation, scaly skin rashes and other skin eruptions, mood swings, irritability, and high cholesterol.

Symptoms of Toxicity—None known with certainty.

Safety Information—Inositol in capsule/tablet form can cause stomach upset. You will probably tolerate lecithin granules better.

Iron

Important Facts—Mineral.

Your body needs iron to produce hemoglobin, the oxygen-carrying pigment that makes red blood cells red, and myoglobin, a similar pigment found in muscle tissues, and as a helper for a variety of important enzyme (chemical) reactions necessary for your good health.

Food Sources—Meat (including beef, veal, chicken, pork, and liver), eggs, fruit, fish, clams, eggs, green leafy vegetables, whole grains, enriched breads and cereals, asparagus, prunes, and raisins.

Functions in the Body—As noted above, you need iron to make healthy blood cells. You will become weak, pale, and fatigued from anemia if you become deficient in iron. But it's not only red blood cells that iron helps to produce; your immune defense cells, the white blood cells, also require sufficient iron for normal production. With iron deficiency, you can become more susceptible to frequent infections.

Studies show that an iron deficiency can have negative effects on learning ability, endurance, and general well-being. Runners who are iron deficient, but not anemic, have been found to have less endurance. A study of college students found that low iron may play a part in faulty attention span. And a study of iron-deficient infants, both anemic and nonanemic, revealed that, when given iron supplementation, these infants showed significant improvement in mental development scores.

Interactions—

• Excess calcium (over 2 grams per day) competes with iron in your intestine for entry into the body. Chronic use of calcium supplements can cause deficiency of iron.

• Taking vitamin C can increase iron uptake by as much as 30%.

• Iron reduces your ability to absorb copper and zinc in their ionic forms, and they return the favor by competing with the iron. For more information, see the discussions on chelation of minerals on pages 30–31 and the ion channel on pages 29–30.

• Food in your stomach reduces your ability to absorb supplemental iron; however, you will absorb the iron contained in red meat best of all.

• Coffee and tea may reduce your ability to absorb iron.

• Reduced stomach acid, from prolonged periods of taking antacids or prescription medications designed to reduce stomach acid (Tagamet, Zantac, Pepcid, Axid), may reduce your ability to absorb iron.

• Milk may reduce your ability to absorb iron.

• Excessive amounts of vitamin E interfere with iron absorption.

• You must have adequate amounts of the B vitamins riboflavin (B_2) and pyridoxine (B_6) in your diet to absorb and use iron properly.

• Deficiency of vitamin A reduces your ability to absorb iron.

• Animal protein enhances your ability to absorb iron while soy protein reduces it.

• Phytates found in cereal grains and dark green vegetables bind iron in your stomach and prevent you from absorbing it.

Recommended Usage—The DRI for men and women is 18 mg. If you take a multivitamin containing iron in a chelated form (such as iron glycinate), this amount of iron should be sufficient to keep you healthy unless you are treating a specific disorder, as listed in this text. Although iron sulfate is the most common and inexpensive form, it can irritate the digestive tract. I recommend iron glycinate or iron fumarate. They are less irritating and less likely to cause constipation. But please remember: Unless you are certain you have an iron deficiency, taking a supplement is not recommended.

Symptoms of Deficiency—Anemia, cracking at the corners of your mouth, inflamed tongue, loss of appetite, fragile bones, sensitivity to cold, constipation, depression and confusion, dizziness, difficulty swallowing, fatigue, brittle nails, fluttering and skipping of your heart with exercise, and stunted growth in children.

Symptoms of Toxicity—Headaches occur from iron excess, but loss of appetite, extreme fatigue, and dizziness occur both with too much iron and too little (see above).

Safety Information—Because iron is an oxidizing substance (which means that it can form free radicals that can damage tissues), you should not take iron in excess of what you need. And you should always take iron along with antioxidants, such as vitamin C and vitamin E. (See discussions concerning oxidation, pages 18–19, free radicals, pages 19–23, and antioxidants, page 20.)

--------------- **K (Vitamin K)** ---------------

Important Facts—Fat-soluble vitamin.

Light and alkaline (soda) solutions destroy this vitamin, which is stored in minute amounts in the liver. Vitamin K appeared on the scene with the discovery in 1934 that a substance in chicken feed containing alfalfa prevented hemorrhage in chicks. The researchers promptly began their quest to uncover the antihemorrhage factor, and by 1940, Henrik Dam of Denmark had isolated and synthesized the compound and given it the name vitamin K for *Koagulationsvitamin* because of its role in blood clotting.[27]

Food Sources—Green leafy vegetables, which provide 50 to 800 *micro*grams of vitamin K per 100 grams of food, contain the highest amounts. Other lesser sources are milk and dairy products, meat, eggs, cereals, fruits, and other vegetables.

Functions in the Body—The vitamin is actually a group of substances—phylloquinone for the K derivatives from plant sources and menaquinone from animal and bacterial sources, and menadione, a vitamin forerunner that your body converts to menaquinone—all of which share a similar action in the body.

Human deficiency, under normal conditions, is almost unheard of it is so rare, because resident bacteria in your colon continuously produce the vitamin in small amounts that you absorb into your bloodstream. Vitamin K also occurs abundantly in a wide variety of vegetable foods. However, because the vitamin is fat soluble, in order to be absorbed properly—whether from a bacterial source or from food—there must be some fat present in your intestine. Therefore, medical conditions that decrease intestinal fat absorption, such as gall bladder stones, could result in secondary deficiency of vitamin K and consequently problems with bleeding.

You could also become deficient if you took prolonged courses of antibiotics that wiped out your colon flora (since the friendly bacteria in your colon provide a goodly portion of your daily vitamin K needs). This effect would be magnified, for example, if you became severely ill, were hospitalized, unable to eat, fed all your nutrition through the vein, and also required large doses of high-potency antibiotic medications. Under such very abnormal circumstances, it may become necessary to supplement vitamin K to prevent bleeding.

On the other side of the coin, if a physician wanted to thin your blood—for example, if you developed blood clots in your legs, lung, heart, or brain, or if you had an artificial heart valve or required coronary artery bypass surgery for atherosclerotic blockages to your heart's blood supply—he or she might use the drug dicumarol (you might be more familiar with this drug by its trade name, Coumadin) to do the job. Coumadin blocks the action of vitamin K, keeps your blood from clotting well, and keeps your blood freely flowing.

As noted above, the function of vitamin K is in maintaining normal clotting of blood. The vitamin may also play a role in normal bone calcification by acting as a cofactor for a critical carboxylating enzyme.

Recent studies reveal other roles for vitamin K. Low levels of the vitamin have been related to osteoporosis. This is due to the fact that vitamin K is essential for the synthesis of osteocalcin, the protein in bone tissue on which calcium crystallizes.

Vitamin K is also helpful in converting glucose into glycogen for storage in the liver, thus promoting healthy liver function.

Preliminary studies reveal that vitamin K may prevent cancers that target the inner linings of the organs.

Interactions—

• Excess calcium intake sufficient to give a ratio of calcium to phosphorus of over 2:1 interferes with vitamin K synthesis or absorption and can cause internal bleeding.

• Large intake (on the order of 2200 IU per day) of vitamin E can reduce absorption of vitamin K from the gastrointestinal tract and can also interfere with vitamin K's effect on proper blood clotting.[28]

Recommended Usage—Basal requirement for vitamin K— that is, that amount needed to prevent deficiency *under normal circumstances*—is 1 *micro*gram per kilogram of body weight per day. There are 2.2 pounds in every kilogram, so in round figures, a 150-pound person would weigh 70 kilograms and would require 70 *micro*grams of vitamin K per day. In the United States, the typical "mixed" diet contains between 300 and 500 *micro*grams of vitamin K per day. Based on that calculation, it's easy to see why deficiency would be rare except when something disrupts normal eating patterns or when interactions from drugs impair absorption of the vitamin. Even without food, a normally functioning population of gastrointestinal bacteria can generate enough vitamin K to at least meet the 70 microgram requirement.

Newborn infants who are exclusively breast-fed risk vitamin K deficiency, because human breast milk contains relatively little of the vitamin, and intestinal flora have not yet populated the infant colon in sufficient numbers to make the vitamin. For this reason, most hospitals now routinely administer vitamin K to newborn infants by injection to prevent deficiency and hemorrhage. And commercial infant formulas contain 4 *micro*grams per 100 calories, which again, under normal circumstances, should be quite sufficient to meet bodily needs.

Symptoms of Deficiency—Free bleeding (hemorrhage) is the only documented symptom of deficiency.

Symptoms of Toxicity—Even in large doses, toxic side effects are rare.

Safety Information—Administration of the menadione (synthetic) form of the vitamin may cause hemolytic anemia, high bilirubin in the blood, and yellowing of the skin and eyes. The phylloquinone form (derived from plants) does not do this.

Linoleic Acid

Important Facts—Essential fat. Macronutrient.

Linoleic acid is the essential fat found in oils extracted from plant sources such as corn oil, safflower oil, sunflower oil, and canola oil. The body absolutely requires this fatty substance because it is the raw material from which your body makes all the prostaglandin chemical messengers. For more information and important facts about this fat source, please refer to the discussion concerning the yin and yang of human health the eicosinoid messengers, and the macronutrients found on page 23.

Food Sources—Plant-derived oils as specified on page 81, plus the supplemental product evening primrose oil.

Functions in the Body—Through production of the good and the bad prostaglandin messengers, linoleic acid regulates both sides of the coin for virtually every important body function: the "good" messengers cause lower blood pressure through relaxing the blood vessels, reduce inflammation, reduce pain, relieve swelling, promote healing, improve blood flow, build lean tissue. And the "bad" ones, basically, do the opposite.

Interactions—Fish oil (omega-3 fatty acids or EPA) help to regulate the flow of prostaglandin messengers toward the "good" side of the equation.

Recommended Usage—For specific dietary recommendations, refer to the discussion entitled "Macronutrients" on page 23.

• One word of caution: Try to use oils that have been derived from the plant or seed by pressing without heat. Heating the oils to high temperatures changes their structure, reducing their quality and usability by your body. Some research even suggests that the altered oils could cause immune system problems that could increase risk for cancer. Cold pressing preserves the healthy qualities of these oils.

Symptoms of Deficiency—Stunted growth, problems with coordination, behavioral problems and learning disabilities, numbness, poor vision, and weakness.

Symptoms of Toxicity—None known.

Safety Information—None applicable.

─────────────── **Magnesium** ───────────────

Important Facts—Mineral.
The bony skeleton contains half or more of the 25 or so grams of magnesium in the adult body, with about 1% in the body fluids and

the remainder in the muscles and soft tissues. This mineral absorbs poorly from the intestine, with as much as 60% to 70% of the amount taken in excreted in the stool; however, this figure changes as intake changes. On diets low in magnesium, you will absorb as much as 75% of what you take in.

Food Sources—Magnesium, because it is a component of plant chlorophyll, occurs in foods at every level of the food chain, such that all unprocessed foods contain some magnesium, although the amount varies widely. The richest sources are whole seeds, such as nuts and legumes, as well as wheat germ and other unprocessed grains, milk and other dairy products, soybeans, meat, and seafood. Be aware that milling of grain (removal of the husk and germ layers) removes up to 80% of the magnesium. Other food sources include green vegetables, spinach, soybeans, peas, molasses, and cornmeal. Some antacids and laxatives also contain magnesium (for example, Milk of Magnesia). Hard water may provide a good supplemental source of magnesium and of calcium; however, the amounts vary widely with location. Soft water is usually quite low in these minerals.

Functions in the Body—Magnesium functions in a critical capacity as a cofactor (or coenzyme) in more than 300 known enzymatic reactions involved in a broad range of metabolic activities. In energy production, the metabolism of glucose, the oxidation of fatty acids, and the activation of amino acids all require magnesium. Magnesium is involved in protein synthesis (the building of new body proteins), in the transmission of the genetic message through production of DNA and RNA (the proteins of inheritance), and in the formation of a compound called cyclic AMP that serves as a "messenger" to tell the cells what to do. Let me digress to explain that a little more fully.

If a gland functions to produce a substance—an enzyme or hormone, for example—the message to initiate the process of making the substance begins with the formation of cyclic AMP within the cell or on the cell membrane. Countless systems throughout the body depend on the message from cyclic AMP to signal when to do their job, and the formation of cyclic AMP depends on there being plenty of magnesium available.

Low magnesium levels are linked with psychiatric problems. In one study, it was discovered that the average magnesium levels in autistic children was well below average. Some evidence suggests that autistic children may improve when given large doses of magnesium along with vitamin B_6.

Magnesium affects the muscle tone of blood vessels, which is why magnesium supplementation has been shown to help control cardiovascular disease.

In addition, magnesium functions in nerve transmission, in helping us adapt to cold, as a structural component of bone and tooth enamel, and in muscular and vascular relaxation.

Interactions—

• Calcium may reduce the absorption of magnesium because the two minerals share a common transport system in the intestine. The ratio of dietary calcium to magnesium should be 2:1.

• A high-fat diet can reduce magnesium absorption because the fat and magnesium combine to form soap-like compounds that the gastrointestinal tract cannot absorb.

• A high-fiber diet can promote loss of some minerals, including magnesium. The mechanism involved in the loss is, again, most likely through preventing adequate absorption or because of combination with oxalates and phytates in fibrous foods to form unabsorbable compounds.

• Supplemental folic acid can increase the demand for magnesium by stepping up the activity of enzymes that require magnesium to work properly.

• Iron may decrease the gastrointestinal absorption of magnesium.

• Cholecalciferol (vitamin D) stimulates the intestinal absorption of magnesium to a degree; however, because its stimulatory effect is stronger for calcium, supplemental vitamin D without extra magnesium can create a relative magnesium deficiency.

• Foods high in oxalic acid, such as almonds, chard, cocoa, rhubarb, spinach, and tea, decrease magnesium absorption.

• A deficiency of vitamin E may reduce magnesium levels in the tissues.

• Alcohol, potassium, and caffeine all increase the loss of magnesium through the kidneys. Alcoholics, because they couple both insufficient dietary intake with excessive urinary output of the mineral, can become quite deficient in magnesium, and it may be this particular deficiency that contributes to the hallucinations (delirium tremens, or DTs) that accompany acute alcohol withdrawal.

• High sugar intake increases your need for magnesium (probably through its interaction in insulin metabolism) as well as by increasing your loss of magnesium in urine.

• High-protein diets increase the demand for magnesium, especially in situations of rapid building of new body tissues, such as growing children, training athletes, pregnant women, and nursing mothers.

• The B vitamins require magnesium to work properly because the mineral is a required cofactor in the formation of thiamine pyrophosphate (TPP), which your body must form before you can make use of thiamine and other B vitamins.

• People taking the drug digitalis can develop heart rhythm disturbances if they become deficient in magnesium.

• Certain diuretics cause an increase in magnesium loss through the kidneys. This group includes the drug furosemide (Lasix).

Recommended Usage—During pregnancy, the needs of the fetus increase magnesium demand by an extra 20 mg per day; nursing mothers need an additional 60 mg per day to keep up with losses in breast milk. DRI figures range from 400 (for adult men and women) to 450 mg (for pregnant and lactating women). Remember that magnesium should be balanced with calcium at a ratio of 1:2.

Physicians routinely prescribe a sustained release form of magnesium, called Slo-Mag, for patients requiring additional magnesium because of medical conditions. However, over-the-counter supplemental forms of magnesium include Milk of Magnesia tablets and gelatin capsules of magnesium sulfate powder (epsom salts) taken in doses of one capsule three to six times per day to combat mild to moderate deficiency states.

Another available source of magnesium is dolomite tablets or powder. A usual dose is $1/2$ to one teaspoon of the powder (or an equivalent dose in pill form) dissolved in water and taken one to four times daily. (See Safety Information.)

Treatment of severe symptomatic deficiencies—such as would usually only occur in eclampsia (the cramping and seizures that sometimes accompany the late stages of pregnancy or labor), in severe, chronic gastrointestinal disorders that prevent adequate absorption of nutrients, or in certain rare inherited disorders in which a person is born without the ability to absorb magnesium— should occur only under the direct supervision of a physician. These cases may require the replacement of magnesium by injection into the vein in heroic (3000 to 4000 mg) doses to correct the problem.

Symptoms of Deficiency—Anemia (caused from red blood cell rupture); loss of appetite; heart rhythm disturbances including rapid heartbeat; mental changes including agitation, anxiety, confusion, depression, disorientation, hallucinations, hyperactivity, irritability, nervousness, restlessness, and exaggerated startle response (jumpiness); neurologic symptoms including numbness and tingling, difficulty balancing with walking, vertigo, and seizures; muscular symptoms including twitches, tremors, pains, and weakness; blood pressure disturbances in both directions (too high and too low); subnormal body temperature; and cold hands and feet.

Symptoms of Toxicity—Toxic symptoms are rare as long as your kidneys function normally. In cases of impaired kidney function, especially in people taking magnesium supplementally, toxic symptoms of excess magnesium may develop. They include: slow heart rate, fatigue, low blood pressure, flushing, dryness of the mouth, muscular weakness, thirst, nausea, and vomiting.

Safety Information—
• If you have any significant degree of kidney disease, please avoid supplemental magnesium intake except under the close and direct supervision of your personal physician or kidney specialist.
• Some brands of dolomite powder or dolomite pills—which provide good sources of both calcium and magnesium—may contain potentially toxic levels of heavy metals including arsenic, lead, cadmium, mercury, and aluminum.

Manganese

Important Facts—Mineral.

Although the first report of manganese poisoning (toxicity) appeared in 1837, its role as a nutrient essential to human good health did not become clear until the 1970s, when while studying vitamin K metabolism medical researchers accidentally created a case of manganese deficiency by failing to add this mineral to the purified diet of one person in their 17-week study. Without manganese for this period, the man developed these symptoms: a mild rash; his black hair took on a reddish hue; growth of his hair, nails, and beard slowed; he suffered occasional bouts of nausea and vomiting; his triglyceride level declined; and he lost weight.

Food Sources—Whole grains and cereals, nuts, seeds, avocados, fruits, green vegetables, dried legumes, tea, ginger, and cloves.

Functions in the Body—Your body needs manganese to properly metabolize fat, to build bones and connective tissues, to produce energy, for healthy nerves and immune system, and to make the cholesterol and the genetic proteins (DNA) required for every living cell to be able to divide—an activity that cells must do to survive.

Interactions—The one important interaction occurs between manganese and iron. If you become deficient in iron, you will absorb more manganese from your diet (with the remote possibility of toxicity from the excess). On the other hand, if you overload iron, you will impair your ability to absorb manganese and possibly create a deficiency.

Recommended Usage—Diets high in refined carbohydrates may not supply adequate amounts of manganese, especially when requirements are increased, as during pregnancy. I recommend that unless you eat large quantities of the foods rich in manganese, you should supplement manganese to 10 mg per day. This figure is above the DRI of 2 mg, but keep in mind that manganese is poorly absorbed and is severely lacking in refined foods. I am not alone in believing the DRI figure is too low. Be sure to take this mineral in chelated form, as manganese aspartate, to prevent possible interference with your absorption of iron and possibly other minerals.

Symptoms of Deficiency—Fragile bones, rashes, sugar intolerance, high cholesterol, nausea, weight loss, a tendency to breast ailments, tremors, rapid pulse, memory loss, hearing problems, eye problems, and reproductive tract (ovary and testes) degeneration.

Symptoms of Toxicity—Loss of appetite, hallucinations, impairment of judgment and memory, sleeplessness, and muscle pains.

Safety Information—At the levels described in this text, the mineral is safe.

--------------------- **Molybdenum** ---------------------

Important Facts—Trace element.

Food Sources—Buckwheat, wheat germ, dark green leafy vegetables, lima beans, soybeans, liver, oats, lentils, barley, and sunflower seeds.

Functions in the Body—This element assists in the metabolism of iron in the liver and is believed to be a critical helper in a number of enzyme (chemical) reactions that the body carries out, most importantly one that prevents gout by helping your body metabolize and remove uric acid. (See Gout, Section II, page 345.) It also promotes normal cell function.

Interactions—Molybdenum may cause an increase in your loss of copper from the urine, even in low doses. A high intake of sulfur may decrease molybdenum levels.

Recommended Usage—No DRI has been set for molybdenum, but I recommend you take 100 *micro*grams of the trace element daily. Estimates of adequate daily intake range from 75 to 250 *micro*grams per day for adults and older children. That is an amount that you can easily get from diet alone if you choose foods rich in this trace element.

Symptoms of Deficiency—Little certain information exists in the medical literature regarding deficiency of this trace mineral, but deficiency *may* cause a higher risk for gout as well as cancer, cavities, and sexual impotence.

Symptoms of Toxicity—In humans, aside from increases in uric acid and gouty attacks at doses of 15 mg per day, no certain symptoms of molybdenum excess have been identified.

Safety Information—Nontoxic in dietary and supplemental amounts specified in this text.

--------------------- **Niacin (Vitamin B$_3$)** ---------------------

Important Facts—Water-soluble vitamin.

Although cooking foods in large amounts of water, then discarding the water, can potentially cause niacin losses from food sources, heat and light do not affect it. Deficiency causes the classic disease pellagra. For a more in-depth discussion and additional important facts about this vitamin, see the Classic Vitamin Deficiency Diseases, pages 10–15.

Food Sources—Milk, meat, poultry, fish, eggs, cheese, dried beans (legumes), sunflower and sesame seeds, tomatoes, peanuts, carrots, broccoli, whole grains, and brewer's yeast.

Functions in the Body—Niacin functions as a required coenzyme in protein metabolism; in the synthesis of genetic material, fatty acids, and cholesterol; in energy production; and it is necessary for proper central nervous system (brain) functions.

A number of studies show that niacin is effective in reducing cholesterol and triglyceride levels in the blood. Because of this, and because of the low cost of the vitamin, it is used in treating patients with elevated cholesterol levels.

Niacin is often used in combination with other medications to help treat mental disorders such as anxiety, nervousness, depression, and even schizophrenia. Niacinamide may also be useful in treating epilepsy, when used with anticonvulsants.

Several studies indicate that niacinamide is effective against several types of carcinogens, making it a possible treatment for cancer.

Interactions—Your body can convert some dietary tryptophan to niacin at a rate such that 60 mg of tryptophan becomes 1 mg of niacin.[29] Nutritional researchers have dubbed the amount of tryptophan that will yield 1 mg of niacin as 1 "niacin equivalent." This conversion allows a diet rich in tryptophan to increase available niacin even in the absence of dietary niacin.

Recommended Usage—DRI recommendation for B_3 is 20 mg.

Symptoms of Deficiency—Loss of appetite, fatigue, weakness, heartburn, depression, and irritability occur early in the developing deficiency. Classic signs of deficiency include a red, inflamed, scaling dermatitis especially prominent on the face, neck, arms, and hands (but present in any sun-exposed areas); diarrhea; painful swallowing from soreness of the mouth and esophagus; psychological symptoms such as depression, disorientation, delusional thoughts and hallucinations; and ultimately, death. Classic deficiency state is termed *pellagra*.

Symptoms of Toxicity—Flushing and itching of the skin, especially of the face and upper trunk, abnormal heart rhythm, and gastrointestinal problems.

Safety Information—Not stored, water soluble. May cause flushing of the skin; however, the niacinamide and nicotinamide forms of the vitamin seem not to cause this symptom as readily as niacin itself. Take note, however, that the niacinamide form of niacin, paradoxically, may cause depression or fatigue in some people.

──────────────── **Nickel** ────────────────

Important Facts—Ultratrace mineral.

The first reports of nickel as a substance toxic to rabbits and dogs appeared in 1826. But by 1936, scientists had begun to suspect that tiny amounts of the mineral might be essential to human health. Even so, not until the 1970s did hard evidence support this theory.

Food Sources—Chocolate, nuts, dried beans, peas, grains, fruits, and vegetables.

Functions in the Body—Although research has yet to conclusively document the precise role for nickel in the human body, there is a growing body of evidence that suggests it may function, as so many ultratrace minerals do, as a critical cofactor, or helper molecule, to certain enzymes that speed up the billions of chemical reactions occurring continually in your body.

Interactions—Nickel needs vary with iron intake. High amounts of iron in your diet increase your need for nickel; low amounts of iron decrease it.

Recommended Usage—Although there is no DRI for nickel yet established, an estimate of human needs based on animal needs puts daily intake in the ballpark of 35 *micro*grams per day. In America, the average dietary intake of nickel is between 170 and 700 *micro*grams, a level more than sufficient to provide you with plenty of dietary nickel without supplementing.

Symptoms of Deficiency—Research has so far not provided us with much information about deficiency in people, probably because the amounts necessary for good health are so small that deficiency rarely if ever happens.

Symptoms of Toxicity—There are no certain signs of toxicity of nickel in humans. Your intestinal tract absorbs so little of the nickel that you consume in foods, it would be unlikely that you would ever take enough by mouth to cause problems. For example, it would take a human dose of 250 mg of nickel to equal the toxic effect (primarily stunted growth) seen from nickel in laboratory animal studies. However, some people develop true allergy to nickel topically—that is, by contact with their skin. In these cases, rashes usually develop to the nickel alloys used to make gold jewelry stronger or to nickel coins in a pocket. Once this kind of skin sensitivity to nickel develops, you could react to nickel you took by mouth, even in small doses.

Safety Information—None applicable.

Phosphorus

Important Facts—Mineral.

Phosphorus is the second most abundant mineral in the body and is a mineral that occurs widely in nature—so widely, in fact, that the average American eats a diet that provides 7 to 10 times the adult requirement.

Food Sources—Milk and other dairy products, meats, poultry, fish, eggs, grains, nuts, dried beans, peas, lentils, and green leafy vegetables.

Functions in the Body—Phosphorus, along with calcium, gives strength to your bones and teeth, which contain 85% of the phosphorus in your body. The remainder assists in a variety of chemical reactions in the body, most importantly in energy production; in metabolism of protein, carbohydrate, and fat; and in building protein. More recently, it has been discovered that many of the B vitamins are effective only when combined with phosphorus. This mineral also maintains the proper pH balance within the body.

Interactions—

• Antacids usually contain either magnesium or aluminum, both of which can interfere with your ability to absorb phosphorus.

• Iron can interfere with your ability to absorb phosphorus.

• Calcium and phosphorous exist in a balance in your bones and teeth. If you eat a diet containing too much phosphorus, your body's tendency to balance these two minerals could cause calcium to be pulled from the bones, weakening them. One study that showed that female athletes who drank phosphorus-rich carbonated beverages had more than twice as many fractures as did those who did not drink these beverages.

• Normal phosphorus metabolism requires sufficient amounts of vitamin D. When phosphorus levels fall, the drop stimulates your body to make more active vitamin D, probably to increase your ability to absorb and use the phosphorus, although the exact connection is unclear.

Recommended Usage—Phosphorus occurs so widely in foods that as long as you can eat, you are not likely to become deficient in phosphorus. Although the richest food sources are of animal origin, even vegetarians can manage to get enough phosphorus if they eat eggs and nuts. Populations that may need to supplement include the elderly, menopausal women, and individuals on restricted diets. The DRI for phosphorus is 1000 mg for adult men and women, 1300 mg for pregnant and lactating women.

Symptoms of Deficiency—Loss of appetite, weight loss, weakness and fatigue, numbness and tingling sensations, bone pain, anxiety, and apprehension.

Symptoms of Toxicity—I know of no documented symptom of phosphorus excess, except in people who suffer from severe kidney disease (renal failure) and cannot rid their body of the excess. Even then, the symptoms are not a consequence of the phosphorus excess as much as the low calcium that occurs because of the excess. These symptoms include: nerve and muscle irritability, muscle spasms, and convulsions. Potentially, this may lead to osteoporosis.

Safety Information—None applicable.

Potassium

Important Facts—Potassium is the major ion in every living cell, which means that you will find it in abundance in fresh foods.

Food Sources—Dairy, fish, legumes, yams, dried apricots, cantaloupe, lima beans, potato, avocado, bananas, broccoli, liver, milk, peanut butter, and citrus fruits.

Nutraceuticals and —— Phytochemicals: Brand-new Terms, Same Old Foods ——

Nutritionally dense foods are not new to the natural food industry—health-food stores have carried lecithin, brewer's yeast, and soy products for over 60 years. What *is* new is the amazing research that points to the disease-preventing abilities of these and other foods. The term *nutraceutical* was coined by Dr. Stephen Felice, director of New York's Foundation for Innovation in Medicine, to describe specific chemical compounds found in foods that may prevent disease. *Phytochemical* is the term now used when discussing the plant source of most of these protective compounds. Right now, these compounds have a "quasi-nutrient" status, so perhaps *phytonutrients* is a more accurate term. But the more common term remains phyto-chemicals.

In the past, phytochemicals were classified as vitamins: Flavonoids were known as vitamin P, indoles and glucosinolates were called vitamin U, and so on. But they lost their status as vitamins because specific deficiency symptoms could not be established. Today, phytochemicals are classified according to their functions as well as individual physical and chemical characteristics of the molecules.

Terpenes

Terpenes make up one of the largest classes of phyto-chemicals. They are found in green foods, soy products, and grains. Terpenes have a role as antioxidants. They protect lipids, blood, and other fluids from free radical oxygen species.

Carotenoids

The most intensely studied terpenes are carotenoids. You've probably heard of beta-carotene. Carotenoids give color to the foods that contain them. The bright yellow, orange, and red pigments found in vegetables comes from carotenoids. Flamingos are pink because of carotenoids; egg yolks owe their yellow hue to carotenoids.

There are more than 600 naturally occurring carotenoids. And although beta-carotene is a precursor to vitamin A, not all carotenoids act in this manner (less than 10% have vitamin A activity). The carotenes have been shown to protect against lung, colorectal, breast, uterine, and prostate cancers. They also protect skin cells against UV radiation.

The other type of carotenoids, xanthophylls, protect vitamins A, E, and other carotenoids from oxidation. Recent evidence suggests that xanthophylls are tissue specific.

Limonoids

Here's another subclass of terpenes. These are found in citrus fruit peels, and seem to be specifically protective of lung tissue.

Phytosterols

Most plants contain sterols. Green and yellow vegetables contain significant amounts, mostly concentrated in their seeds. Most of the research done in this area has focused on the seeds of pumpkins, yams, soy, rice, and herbs. Phytosterols block the uptake of cholesterol and help excrete it from the body, thus making these phytochemicals valuable in preventing cardiovascular disease. Research indicates that phytosterols also halt the development of tumors in colon, breast, and prostate glands, though *why* they do this is unclear.

Phenols

Another widely studied phytochemical class is phenols. Phenols protect us from oxidative damage. The blue, blue-red, and violet pigments found in berries, grapes, and eggplant come from to their phenolic content. Phenols have the ability to block the enzymes that cause inflammation. They also protect platelets from clumping.

Flavonoids

This phenol subclass enhances the effects of vitamin C. Although there are over 1500 flavonoids, some of the more "popular" ones include flavones, flavonols (quercetin, ginkgo, rutin), and flavanones.

Flavonoids fight against allergies, inflammation, free radicals, ulcers, viruses, and tumors. They also inhibit specific enzymes that cause health problems. For example, they block the enzyme that raises blood pressure. This, in combination with their ability to protect the vascular system and strengthen the capillaries that carry oxygen and essential nutrients to all cells, makes flavonoids essential in the prevention of many cancers and cardiovascular diseases.

Flavonoids also reduce the risk of estrogen-induced cancers by blocking the enzymes that produce estrogen.

And finally, these little wonders also seem to retard the development of cataracts in people with sugar metabolism disorders, such as diabetes. Experts don't fully understand how they do this, but it is suspected that flavonoids prevent cataracts by blocking a digestive enzyme that converts the sugar galactose into the potentially harmful form of galacticol.

Anthocyanidins

This group of flavonoids is technically known as "flavonals." They provide bridges that connect and strengthen the strands of collagen protein. Collagen health is vital because collagen makes up soft tissues, tendons, ligaments, and bone matrix. Collagen strength depends on the maintenance of those cross-links. Anthocyanidins also act as free radical scavengers. This is of great importance to anyone who exercises, since exercising generates massive amounts of free radicals.

Isoflavones

Isoflavones are found in beans and other legumes. They are much like flavonoids in the way they block enzymes that promote tumor growth. Soy products are high in isoflavones, and it has been shown that people who consume high amounts of soy foods significantly lower their risk of breast, uterine, and prostate cancer.

Glucosinates

These phytochemicals are found in cruciferous vegetables and help detoxify the liver. They also regulate white blood cells and cytokines. White blood cells scavenge the immune system while cytokines act as messengers, coordinating the activities of all immune cells. Glucosinates block enzymes that promote tumor growth, especially in the breast, liver, colon, lung, stomach, and esophagus.

Allylic Sulfides

You know these phytochemicals as garlic and onion. Leeks, shallots, and chives are also included in this category. As a group, these allylic sulfides possess antimutagenic and anticarcinogenic properties as well as immune and cardiovascular protection. Research indicates they also offer antigrowth activity for tumors, fungi, parasites, cholesterol, and platelet/leukocyte adhesion factors.

Indoles

The vegetables that contain indoles also contain significant amounts of vitamin C, so it's no surprise that some of the indoles interact with vitamin C. Indole complexes activate detoxification enzymes, particularly in the gastrointestinal tract.

Isoprenoids

These phytochemicals neutralize free radicals. However, rather than neutralize them themselves, they grab the free radicals and pass them off to other antioxidants.

Tocotrienols and Tocopherols

These two are cousins and occur in grains and palm oil. Tocotrienols seem to inhibit breast cancer cell growth, though they have been most widely studied for their ability to lower cholesterol.

Lipoic Acid and Ubiquinone

Lipoic acid and ubiquinone (more commonly known as coenzyme Q_{10}) are antioxidants that work to extend the effects of other antioxidants. Lipoic acid protects vitamin E and C as well as SOD (catalase and glutathione), all of which are important in liver detoxification activity. Other unproven but speculated benefits include improved heart-muscle metabolism, lowered blood pressure, treatment of chest pain caused by coronary insufficiency, treatment of congestive heart failure.

Functions in the Body—Although the vast majority of potassium remains inside the cells that make up your body, it is in a constant state of balance with a small amount that remains outside. That small amount, however, is of critical importance in contributing to the passage of electrical nerve impulses throughout your body, controlling the contraction of muscles including the heart muscle, and helping to maintain your blood pressure in the normal range.

It is becoming more evident that low levels of potassium are associated with high blood pressure. Some researchers believe that low potassium may play a more significant role in hypertension than high sodium does. In many studies, for example, potassium supplementation significantly lowered blood pressure without sodium restriction. Further studies show that potassium lowers the rate of fatal strokes by reducing blood pressure.

Your kidneys, primarily, regulate the loss of potassium from your body, although you do lose some in stomach acid secretions and in sweat. If you suffer a prolonged period of vomiting and diarrhea, you can also become deficient in potassium. The most common cause of low potassium, however, is the overuse of diuretic medications ("water" pills).

Interactions—

• Certain diuretic medications cause your kidneys to rid you of excess fluid by making you waste sodium. Where sodium goes, so goes body water; so if your kidneys rid you of sodium, water will follow. The removal device that the kidney uses to get rid of sodium is called the sodium-potassium pump. Diuretic medications—such as the thiazides (hydrochlorothiazide) and furosemide (Lasix, Bumex)—cause a pumping not only of sodium, but also of potassium. Their use requires you to supplement with potassium to keep up with the loss.

• Tobacco inhibits potassium uptake.

• Caffeine causes you to waste more potassium through your kidneys and may cause you to become deficient.

• If you are deficient in magnesium, you will find it difficult to correct low potassium, and you must first correct the low magnesium before supplemental potassium will do much good.

• Certain diuretic and heart/blood pressure medications have been designed to "spare" the loss of potassium you would normally suffer from their use. Taking extra potassium while also taking the following medications could cause you to develop toxic symptoms from too much potassium: Dyazide, Maxzide, and the ACE inhibitors (such as Zestril, Capoten, and Vasotec).

Recommended Usage—It is estimated that the average American diet contains 2 to 6 grams of potassium daily. This is sufficient for a healthy adult. However, deficiency can result from alcoholism, anorexia/bingeing/purging, illnesses that interfere with appetite, and use of diuretics, steroids, or laxatives. What's more, potassium must exist in balance with sodium. High-sodium foods include canned goods, lunch meats, sausages, processed foods, and many frozen foods. The best way to avoid a potassium deficiency is to eat a variety of fresh foods. There is no DRI for potassium.

Symptoms of Deficiency—Acne, constipation, salt and fluid retention, stunted growth, low blood pressure, fatigue, insomnia, muscle weakness and cramping, thirst, depression, nervousness, clouded thinking, sugar intolerance, high cholesterol, extremely dry skin and mouth, and heart palpitations.

Symptoms of Toxicity—Clouded thinking (yes, this symptom occurs from both too much and too little potassium), irregular heartbeat, possible heart failure, muscle fatigue, difficulty speaking, and weakness. Keep in mind that toxicity is seen only when daily intake exceeds 18 grams, an amount highly unlikely when ingested through food.

Safety Information—With normal kidneys, supplemental potassium almost never causes problems. People with severe kidney impairment (renal failure) cannot handle extra potassium and should add potassium only under the direct supervision of their personal physician or kidney specialist.

——— Riboflavin (Vitamin B₂) ———

Important Facts—Water-soluble vitamin.

Because the vitamin is destroyed by light and heat, food kept in clear containers or sun-dried foods may lose significant amounts of riboflavin. The name *riboflavin* takes its root from the Latin word *flavius,* meaning yellow, the basis for which is readily apparent in the rich yellow color the vitamin imparts to urine.

Food Sources—Found in animal protein sources: eggs, meat, fish, poultry, liver, and dairy products. Not found at high levels in natural grains, but enriched or fortified grains, cereals, and bakery products as well as yeast extract contain high amounts. Broccoli, turnip greens, asparagus, and spinach are good green vegetable sources.

Functions in the Body—Riboflavin functions in metabolism as a coenzyme in oxidation and reduction reactions (see oxidation, pages 18–19) and is needed for proper conversion of tryptophan to niacin and for transformation and activation of a number of other vitamins, notably pyridoxine, folic acid, and vitamin K. It is necessary for the breakdown of fat and for the synthesis of corticosteroids, red blood cells, and glycogen.

Animal studies show that riboflavin deficiency may increase the susceptibility of tissues of the esophagus to cancer. A deficiency also reduces the body's ability to produce antibodies, thus making this vitamin an immune booster.

Eye health depends on riboflavin. This vitamin enables the eyes to adapt to light. Riboflavin is used by many practitioners as a treatment in the early stages of cataracts. The positive results indicate that this vitamin may actually prevent or at least delay the progress of cataracts.

Because riboflavin is helpful to people with carpal tunnel syndrome, researchers believe it is useful for neurological problems.

Interactions—
• Sunlight destroys riboflavin.
• Facilitates iron absorption, mobilization, and retention.[30]

• Increases in exercise and in physical work increase riboflavin requirements, but precise need for excess supplementation in these situations has yet to be determined.

• Thyroid hormone enhances the conversion of riboflavin to its active coenzyme forms.

• Aldactone (a blood pressure drug) increases the conversion of riboflavin to its coenzyme forms. Spironolactone (an aldosterone antagonist also used to treat high blood pressure) blocks the conversion.

• Chlorpromazine (used in depression and psychoses) inhibits the conversion of riboflavin to one of its coenzyme forms.

• The tricyclic antidepressants imipramine and amitriptyline inhibit riboflavin metabolism, especially in the heart tissue.

• Boric acid increases excretion (or loss) of riboflavin. (And treatment with riboflavin has been used clinically to reverse boric acid intoxication.)

• Antibiotics and alcohol destroy riboflavin.

Recommended Usage—The DRI for riboflavin is 1.7 mg for adult men and women and 2.0 mg for pregnant and lactating women.

Symptoms of Deficiency—Alopecia (spotty hair loss); depression and deterioration of personality; lesions of the lining of the mouth, sores of the angle of the mouth, and glossitis (smooth, red, painful tongue); a seborrheic scaling dermatitis around the nose and mouth, on the body as a whole, and in particular itchiness and inflammation of the skin of the external genitalia in men and women; redness, itching, burning, and light-sensitivity of the eyes, blurred vision, and even cataract formation; and dizziness. In experimental animals, deficiency of riboflavin causes congenital malformations.

Symptoms of Toxicity—None known.

Safety Information—None applicable.

Selenium

Important Facts—Mineral. Antioxidant.

Selenium first entered the nutritional scene in the 1930s, not as a deficiency as most nutrients did, but as a toxicity in animals. Cows grazing on plants and grasses grown in a high-selenium–containing soil developed chronic poisoning called alkali disease (with hair loss, liver cirrhosis, hoof malformations, and muscle loss). The importance of this trace element in human nutrition did not become clear until 1979, when scientists in China discovered that they could prevent a serious heart disease (a cardiomyopathy or heart-muscle–weakening disease) afflicting young women and children by giving them selenium. Since that time, a flurry of research activity has documented its role as an antioxidant assisting vitamin E and vitamin C in protecting us from diseases such as cancer and our tissues from aging damage by free radicals. (Please refer to the discussions concerning oxidation, free radicals, and antioxidants on pages 18–23.)

Food Sources—Seafood, kidney, liver, and muscle meats contain high amounts of selenium. Grains and seeds may contain a good amount of selenium, but it depends on the selenium content of the soil in which they were grown. Fruits and vegetables contain little selenium.

Functions in the Body—Your body requires selenium, along with vitamin E, to produce its own natural free radical scavenger and potent antioxidant, glutathione. This body chemical works to promote a healthy immune system. Because your immune system defends you from infection, from developing cancer, and possibly from aging, you require selenium to maintain good health.

In its role as an antioxidant, selenium is an anticancer mineral. Researchers have found that people living in areas with selenium-rich soil have a significantly lower risk of cancer, as do people with a high-selenium food supply and people with higher blood levels of selenium. Studies indicate it is especially protective against tumors of the ovaries, cervix, rectum, bladder, esophagus, pancreas, skin, liver, and prostate, as well as leukemia.

A Finnish study of 12,000 people indicated that the risk of fatal cancer in people with the lowest levels of serum selenium was almost six times higher than that in people with the highest selenium concentrations. But selenium cannot do its work alone. When combined with vitamin E, and perhaps with vitamin A, as well, selenium's antioxidant properties are enhanced. The National Cancer Institute is conducting ongoing chemopreventive trials of several nutrients, including selenium, vitamin E, and vitamin A.

People who have selenium deficiencies have also been found to suffer from heart problems that respond to selenium supplementation.

Selenium seems to play a role in the war against aging. Another Finnish study on elderly patients revealed that participants who were given large doses of selenium and vitamin E for one year enjoyed enhanced mental well-being, including less fatigue, depression, and anxiety; increased mental alertness; and increased abilities for self-care.

Interactions—
• Vitamin E works with selenium to produce glutathione, and therefore, deficiency of vitamin E can impair your ability to use selenium to your benefit.
• Vitamin C, another powerful antioxidant, assists in the normal metabolism of selenium, and therefore, deficiency in vitamin C can undermine your body's use of selenium.

Recommended Usage—The DRI for selenium is 70 *micro*grams for all men and women. If possible, try to find a selenium supplement as an amino acid chelate, such as L-selenomethionine. This form is the least toxic and most easily absorbed. I recommend taking 100 to 200 *micro*grams per day. Sodium selenate in the same dose will suffice.

Symptoms of Deficiency—High cholesterol, stunted growth, frequent infections, poor function of the liver and the pancreas, muscular weakness, and sterility in men.

Symptoms of Toxicity—Alopecia (spotty hair loss), arthritis, brittle nails, diabetes mellitus, garlic breath odor and metallic taste in the mouth, muscle pains, irritability, poor immune function, poor kidney and liver function, yellow tinge to the skin, rashes, and pale complexion.

Safety Information—In the form selenite, this mineral can interact with oxygen to produce free radicals that can damage your tissues. Sodium selenate is less toxic and more easily removed by your kidneys. If possible, purchase selenium as an amino acid chelate (also called organic selenium) in the form L-selenomethionine, which your body rapidly and completely absorbs and which has fewer side effects.

Silicon

Important Facts—Ultratrace mineral.

Although silicon, the most abundant element on earth, was identified as early as 1848, it was not until 1972 that scientists came to believe it played a role in animal and human health. It is the major constituent in sand, hence its abundance.

Food Sources—Whole grains, alfalfa, brown rice, soybeans, leafy green vegetables, bell peppers, root vegetables, unrefined cereal products, and the skin of chicken.

Functions in the Body—Silicon is chemically much like its "sister" element, carbon. Its most important function (probably because very little research into its actions in human beings has been done) is in a chemical reaction that hooks the tiny subunits of fibrous body tissues, collagen and elastin, tightly together, giving them their resilience and strength. It also plays a role in bone calcification, although we don't yet know how.

Because it counteracts the effects of aluminum on the body, it is important in the prevention of Alzheimer's disease and osteoporosis.

Silicon inhibits the aging process and is needed in larger amounts in the elderly population.

Interactions—Boron, calcium, magnesium, manganese, and potassium enhance the absorption of silicon.

Recommended Usage—There is no hard information yet available for a recommendation for this nutrient. A ballpark estimate for intake—and it truly is that, an estimate—is 20 to 45 mg per day for adults. No studies have been done in infants or children. You should be able to get that amount from food without any problem.

Symptoms of Deficiency—In people, there's really very little information; however, deficiency in animals causes abnormal bone formation and weak fibrous tissues. There's no reason to assume the same problems would not also occur in people—especially growing people—if they were to become deficient, but the data simply aren't there yet to say.

Symptoms of Toxicity—Nontoxic.

Safety Information—Not applicable.

Sodium

Important Facts—Mineral. Electrolyte.

Sodium is the major ion in the fluids of the body outside the cells (inside the cell, its partner potassium rules the roost). It maintains proper water balance and blood pH. Sodium, combined in its most common form with chloride, is table salt.

Food Sources—Table salt, soy sauce, and salty foods (pickles, bouillon, cured meats, and sauerkraut); virtually all foods contain some sodium.

Functions in the Body—The sodium content of your body fluids determines your water balance—that is, how much fluid your body holds. But sodium also helps to regulate the passage of substances (such as blood sugar) into and out of each cell, to generate normal electrical nerve signals, and for muscle contraction.

Your kidneys help to keep the amount of sodium in your blood and body fluids at a pretty constant level—wasting some if you eat too much, hanging on more tightly to it if you don't get enough—and under normal conditions, you should not become deficient in sodium. However, in some situations, your body can lose more sodium (or salt) than normal; exercise in extreme heat, heavy persistent sweating, fever, chronic diarrhea, or a prolonged bout of vomiting and diarrhea can cause you to need extra sodium.

Interactions—

• Diuretic medications (water or fluid pills) make you shed water through your kidneys by making your body waste sodium. Chronic use of these medications can cause your body to become depleted in sodium.

• A diet high in sodium may cause you to lose more calcium and magnesium in your urine, possibly leading to deficiencies in these minerals.

• To ensure good health, there must exist a balance of potassium and sodium. Since most people consume too much sodium, they need more potassium as well. An imbalance can lead to heart disease.

• Caffeine promotes loss of sodium and, consequently, water from your kidneys—that is, caffeine acts as a weak diuretic.

Recommended Usage—DRI for sodium is 6 grams per day in adults living in temperate climates under normal conditions. However, the American Heart Association recommends a daily intake of no more than 3 grams. During physical activity (work or play) in extreme heat (temperatures over 100 degrees F with humidity) for prolonged periods, you may need to increase that recommendation by several grams, but your chief need in these circumstances will be water. Replenishing your fluid losses with a beverage containing sodium, along with its closely allied electrolyte buddies potassium and chloride, will easily make up the difference in loss through sweat.

Symptoms of Deficiency—Loss of appetite, loss of sense of taste, weight loss, nausea and vomiting, stomach cramping, gaseousness, difficulty balancing to walk, fatigue, lethargy, muscle weakness, dizziness, confusion, hallucinations, problems with memory, skin rashes, headache, depression, flatulence, poor coordination, mood swings and tearfulness, frequent infections, and seizures.

Symptoms of Toxicity—Cloudy thinking, fluid retention (edema), hypertension, muscle and nerve irritability, muscle tremors, thirst and increased fluid intake, frequent urination, congestive heart failure, potassium deficiency, and (as with too little sodium) loss of appetite.

Safety Information—Not applicable.

Sulfur

Important Facts—Mineral.
Sulfur is a yellowish powder that in certain forms (combined with hydrogen to make hydrogen sulfide) smells like rotten eggs; and, in fact, the yolks of eggs are quite rich in sulfur. You're greeted by this same sulfurous smell when you strike a match or get a whiff of the emissions from a catalytic converter on your automobile. These examples sound so unappetizing you may not be too keen on adding sulfur to your nutritional armamentarium, but press on, because sulfur really is important to your health.

Food Sources—Egg yolks, garlic, onion, high-protein foods (such as meat, poultry, and seafood), beans, and asparagus.

Functions in the Body—Sulfur plays roles in energy production, in blood clotting, and in the production of collagen, the chief protein that forms the framework for bones, fibrous tissues, skin, hair, and nails, and in building enzymes (the tiny helpers that speed up the billions of chemical reactions that take place in your body all the time). It also helps maintain the oxygen balance necessary for proper brain function.

Sulfur protects the body against toxins and is therefore effective in reducing the harmful effects of radiation and pollution, making it an antiaging mineral.

Sulfur stimulates bile secretion.

Recent research also suggests that the beneficial effects of garlic (a much-touted remedy for curing almost anything that ails you by some accounts) in reducing elevated blood cholesterol, blood pressure, and blood sugar are from its sulfur content.

Interactions—Moisture and heat can destroy and change the action of sulfur in the body.

Recommended Usage—There is no DRI listing for this nutrient; however, an estimate of reasonable daily intake for adults would be in the range of 500 to 1000 mg per day. That is an amount you can get easily from food unless you are a strict vegetarian. Even then, if you are able to eat plenty of garlic and onions, you should have no trouble meeting the daily requirement by food alone. Generally, a diet sufficient in protein is sufficient in sulfur.

The few strict vegetarians who cannot eat onion or garlic, can supplement the 500 to 1000 mg of sulfur using "flowers of sulfur" powder available at most health and nutrition stores.

Symptoms of Deficiency—Little is known with certainty; however, there is speculation in the medical community that deficiency of sulfur can cause painful joints, high blood sugar, and high blood fat levels.

Symptoms of Toxicity—None documented in the medical literature.

Safety Information—Some people have severe allergies to sulfur and sulfur-containing substances, which could include foods or medications (such as sulfamethoxizole, Bactrim, or Septra). If that is your situation, you should not use over-the-counter sulfur supplements, such as "flowers of sulfur."

—————————— **Taurine** ——————————

Important Facts—Vitamin-like molecule, usually classified with the amino acids.

Researchers first isolated the amino acid taurine from ox bile in 1827, but interest has focused in recent years on its probable role as an essential nutrient for good health. It is abundant in the tissues of the heart, the skeletal muscles, and the central nervous system. As with carnitine, your body can produce taurine by remodeling other amino acids, especially cysteine and methionine.

Food Sources—Shellfish, especially clams and oysters; muscle meats, such as beef, chicken, and pork; milk; and eggs. Vegetables contain almost no taurine.

Functions in the Body—A growing infant requires taurine for normal development of its nervous system, its retina (the screen of the back of the eye onto which visual images focus), and its muscles. Taurine also improves the vigor of the heart muscle, improves the "swimming" action of sperm, enhances growth, is important in the production of bile needed for normal digestion of fats, and improves the action of insulin.

Because it controls serum cholesterol levels, taurine is useful for people with edema, hypoglycemia, hypertension, atherosclerosis, and heart disorders. It is also important in the prevention of cardiac arrhythmias because it plays a role in preventing the loss of potassium from the heart muscle.

Taurine protects the brain, especially when it is dehydrated. It is used to treat anxiety, epilepsy, hyperactivity, poor brain function, and seizures.

When used in combination with zinc, taurine maintains healthy eye function and helps prevent macular degeneration.

Interactions—

• Vitamin B_6 is needed to convert the amino acids cysteine and methionine into taurine.

• Excessive consumption of alcohol is associated with high urinary losses of taurine. This overconsumption also causes the body to lose its ability to utilize taurine properly.

• Diabetes increases the body's requirement for taurine.

Conversely, taurine taken in combination with cystine may reduce the need for insulin.

Recommended Usage—Because this nutrient is not considered essential yet, there is no DRI listing even for infants. Based on medical research done to date, your requirement for taurine is quite small, and except in strict vegetarians, you should get plenty of taurine in your diet if you meet your daily requirement for lean protein. See the discussion of Macronutrients, found on page 23, for more information about calculating your daily protein needs. If you do decide to supplement, take up to three 500 mg capsules daily, with juice or water, half an hour before meals.

Symptoms of Deficiency—None identified in people.

Symptoms of Toxicity—None identified in people.

Safety Information—From food sources, taurine is safe.

———— Thiamine (Vitamin B₁) ————

Important Facts—Water-soluble vitamin.

Cooking in water leeches much of the thiamine content out of foods. Deficiency of this vitamin caused one of the classic deficiency diseases of history—beriberi—which I have discussed fully in a section devoted to these deficiency disorders. Please refer to that section, beginning on page 10, for more important information about thiamine.

Food Sources—Beans, grains and seeds, meat (especially liver), pork, soybeans, brown rice, egg yolks, fish, wheat germ, and brewer's yeast.

Functions in the Body—Thiamine functions in your body as a required coenzyme or helper molecule in the metabolism of protein, carbohydrate, and fat for energy production. You also need this vitamin to be able to produce the copies of genetic material that must pass from one cell to another when cells divide—an activity that all living cells must regularly do. Thiamine is a key player in the conversion of fatty acids into steroid hormones such as cortisol and progesterone. Healthy skin also depends on sufficient amounts of this vitamin. Like other B vitamins, there is indication that thiamine plays a role in our ability to resist disease. And finally, thiamine is necessary for proper transmission of electrical nerve signals.

Interactions—

• Adequate magnesium is necessary to convert thiamine into its active form (see also Magnesium).

• Sugar, alcohol, and tobacco consumption deplete your thiamine stores.

• Tea leaves and raw fish contain an enzyme (thiaminase) that can destroy thiamine. Cooking or boiling inactivates the enzyme; therefore, cooked fish or boiled tea leaves do not present a problem in contributing to thiamine deficiency, but beware of too much sushi!

• It is believed that heavy tea and coffee drinkers may have symptoms of nervous disorders associated with thiamine deficiency, but have either failed to seek help or have been misdiagnosed.

• Schizophrenics tend to have low levels of thiamine. One survey of psychiatric patients showed 30% of patients to be deficient in thiamine, although only one patient showed clinical symptoms of deficiency. Thiamine is often used in combination with other B vitamins to treat various emotional and psychiatric illnesses.

Recommended Usage—The DRI for vitamin B_1 is 1.5 mg for men and women and 1.7 mg for pregnant and lactating women. However, in treating specific deficiency states, orthomolecular physicians (those practitioners who specialize in treating diseases with large doses of vitamins) prescribe doses of 500 to 6000 mg per day without consequence. Increased need occurs in illnesses with fever because of the increased rate of metabolism associated with higher body temperature.

Symptoms of Deficiency—Loss of appetite, clouded thinking, sluggish bowel, lack of coordination, mental or emotional depression, fatigue, irritability, memory problems, muscle weakness or wasting, nervousness, numbness or burning of hands and feet, decreased pain tolerance, shortness of breath, and fluid retention in the hands and feet. The classic deficiency syndrome is called beriberi.

Symptoms of Toxicity—None known.

Safety Information—Not stored, quickly excreted, little or no risk of toxic buildup if taken orally. Take care with other routes of administration, however, because thiamine by injection can cause potentially fatal allergic reactions.[31]

────────────────── **Vanadium** ──────────────────

Important Facts—Ultratrace mineral.

Vanadium first gained notice in an 1876 report of its toxicity to people. However, through the next 100 years, researchers have alternately supported and refuted its role as a nutrient essential to human health. In 1974, scientists settled on a "yes" answer to the question "Is it necessary for good health?" based on laboratory testing that showed that vanadium is quite active in a number of chemical reactions that take place in the body.

Food Sources—Black pepper, shellfish, mushrooms, dill seed, parsley, soy, corn, olives, olive oil, and gelatin.

Functions in the Body—Vanadium reduces the production of cholesterol, which makes it potentially useful in treating atherosclerosis and heart disease. It could reduce the risk of heart attack.

Some experts recommend vanadium in the treatment of diabetes and neurasthenia, perhaps because of the mineral's ability to mimic insulin.

Interactions—Very little information exists.

• Although the connection is a sketchy one, your body absorbs vanadium using the same helper molecules that transport iron. Levels of these molecules vary with iron intake, so being deficient in iron could affect your ability to absorb vanadium.

• Tobacco use decreases the absorption of vanadium.

• There is a possible interaction between vanadium and chromium. If you take supplements for these, do so at different times of the day.

Recommended Usage—There is no DRI listing for vanadium. Because it is an ultratrace mineral, your requirement for it is very small. Estimates of the average American dietary intake—20 to 30 *micro*grams per day—probably suffice to provide you with vanadium, but there's simply no hard science to hang a number on yet. This mineral really does not need to be supplemented; a good fish dinner will boost your supply.

Symptoms of Deficiency—Research to date has not provided us with many hard facts about human vanadium deficiency. There is suspicion that a deficiency can increase your risk of heart disease and cancer. In animal studies, deficiency caused problems with reproduction and bone development.

Symptoms of Toxicity—Again, not much research exists examining toxicity in humans; however, in laboratory animals, researchers believe that this mineral can be toxic to nerve tissues, kidney, liver, and blood-producing tissues. Signs of toxicity in animals include: stunted growth, diarrhea, loss of appetite, and, ultimately, death.

Safety Information—Because your need for this mineral is so small, and because of potential toxicity, I do not recommend supplementation. Diabetics are especially susceptible to toxicity from this mineral.

Zinc

Important Facts—Mineral.
The first recognition of zinc as an element occurred in 1509, but not until 1934 did a researcher prove a role for zinc as essential to animals. By 1956, research had proven health consequences in people from zinc deficiency.

Food Sources—Beef, liver, poultry (especially dark meat), seafood (such as oysters, herring, and clams), wheat germ, eggs, whole grains, carrots, peas, bran, oatmeal, and nuts.

Functions in the Body—Zinc is necessary for proper growth of skin, hair, and nails and in healing wounds because of its role in the production of body proteins and copying the genetic material that must pass from one cell to another each time your cells divide and grow. This role also means that you require zinc for a healthy immune system to fight off diseases and cancer. Low zinc levels, often accompanied by high copper levels, have been reported in people with many types of cancer. Zinc acts as a critical cofactor or helper in over a dozen chemical reactions essential to human health, one of these being the enzyme gustin, which allows you to perceive the sense of taste. Finally, zinc acts as a detoxifier, aiding in removing excess carbon dioxide from your body and in helping you to detoxify alcohol.

Research reveals that there exists a link between low zinc levels and anorexia nervosa. Scientists believe that deficient levels of zinc somehow trigger the development of the disease, which further depletes zinc levels, which worsens symptoms, and so on. It is a vicious cycle.

The prostate gland has one of the highest concentrations of zinc in the body. Low levels of this mineral have been associated with diseases of the gland. What's more, zinc inhibits the binding of androgens to receptors in the prostate gland, which may prevent prostate cancer and other diseases of the gland.

Interactions—In its ionic form, zinc can cause you to become deficient in other minerals, notably copper, because the two compete with each other for absorption from your intestine. Both must pass into the cells through the ion channel (see the discussion of Single Ion Channel Theory, on pages 29–30). For that reason, you should always take zinc in its chelated form (see chelation, pages 30–31).

Alcohol, diuretics, and oral contraceptives interfere with zinc absorption and metabolism.

Impotency has been linked to zinc deficiencies.

Recommended Usage—The DRI for this substance has been set at 15 mg per day for adults. Except when you need higher amounts to treat specific disorders as specified in this text, 15 to 20 mg of chelated zinc per day should be sufficient for adults and 5 to 10 mg per day for children.

Symptoms of Deficiency—Acne, spotty hair loss, loss of appetite, loss of taste and smell, brittle nails, white spots on nails, scaly skin rashes, frequent infections, poor growth, delayed puberty, impotence and male infertility, irritability, night blindness, amnesia and memory loss, paranoid feelings, poor wound healing, high cholesterol, diarrhea, and fatigue.

Symptoms of Toxicity—Stomach irritation and vomiting have occurred on doses of 2 grams (that's 2000 mg) per day.

Safety Information—Taken in the chelated form and in the doses specified in this text, zinc is quite nontoxic.

—— Adult Supplementation, General ——

What to Take

A multivitamin and chelated mineral supplement that approximates the following combination will provide everything that healthy men and women, weighing 200 or more pounds, require:

vitamin A	10,000 IU	beta-carotene	15,000 IU
vitamin B_1	30 mg	choline	200 mg
vitamin B_2	30 mg	inositol	150 mg
vitamin B_3	250 mg	folic acid	2 mg
vitamin B_5	150 mg	biotin	300 mcg
vitamin B_6	50 mg	calcium	500 mg
vitamin B_{12}	250 mcg	magnesium	200 mg
vitamin C	4000 IU	potassium	99 mg
vitamin D_3	20 IU	chromium	200 mcg
vitamin E	400 IU	selenium	100 mcg
		iodine	150 mcg
		molybdenum	100 mcg

Adult men and women weighing less than 200 pounds should take the following amounts:

vitamin A	5,000 IU	beta-carotene	15,000 IU
vitamin B_1	30 mg	choline	200 mg
vitamin B_2	30 mg	inositol	150 mg
vitamin B_3	250 mg	folic acid	2 mg
vitamin B_5	100 mg	biotin	300 mcg
vitamin B_6	50 mg	calcium	500 mg
vitamin B_{12}	125 mcg	magnesium	200 mg
vitamin C	2000 IU	potassium	99 mg
vitamin D_3	10 IU	chromium	200 mcg
vitamin E	400 IU	selenium	100 mcg
		iodine	150 mcg
		molybdenum	100 mcg

You should take all minerals in chelated form (see discussion of chelation of minerals on pages 30–31) to prevent your becoming deficient in any mineral because of competition between them for entry into your body.

— Children's Supplementation, General —

What to Give

In otherwise healthy children, I recommend a multivitamin supplement containing approximately these amounts for children 2 to 4 years, double these amounts for children 4 to 7 years, and triple these amounts for children over 7 years:

vitamin A	2500 IU	niacinamide	18 mg
vitamin C	100 mg	pantothenic acid	5 mg
vitamin D_3	100 IU	thiamine	1.5 mg
vitamin E	20 IU	folic acid	300 mcg
vitamin B_6	1.5 mg	biotin	35 mcg
vitamin B_{12}	6 mcg	calcium glycinate	15 mg
zinc gluconate	2 mg	magnesium glycinate	15 mg
iron glycinate	2 mg	manganese aspartate	500 mcg
copper (chelated)	100 mcg	potassium iodide	70 mcg

Notes

1. H. L. Newbold, *Mega-Nutrients: A Prescription for Total Health* (Los Angeles: The Body Press, 1987), 152.

2. Eleanor Williams, *Nutrition: Principles, Issues, and Applications* (New York: McGraw-Hill Inc., 1984), 284.

3. *Recommended Dietary Allowances,* 10th ed. (Washington, D.C.: Food and Nutrition Board, Commission on Life Sciences, National Research Council, National Academy Press), 146.

4. Newbold, 221.

5. Melvyn Werbach, *Nutritional Influences on Illness: A Sourcebook of Clinical Research,* 2nd ed. (Tarzana, Calif.: Thirdline Press, 1993), 639.

6. Newbold, 160.

7. J. A. Vinson and P. Bose, "Comparative Bioavailability to Humans of Ascorbic Acid Alone or in a Citrus Extract," *American Journal of Clinical Nutrition* 48 (1988): 601–604.

8. Williams.

9. Werbach, 640.

10. Robert Olson, ed., *Present Knowledge in Nutrition,* 5th ed. (Washington, D.C.: The Nutrition Foundation, 1984), 350–351.

11. Linus Pauling, "Vitamin C: An Historical Perspective"

(paper delivered at the Adjuvant Nutrition in Cancer Treatment Symposium, Tulsa, Oklahoma, November 1992).

12. R. F. Cathcart, "The Third Face of Vitamin C," *Journal of Orthomolecular Medicine* 7 (1992): 197–200.

13. Linus Pauling, *How to Live Longer and Feel Better* (New York: Avon Books, 1986), 156–158.

14. L. H. Allen, "Calcium and Osteoporosis," *Nutrition Today* 21 (1986): 6–10.

15. Newbold, 188.

16. M. T. Childs, et al., "The Contrasting Effects of Dietary Soya Lecithin and Corn Oil on Lipoprotein Lipids in Normolipidemic and Familial Hypercholesterolemic Subjects," *Atherosclerosis* 38 (1981): 217–228.

17. Olson, 389.

18. *Diet and Health: Implications for Reducing Chronic Disease Risk* (Washington, D.C.: Committee on Diet and Health, Food and Nutrition Board, National Academy Press, 1989), 312.

19. Newbold, 275.

20. Pauling, *How to Live Longer and Feel Better,* 338.

21. Maurice E. Shils and Vernon Young, eds., *Modern Nutrition in Health and Disease,* 7th ed. (Philadelphia: Lea & Febiger, 1988), 352.

22. M. Fariss, "Oxygen Toxicity: Unique Cytoprotective Properties of Vitamin E Succinate in Hepatocytes," *Free Radical Biology and Medicine* 9 (1990): 333–343.

23. Werbach, 640.

24. *Recommended Dietary Allowances,* 10th ed., 155.

25. *Recommended Dietary Allowances,* 10th ed., 152.

26. Werbach, 633.

27. John Yudkin, *The Penguin Encyclopedia of Nutrition* (Middlesex, England: Penguin Books, Ltd., 1986), 376.

28. Werbach, 669.

29. *Diet and Health: Implications for Reducing Chronic Disease Risk,* 330.

30. Werbach, 660.

31. Newbold, 147.

HERBAL ENCYCLOPEDIA

---------------- **Alfalfa** ----------------

Medicago sativa

Forms—seeds, sprouts, solid extractions, fluid extractions, and tinctures; teas and tablets may not deliver enough active ingredient to be effective.

Nutritional value—The leaves of the alfalfa plant are rich in calcium, magnesium, potassium, phosphorus, carotene, and all known vitamins. Because all the minerals are in a balanced form, they can be readily absorbed. Alfalfa has long been appreciated as a food for livestock, but has also come to be considered a health food with medicinal value. It contains three major phytoestrogens: coumestrol, genistein, and formonetin; and two less important ones: diadzein and biochanin A.

Medicinal uses—

• Phytoestrogens are important because they have the ability to alter the biological response to estrogen. Thus, they are useful in treating symptoms of menopause and in the prevention of osteoporosis. Alfalfa may also be used by breast-feeding mothers to increase production of milk.

• Alfalfa will decrease estrogenic stimulation (it decreases the amount of estrogen produced in the body. This is good for those disorders listed, which are linked directly with an overproduction of estrogen. Too much estrogen throws the hormonal balance off) and may benefit women with fibrocystic breasts, breast cancer, and PMS.

• Many autoimmune diseases such as AIDS, HIV, and multiple sclerosis are aggravated by estrogens. Alfalfa's hypoestrogenic effects (like estrogen) could improve these conditions. See Contraindications section below.

• Research supports the idea that alfalfa lowers total cholesterol by lowering triglycerides, LDLs, and VLDLs, while not significantly lowering the desirable HDLs. All parts of the plant (seed, root, meal) were used in these studies, and the results were virtually the same. Lowering cholesterol levels is an important factor in reducing your risk of cardiovascular disease.

• Since the sixth century, the Chinese have been using alfalfa to treat kidney stones and relieve fluid retention and swelling.

• Alfalfa is rich in chlorophyll, which is well known for its cleansing qualities. It is used to treat intestinal ulcers, gastritis, liver disorders, eczema, hemorrhoids, asthma, high blood pressure, anemia, constipation, body and breath odor, bleeding gums, infections, burns, athlete's foot, and cancer.

Contraindications—Two forms of alfalfa—seeds and sprouts—should not be used to treat autoimmune diseases. They contain canavanine, which has been shown to destroy T-suppressor activity. People suffering from autoimmune diseases should use only the mature tops of the plant for treatment.

Aloe

Aloe vera (there are more than 200 species)

Forms—gel, juice, dried gel powder, capsules.

Nutritional value—This desert succulent contains amino acids as well as some vitamins and minerals.

Medicinal uses—

• Although the FDA claims there is "insufficient evidence" that aloe is useful for burns, it has been used for centuries by many cultures for just that purpose. The inside of the leaf has a gel that soothes, and many people claim it reduces inflammation and blistering. This would make sense, as the gel contains enzymes that also decrease redness and swelling. Scientists are not sure how aloe speeds healing. However, aloe does increase the amount of blood flowing to areas of burned tissue, causing more of the body's healing resources to concentrate on the affected area. What's more, aloe gel has antibacterial and antifungal properties, which prevent burns from getting infected.

• The gel is also effective for relieving the pain from cuts, insect stings, bruises, acne and blemishes, poison ivy, welts, skin ulcers, and eczema.

• Aloe contains an immune-stimulating compound called acemannan that has been beneficial in treating AIDS. Test-tube studies have shown the compound to be active against HIV because it boosts T-lymphocyte cells that aid natural resistance. Any of the forms of aloe are effective for this treatment, though most juices are not pleasing to the palate. I recommend George's Aloe Vera Juice from Warren Laboratories, which tastes like plain water.

• Aloe vera that is almost pure (98 to 99%) can be taken internally to aid in the healing of stomach disorders, ulcers, constipation, hemorrhoids, rectal itching, colitis, and all colon problems. It also helps varicose veins, skin cancer, and arthritis.

Contraindications—It is possible to develop a tolerance to aloe vera juice, thus reducing its effectiveness, so don't take it on a regular basis.

Although rare, some people are allergic to this herb. Apply a small amount behind the ear or on the underarm. If stinging or rash occurs, do not use.

Astragalus

Astragalus membranaceus

Forms—tincture, tea made from dried herb, injections.

Nutritional value—Choline, dimethoxyisoflavone, and sucrose. Astragalus is known as an immune stimulant. It works by stimulating the body's production of interferon (antiviral compounds) and by restoring red blood cell formation in bone marrow.

Medicinal uses—

• Because it stimulates the immune system, astragalus is being used to treat HIV, viral infections, pneumonia, and cardiac arrhythmia.

• In one study, 10 people with serious viral infections showed low levels of natural killer cells in their bodies. The participants were given injections of astragalus for four months. Compared with study participants who did not receive the injections, their natural killer cell activity increased significantly, other components of their immune system were restored, and their symptoms improved.

• This herb originated in China and has long been used there to treat viruses. In one small Chinese study, 10 people whose heart muscles were infected by a virus that causes heart inflammation received injections of astragalus for three to four months. The activity of their natural killer cells rose 11 to 45%. They also showed increased levels of interferon, and their symptoms improved. European studies suggest that many of the immune-stimulating compounds are active when taken orally, as well.

• Astragalus is known as the Asian equivalent to our own echinacea. Both can be used in treating pneumonia.

• Herbalists claim that the immune-stimulating properties of astragalus also help prevent and treat arrhythmia and suggest drinking a tea made with one to two teaspoons of dried herb steeped in boiling water.

Contraindications—Do not take astragalus if you have a fever.

Bilberry

Vaccinium myrtillus

Forms—tea, juice, fruit, capsules.

Nutritional value—This fruit and its relatives, blueberry, cranberry, huckleberry, blackberry, grape, plum, and wild cherry, contain potent antioxidants, including beta-carotene.

Medicinal uses—

• Bilberry is valuable for its ability to treat eye disorders. Research shows it works by improving the circulation and regeneration of retinal purple, a substance necessary for good eyesight. This was discovered when British Royal Air Force pilots during World War II ate bilberry preserves before night missions and discovered that their night vision was drastically improved afterward.

• Bilberry is also used to treat retinitis pigmentosa, macular degeneration, glaucoma, and myopia. Anthocyanin is a natural antioxidant found in bilberry. This antioxidant enhances the health of collagen structures in the blood vessels of the eyes.

• This herb may also be helpful in treating certain digestive disorders. It stimulates the production of mucus that protects the stomach lining from digestive acids. Animal studies show that bilberry offers significant protection against ulcers.

• The tannins and pectin found in bilberry make it useful in treating diarrhea. Tannins cause mucous membranes to thicken and restrict secretions. Pectin is a soluble fiber that adds bulk to stool and soothes the gut.

• The anthocyanidins in bilberry have muscle-relaxant properties, which help relieve menstrual cramps. Herbalists suggest taking 20 to 40 mg of concentrated bilberry extract three times daily. A half-cup of fresh bilberries is a good alternative. Bilberries can be found at natural and health-food stores.

• Bilberry strengthens capillary walls and increases the overall health of the circulatory system, and so is an effective treatment for varicose veins. Eat whole berries if possible; capsules are an acceptable alternative.

Contraindications—This herb interferes with the absorption of iron when taken internally.

Black Cohosh

Cimicifuga racemosa

Forms—The root is used to make tea and tincture.

Nutritional value—Oleic acid, estrogenic substances, triterpenes, pantothenic acid, phosphorus, vitamin A.

Black cohosh, also known as black snakeroot, bugbane, rattleroot, rattleweed, and squawroot, is a powerful relaxant and a normalizer of the female reproductive system.

Medicinal uses—

• This herb is useful in relieving the pain of dysmenorrhea (painful menstruation). It can also be used to help restore suppressed menses, as it promotes menstrual discharge.

• Black cohosh can be used to treat infertility because it improves the functional power of the uterus.

• For years, the herb ergot was used to promote contractions during labor and delivery. Black cohosh, however, is a better choice because it produces natural, intermittent uterine contractions. The contractions produced by ergot are constant, which endangers the life of the baby and increases the risk of rupture of the uterus. Black cohosh is also used as a diagnostic agent because it is able to differentiate between "false" and real labor pains. Once detected, it can increase the latter or cause the former to dissipate. It is also an effective pain reliever for after-birth discomfort.

• Headaches are relieved by black cohosh, as are fevers, runny and stuffy noses, sore throats, and other symptoms brought on by colds or respiratory disorders.

• Black cohosh calms the nervous system by nourishing blood vessels. It has been used successfully as an antispasmodic in hysteria, asthma, periodic convulsions, nervous excitability, pertussis, and other spasmodic afflictions. Inflammation can be controlled using black cohosh.

• Because it balances hormones by binding to estrogen receptors, this herb is useful in treating the symptoms of menopause.

• Few herbs are as useful as black cohosh in treating rheumatism and neuralgia. Its relaxant properties help ease the pain of these disorders.

Contraindications—For black cohosh to be of any medicinal value, it must be prepared from recently dried roots.

———————— Blue Cohosh ————————

Caulophyllum thalictroides

Forms—The root is used to make tea and tincture.

Nutritional value—Calcium, folic acid, inositol, iron, magnesium, pantothenic acid, phosphoric acid, phosphorus, potassium, silicon, vitamins B_3 and E. Blue cohosh is used primarily to support function of the female reproductive system. It is a powerful emmenagogue (stimulating the menstrual process) that also acts as a diuretic and expectorant. Its uses are almost identical to those of black cohosh.

Medicinal uses—

• Because of its antispasmodic action, blue cohosh eases false labor pains and dysmenorrhea. Given right before birth, it will help ensure an easy delivery. Do not use during the first two trimesters of pregnancy.

• As a relaxant, this herb is effective in treating the discomfort of endometriosis, ovaritis, dysmenorrhea, urethritis, vaginitis, thrush, restlessness during pregnancy, and menopausal pains and discomfort.

• Its expectorant properties make blue cohosh a logical treatment for bronchitis and whooping cough.

• To strengthen and tone the uterus, blue cohosh can be combined with yarrow, motherwort, or false unicorn.

Contraindications—None.

Burdock

Arctium lappa

Forms—The roots are used to make tea and tincture.

Nutritional value—Copper, essential oils, iron, manganese, sulfur, zinc, vitamins B_1, B_6, B_{12}, and E. Burdock is a natural blood purifier and detoxifier.

Medicinal uses—

• Burdock is especially useful for the treatment of skin disorders that result in dry, scaly skin. If used over a long period of time, it may be effective for psoriasis. Other skin disorders that can be improved by this herb include boils, dermatitis, and eczema. It is most effective when combined with yellow dock and red clover.

• Burdock restores liver and gall bladder functions and is useful in treating gout, rheumatism, and sciatica.

• Because it increases digestive juices and bile secretion, it aids digestion and appetite, making it an effective component in the treatment of anorexia nervosa and similar conditions.

Contraindications—When taken internally, burdock interferes with iron absorption.

Cat's Claw

Uncaria tomentosa

Forms—The inner bark is used to make capsules, extract, liquid, and tablets.

Nutritional value—Polyphenols, plant sterols, oxindole alkaloids, triterpenes. Also called *una de gato,* cat's claw is a woody vine that grows in the tops of trees in Peruvian rain forests. It is a favorite for stimulating the immune system. Many of the single chemicals found in this powerful herb have been patented for use in treating AIDS, cancer, arthritis, and other diseases. However, using the whole plant can be more potent than any one isolated ingredient.

Medicinal uses—

• There are six alkaloids prevalent in cat's claw bark. These are what give this herb its incredible healing power. These alkaloids are antiviral, anti-inflammatory, immuno-stimulating, and antioxidant. Though they probably didn't know the term *antioxidant,* the ancient Incas used una de gato as a healing tonic for centuries, relying on its ability to cleanse the intestinal tract and provide relief from stomach and bowel disorders. People suffering with colitis, gastritis, Crohn's disease, and even ulcers have benefited from this herb. Dr. Satya Ambrose, cofounder of the Oregon College of Oriental Medicine, claims to have noticed a significant improvement in patients suffering from Crohn's disease, ulcers, asthma, arthritis, iritis, shingles, dysbiosis, and chronic fatigue syndrome. Since the 1970s, research clinics in Peru, Austria, Germany, England, Hungary, and Italy have validated these findings.

• The symptoms of immune diseases such as AIDS and cancer are improved by cat's claw due to four of the six alkaloids, which enhance the white blood cell functions.

Contraindications—

• This herb should not be used during pregnancy. Be sure the supply of cat's claw that you purchase was harvested from the bark only, not the root. The Peruvian government claims that the inner bark contains all the components of the root and can regrow as long as the root is not disturbed. Like any other herbal found in the rain forest, una de gato is in danger of becoming extinct.

• It is equally important that you purchase the true una de gato, called *Uncaria tomentosa.* Other herbs are informally called cat's claw, and there is a vine of una de gato from the Peruvian lowlands; these do not contain the same alkaloids as the genuine herb.

——————— **Cayenne** ———————

Capsicum minimum

Forms—Berries are used to make capsules, topical preparations, and powder.

Nutritional value—Capsaicin, cobalt, folic acid, pantothenic acid, zinc, vitamins A, B_1, B_2, B_3, B_6, and C. Cayenne is a pepper well known for its benefits to the circulatory system.

Medicinal uses—

• Because it stimulates blood flow, cayenne is used to strengthen the heart, arteries, capillaries, and nerves.

• Cayenne enhances the body's utilization of other herbs, and so is especially effective when used in herbal combinations. For example, when mixed with myrrh to form a gargle, it relieves the discomfort of laryngitis. Mixed with lobelia, it enhances nervous system function.

• Cayenne contains salicylic acid, which helps inhibit the production of compounds in our bodies responsible for pain. Aspirin is made from salicylic acid. This acid, when combined with a chemical called capsaicin (also found in cayenne), thins the blood and facilitates even blood flow while alleviating pain. For this reason, cayenne is effective in treating cluster headaches. In one double-blind study, patients received either capsaicin ointment or a placebo intranasally for seven days. Researchers recorded the headache severity of the subjects for 15 days. Headaches on days 8 to 15 were significantly less severe in the capsaicin group versus the placebo group.

• An infusion of cayenne can be used to effectively treat the symptoms of colds, hoarseness, sore throats, and sinus infections.

• Topically used, cayenne relieves the symptoms and discomfort of arthritis and rheumatism.

• Cayenne contains six pain-relieving compounds and seven that are anti-inflammatory. Because of these substances, this herb is an effective treatment for carpal tunnel syndrome.

• Several teaspoons of powdered cayenne added to a quarter-cup of skin lotion can be rubbed onto the wrists.

Contraindications—

• Pregnant women should never use cayenne, as studies on lab animals indicate it promotes uterine contractions.

• In large doses, it can cause vomiting, purging, pains in the stomach and bowels, heat and inflammation of the stomach, giddiness, and a decrease in nervous system function.

• Some people are very sensitive to this herb. If you plan to apply it topically, test it on a small patch of skin before using it on a larger area.

Celery Seed

Apium graveolens

Forms—The juice, roots, and seeds are used to make tea and tincture.

Nutritional value—Vitamins A, C, and B-complex, iron. Celery seeds are used mainly in the treatment of rheumatism, arthritis, and gout.

Medicinal uses—
• Gout is treated with celery because it keeps uric acid levels below critical levels.
• Traditional Chinese medicine recommends using celery to treat high blood pressure. In one study, lab animals injected with celery extract experienced significantly lower blood pressure. Eating as few as four stalks of celery daily can have the same results in humans.
• The diuretic properties of celery may be helpful in treating rheumatic conditions, as may the herb's urinary antiseptic properties. For these conditions, this herb seems to work even better when teamed with dandelion.

Contraindications—Do not use in large amounts during pregnancy.

Chamomile

Matricaria recutita

Forms—The flowering top is used to make fresh and dried herbs, teas, tinctures, and essential oils.

Nutritional value—Calcium, essential oils, iron, magnesium, manganese, potassium, tannic acid, vitamin A.

Chamomile is probably the most widely used relaxing herb in the

Western world. It relaxes and tones the nervous system, and is especially useful in the treatment of anxiety, tension, and the resulting symptoms such as gas, colic pains, and ulcers.

Medicinal uses—

• Because it relaxes the nervous system, chamomile is an excellent remedy for insomnia. For the same reason, it is effective in treating infants who are teething.

• Its antispasmodic properties work on the peripheral nerves and muscles, indirectly relaxing the entire body. This can help prevent or ease muscle cramps.

• Chamomile is rich in essential oil, which enhances proper functioning of the digestive system. It soothes the walls of the intestines and helps eliminate gas. When taken internally, its anti-inflammatory properties help the digestive and respiratory systems.

• Using the essential oil as a steam inhalation relieves inflamed mucous membranes in the sinuses and lungs. This improves head colds and allergies.

• Taken by mouth or used as an enema, chamomile is especially helpful in colitis and irritable bowel syndrome.

• Tattoos often "weep" where the skin has been abraded. A recent German study shows that by applying chamomile topically to the tattoo during the drying and healing process, the amount of weeping is minimized.

Contraindications—Though this herb can relieve allergy and cold symptoms, it should not be used for long periods of time, as it may lead to an actual ragweed allergy. Those who are allergic to ragweed should not use chamomile at all.

Cranberry

Vaccinium macrocarpon

Forms—Berries are used to make juice and capsules.

Nutritional value—Vitamin C, alpha D-mannopyranoside. Cranberry acidifies the urine and prevents bacteria from adhering to the bladder.

Medicinal uses—

• In unsweetened, pure form, cranberry is effective in treating infections of the urinary tract.

• Because it is high in vitamin C and contains four antiasthmatic compounds, this herb is beneficial in the treatment of asthma.

Contraindications—None known.

Echinacea

Echinacea spp.

Forms—The root and leaves are used to make fresh, dried, freeze-dried, or alcohol-based extract, liquid, tea, capsules, or salve.

Nutritional value—Copper, enzymes, fatty acids, glucose, iron, potassium, protein, sulfur, tannins, vitamins A, C, and E. Used topically, echinacea repairs skin wounds. Taken internally, it enhances the immune system. It stimulates certain white blood cells and has anti-inflammatory and antiviral properties. The constituents in echinacea that are believed to enhance the immune system are known as polysaccharides.

Medicinal uses—
• Echinacea is especially useful for treating infections of the upper respiratory tract such as laryngitis and tonsillitis, and conditions of the nose and sinus.
• To help treat gingivitis, the tincture can be used as a mouthwash.
• Because echinacea is a blood purifier, it is an effective treatment for skin problems such as acne, boils, and abscesses.
• Taking echinacea as soon as flu or cold symptoms are noticed can help relieve symptoms and prevent further progress of the infection.
• This herb has antitumor activity. Taken in combination with yarrow, it stops cystitis.

Contraindications—
• Anyone allergic to plants in the sunflower family should not take echinacea.
• For internal use, the freeze-dried form or alcohol-free extract is recommended.
• Although many people use this herb daily as an immune support, Dr. Daniel Mowrey warns against this: "During cold and flu season, two to four capsules per day is sufficient. In the presence of acute infection, that dosage may be increased, without danger, to

more than 8 capsules. In the presence of chronic infections . . . echinacea may be used continuously for several months. However, for the maintenance of a healthy immune system, echinacea is most wisely used periodically—a few weeks on, and a few weeks off, throughout the year. . . . During breaks, the immune system will adapt and increase in natural strength."

———————————— **Garlic** ————————————

Allium sativum

Forms—The bulb is made of cloves to be eaten, used as is, or to make capsules, oil, and powder. Aged garlic extract is the best.

Nutritional value—Calcium, copper, essential oils, germanium, iron, magnesium, manganese, phosphorus, phytoncides, potassium, selenium, sulfur, zinc, vitamins A, B_1, B_2, and C. Garlic is universally recognized as an herb that supports the body in ways no other herb does. It is one of the most effective antimicrobial plants, acting on bacteria, viruses, and parasites. It acts as a natural antibiotic and immune enhancer, and is the best herb known for thinning blood. In short, it is beneficial for treating just about any disease or infection.

Medicinal uses—
• The volatile oil contained in garlic is largely excreted through the lungs, making this herb effective in treating chronic bronchitis, recurrent colds, asthma, whooping cough, and influenza.
• Garlic lowers blood pressure and improves circulation. It also lowers cholesterol levels. For these reasons, it is a major factor in preventing heart conditions.
• The list of disorders that can be treated with garlic is virtually endless. Among those disorders we can include are cancer, stroke, arthritis, breast-feeding problems, burns, diabetes, earache, headache, HIV infections, Lyme disease, Raynaud's disease, sore throat, tonsillitis, ulcers, yeast infections, and digestive problems.

Contraindications—
Because garlic is an anticlotting herb, people concerned about hemorrhagic stroke or other blood-clotting disorders should avoid it.

Feverfew

Tanacetum parthenium

Forms—It is preferable to use fresh leaves, but tincture, capsules, and tablets made from the leaves, bark, and dried flowers are adequate.

Nutritional value—Camphor, parthenolide, pyrethrins, terpene. Feverfew is best known for its ability to relieve migraine headache pain.

Medicinal uses—
• Studies published in the *British Medical Journal* claim that taking feverfew regularly prevents migraine attacks. An article in the *Harvard Medical School Health Letter* agrees: "Eating feverfew leaves has become a popular method for preventing migraine attacks in England." Feverfew promotes menses and so is useful in treating amenorrhea.
• This herb is helpful for treatment of colitis, arthritis, fever, and muscle tension and pain.

Contraindications—
• Pregnant women should not use feverfew because of its ability to stimulate uterine contractions.
• Nursing mothers should avoid this herb so as not to pass it to their infant.
• Although chewing the leaves of this plant is one of the most effective ways to benefit from its healing properties, doing so can cause mouth sores.
• Long-term use can have a tranquilizing effect.

Ginger

Zingiber officinale

Forms—The roots and rhizomes are used to make juice, powder, capsules, and dried herb.

Nutritional value—Choline, essential oils, folic acid, inositol, manganese, pantothenic acid, silicon, vitamin B_3. This nutritional herb is a strong antioxidant and useful in the treatment of many disorders.

Medicinal uses—
• Ginger is well known for its anti-inflammatory properties. Indian and Scandinavian studies have consistently shown that this herb is useful for treating most forms of arthritis. The more than 12 antioxidants present in ginger neutralize the free radicals that aid in causing inflammation.

• Thousands of years ago, Chinese sailors chewed gingerroot to combat seasickness. One modern study of 80 naval cadets showed that taking a half-teaspoon of powdered ginger shortly before shipping out reduced symptoms of seasickness, including dizziness, by 38%. Earlier studies indicated that one gram of ginger relieved vertigo and motion sickness in 18 healthy subjects.

• Ginger is used in a wide range of cultures to induce menstruation. It can also reduce the pain of menstrual cramps because it contains at least six pain-relieving compounds and six anticramping compounds.

• Ginger also helps bowel disorders, circulatory problems, fever, hot flashes, and indigestion.

Contraindications—If taken in large doses, ginger can cause stomach distress.

───────────────── **Ginkgo** ─────────────────

Ginkgo biloba

Forms—The leaves are used to make capsules.

Nutritional value—Ginkgolides are heterosides. Ginkgo is one of the most highly studied herbs. With powerful antioxidant properties, ginkgo is very effective in minimizing the effects of aging.

Medicinal uses—
• Ginkgo's ability to increase blood flow to the brain has been shown to benefit people as they age. It improves alertness, memory, and the ability to concentrate. It also elevates mood and relieves tinnitus (ringing in the ears), dizziness, and anxiety.

• Asian healers have used ginkgo for thousands of years to treat asthma, allergies, bronchitis, and coughs. Ginkgo helps these disorders, especially asthma, because it interferes with platelet-activating factor, a protein in the blood that works to trigger bronchospasms.

• This herb is also a favorite Chinese heart tonic. It can help reduce shortness of breath and chest pain, making it a beneficial treatment for cardiac arrhythmia.

Contraindications—

• The active constituents in ginkgo—ginkgolides—are present in very low concentrations in the tree's leaves, making it difficult to get one effective dose. The best way to take this herb is to buy a 50:1 extract (50 lbs. of leaves yield one pound of extract).

• Most natural foods stores carry ginkgo extracts. This herb must be taken for at least two weeks for best results.

• Taken in high doses (higher than 240 mg daily), ginkgo can cause diarrhea, irritability, and restlessness.

Ginseng

Panax spp.

Forms—The root can be chewed or made into powder.

Nutritional value—Calcium, camphor, iron, resin, starch, vitamins A, B_1, B_{12}, and E. Ginseng nourishes the circulatory system and enhances mental alertness and stamina. It has long been used to enhance the immune system and increase long-term energy. Although there are three species of the herb—Siberian, American, and Korean—all have similar uses.

Medicinal uses—

• Asians revere this herb as the fountain of youth. It tones the skin and muscles and helps improve appetite and digestion. It also enhances sexual energy. It is a beneficial herb to the aging and chronically ill.

• The symptoms of chronic fatigue syndrome can be alleviated with ginseng. Commission E, a group of scientists in Germany, endorses the herb "as a tonic to combat feelings of lassitude and debility, lack of energy and the ability to concentrate."

• Athletes use ginseng for overall body strengthening, though it takes up to a month of regular use to notice the benefits.

• People suffering from drug withdrawal can find relief with ginseng.

Contraindications—

• This herb should not be used if you suffer from hypoglycemia, high blood pressure, or heart disorder. High doses (above 500 mg) may result in increased blood pressure, diarrhea, skin eruptions, or insomnia.

• Pregnant women should avoid this herb.

• Ginseng may interact with the hormonal system and have some estrogenic activity; this could cause problems in women with fibrocystic breast disease.

Goldenseal

Hydrastis canadensis

Forms—The root and rhizome are used to make powder and tincture.

Nutritional value—Albumin, B-complex vitamins, biotin, calcium, chlorine, choline, essential oils, fats, inositol, iron, manganese, phosphorus, potassium, resin, starch, sugar, vitamins A, C, and E. The nutritional properties of goldenseal help the body fight infections both internally and externally. Much of its value is due to the tonic effects it has on the mucous membranes of the body.

Medicinal uses—

• Because of its cleansing effect on mucous membranes, this herb is helpful in all digestive problems, from peptic ulcers to colitis.

• Goldenseal is effective in treating colds and flu because it is an antiseptic and immune stimulator. It increases the blood supply to the spleen, which is the staging area for the immune system's fighting cells. It can literally stop a cold, flu, or sore throat from developing.

• Berberine, a powerful antifungal and antibacterial compound, is found in goldenseal. This makes it effective in treating disorders such as athlete's foot, canker sores, vaginitis, yeast infections, and any other viral or fungal infection.

• Goldenseal promotes liver, colon, pancreas, spleen, and lymphatic and respiratory system function.

Contraindications—

• This herb should not be used during pregnancy.

• Do not use for prolonged periods of time.

• People suffering from cardiovascular disease, diabetes, or glaucoma should use goldenseal only under the supervision of a health professional.

• The alcohol-free extract is the best form of this herb.

Green Tea

Camellia sinensis

Forms—The leaves are used to make tea.

Nutritional value—Bioflavonoids, fluoride, polyphenols, tannins, vitamin C. Green tea has antioxidant properties that make it useful in slowing the aging process and protecting against heart disease.

Medicinal uses—

• Green tea is useful in treating cancer because it counters the effects of radiation, keeps the pH of the blood balanced, and is high in antioxidants. The polyphenolic catechins found in green tea are actually more powerful than vitamin E in fighting free radicals.

• Although green tea contains caffeine, the amount is minuscule. But the presence of caffeine in the herb makes it an energy enhancer that creates a cooling sensation and alleviates sharp menstrual pains.

• This herb combats mental fatigue, possibly due to the presence of caffeine in the leaves.

Contraindications—

• Pregnant and nursing women should not consume green tea in large quantities.

• People with anxiety disorder or irregular heartbeat should limit their intake to two cups daily.

Hawthorn

Crataegus spp.

Forms—The berries, flowers, and leaves are used to make powder and tea.

Nutritional value—Choline, citric acid, flavonoids, folic acid, inositol, pantothenic acid, purines, sugar, vitamins B_1, B_2, B_3, B_6, B_{12}, and C. This herb is a traditional heart tonic that nourishes the blood and improves circulation.

Medicinal uses—Because hawthorn dilates the coronary blood vessels, lowers cholesterol levels, and restores heart muscle, it is useful in treating cardiovascular disorders such as arrhythmia, angina, heart disease, and high blood pressure. According to Varro Tyler, Ph.D., and author of *Herbs of Choice,* hawthorn's heart benefits are due to special compounds in the plant—oligomeric procyanidins.

Contraindications—None known; safe for long-term use.

Horsetail

Equisetum arvense

Forms—The stems are used to make dried herb, powder, and tincture.

Nutritional value—Calcium, copper, fatty acids, fluorine, pantothenic acid, silica, sodium, starch, and zinc. Horsetail is rich in the vital nutrients that nourish the nails, skin, hair, bones, and the body's connective tissue.

Medicinal uses—
• Because of its rich supply of nutrients, horsetail helps heal fractured bones.
• This herb is an astringent for the genitourinary system that reduces hemorrhage caused by heavy menstrual cycles and heals wounds that occur with certain bacterial, viral, and sexually transmitted diseases due to its high silica content.
• Horsetail is often combined with hydrangea in the treatment of prostate troubles.
• Because of its high silica content, horsetail has been used in preventing osteoporosis. Make a tea from the herb and add a teaspoon of sugar, which will pull even more silicon from the plant.
• Horsetail increases urinary output and is recommended by Commission E, the German government's nutrition experts, for the treatment of kidney stones and general health of the urinary tract.
• This herb strengthens the heart and lungs and acts as a diuretic.

Contraindications—None known.

Kava Kava

Piper methysticum

Forms—The roots are used to make dried herb, tablets, tinctures, and capsules.

Nutritional value—Demethoxyangonin, kawain, methysticin, starch, yangonin. This member of the pepper family has been widely used as a social relaxant in South Pacific societies for more than 3000 years. It has also been used in ceremonies and rituals to reach a higher level of consciousness. More recently, the herb has been described by researchers as a narcotic, hypnotic, and sedative. Users commonly experience mild euphoria characterized by elevated mood, lively speech, and an increased sensitivity to sound.

Medicinal uses—
• Kava kava reduces anxiety, relaxes muscle tension, produces analgesic effects, acts as a local anesthetic, and has a potential antibacterial benefit. It is helpful in treating anxiety, depression, insomnia, and stress-related disorders.

• Because it acts as a diuretic, this herb is effective in treating urinary tract infections, gout, and incontinence.

• Kava kava has been used for more than a century to successfully treat gonorrhea, vaginitis, and other diseases of the genitourinary tract.

• As a muscle relaxer, this herb is effective in relieving the pain of menstrual cramps.

• Kavalactones, the active ingredient in kava kava, change brain activity without sedation. A 1993 report in the *British Journal of Phytotherapy* referred to kava as one of the few herbs that can safely relax the skeletal muscle.

• A 1996 double-blind study showed that the herb significantly reduces anxiety in humans. Two groups of 29 people with normal anxiety were treated for four weeks with three daily doses of 100 mg of kava extract or a placebo. After one week, members of the kava group had significantly lower anxiety levels compared with that of the placebo group. The difference between the two groups increased with time.

Contraindications—
• Can cause excessive drowsiness if taken in large doses. Do not use this herb during pregnancy, nursing, bouts of depression, or while driving or operating machinery.

• Commission E warns against using kava kava with alcohol, antidepressants, and other substances that may act on the central nervous system.

• Long-term, heavy use can cause temporary yellowing of the

skin, hair, and nails, as well as itching, sores, and vision disturbances.

• A 1995 report described four patients who experienced unpleasant side effects from using various kava preparations. Symptoms ranged from spasms in the neck and eye muscles lasting for 40
minutes to impaired movement in a Parkinson's disease patient. Two
of the four patients were over 60. The study's authors suggest that
kava be used cautiously, especially with elderly patients.

• There is no scientific evidence to date that proves this herb is
addictive.

Licorice

Glycyrrhiza glabra

Forms—The roots are used to make dried herb, powder, and tea.
The fresh root is sometimes chewed.

Nutritional value—Biotin, choline, fat, folic acid, inositol,
lecithin, manganese, pantothenic acid, pentacyclic terpenes, phosphorus, protein, sugar, yellow dye, vitamins B_1, B_2, B_3, B_6, and E.
Licorice root nutritionally supports the respiratory and gastrointestinal systems, heart, and spleen. It soothes irritated mucous membranes and helps the body get rid of unwanted mucus with its
expectorant properties. Licorice has properties similar to estrogen
and cortisone. It also helps the body cope with stress.

Medicinal uses—

• Licorice root acts upon mucous surfaces, lessening irritation.
For this reason, it is useful in treatment of coughs, irritation of the
urinary organs, and pain of the intestines due to diarrhea. Extract in
the form of a lozenge is useful for coughs.

• Licorice tea soothes the throat and is useful in treating asthma.

• When combined with willow and garlic, licorice is useful as an
anti-inflammatory in treating arthritis. It is used in this combination
because willow bark can upset your stomach, but licorice helps treat
gastrointestinal problems.

• Licorice has more anitdepressant compounds than any other
herb but, strangely enough, is not used to treat depression as often
as St. John's wort.

• Because of its expectorant and antioxidant properties, licorice
is effective in treating emphysema.

• Licorice inhibits liver cell injury caused by chemicals. It is used in the treatment of cirrhosis and chronic hepatitis.

• People with HIV can benefit from licorice. Glycyrrhizin, the active constituent, can inhibit a number of processes involved in viral replication. Studies and clinical trials indicate that glycyrrhizin inhibits the growth of HIV in the test tube. It also seems to reduce the side effects of AZT.

• In Europe, licorice derivatives have been recommended as a standard support for ulcer sufferers. Licorice contains several anti-ulcer compounds.

Contraindications—Long-term use can result in headache, lethargy, sodium and water retention, excessive loss of potassium, and high blood pressure.

Lobelia

Lobelia inflata

Forms—The flowers, leaves, and seeds are used to make dried herb.

Nutritional value—Alkaloids, chelidonic acid, lobelic acid, selenium, sulfur. Lobelia has traditionally been used to nourish the nervous system. It also enhances the respiratory system and has antispasmodic effects.

Medicinal uses—

• This herb is beneficial in the treatment of asthma and bronchitis as well as whooping cough, spasmodic croup, and membranous croup because lobeline, an alkaloid, is a powerful respiratory stimulant, while isolobelanine is a respiratory relaxant. This combination stimulates mucus secretion while relaxing the muscles of the respiratory system.

• The expectorant properties of lobelia make it an effective treatment for coughs.

• Lobelia reduces the symptoms of cold and flu, including fever.

Contraindications—None known.

Milk Thistle

Silybum marianum

Forms—The fruit, leaves, and seeds are made into dried herb, capsule, and tincture.

Nutritional value—Silymarin, a unique type of flavonoid with antioxidant ability. This herb was used in the eighteenth century to prevent obstructions of the liver and spleen, and in the nineteenth century for liver congestion as well as varicose veins, menstrual disorders, and other conditions now known to be associated with liver disorders. More recently, the toxicity of alcohol abuse, drug use, coffee, and pesticides have been shown to respond to milk thistle, which tonifies and helps rebuild the liver. Milk thistle fortifies the liver cell walls with proteins so that toxins cannot enter so easily.

Medicinal uses—
• Recent studies show that the silymarin and silybin found in milk thistle work as antioxidants. These studies suggest that they protect against genetic damage, increase liver cell protein synthesis, decrease the activity of tumor promoters, stabilize allergenic mast cells, chelate iron (for more information on chelation, see pages 30–31), and slow calcium metabolism. In short, nature has provided an effective way to combat the many liver-damaging compounds present in modern life.
• This herb promotes milk production and is of benefit to breast-feeding mothers.
• Milk thistle contains at least eight anti-inflammatory compounds that act on the skin, making it effective treatment for many skin disorders, including psoriasis.

Contraindications—None known.

Nettle

Urtica dioica

Forms—The flowers, leaves, and roots are used to make dried herb and tincture.

Nutritional value—Calcium, chlorine, chlorophyll, iodine, iron, magnesium, potassium, silicon, sodium, sulfur, tannin, vitamins A and C. Nettles strengthen and support the whole body.

Throughout Europe they are used as a tonic and general detoxifying remedy. Nettles, also referred to as stinging nettles, contain vital minerals that are essential in the treatment of many disorders.

Medicinal uses—

• Nettles are beneficial in treating all the varieties of eczema, especially nervous eczema and childhood eczema. They are most effective for this disorder when used in combination with figwort and burdock.

• As an astringent, nettles are useful in stopping nosebleeds and in relieving the symptoms of hemorrhage anywhere in the body.

• Boron plays a role in helping bones retain calcium. It also has a positive influence on the body's endocrine system, which helps maintain healthy bones and joints. USDA scientists analyzed nettle and found it to contain 47 parts per million of the mineral boron, figured on a dry-weight basis. So a 100 gram serving of nettle, prepared by steaming the leaves, could easily contain more than the recommended 3 mg of boron necessary in relieving the pain and inflammation of arthritis.

• Nettle has proven beneficial to a number of other disorders, including anemia, hay fever and other allergic conditions, kidney problems, goiter, inflammatory conditions, and mucous conditions of the lungs.

Contraindications—None known.

——————————— **Parsley** ———————————

Petroselinum crispum

Forms—The tap root, leaves, and seeds are used to make tincture.

Nutritional value—Calcium, fatty oil, essential oils, iodine, iron, mucilage, petroselinic acid, phosphorus, potassium, vitamins A and C (more vitamin C than oranges, by weight). Parsley has three main medical uses: It is an effective diuretic, ridding the body of excess water; it is an emmenagogue, stimulating the menstrual process; and it eases flatulence and the colic pains that may accompany it.

Medicinal uses—

• Parsley contains high levels of boron, which nourishes bones by helping them retain calcium. This herb is an effective component of osteoporosis treatment.

• Parsley contains compounds that act much like calcium channel blockers. These blockers are standard antiangina drugs.

• Tradition credits parsley with easing breast tenderness in nursing mothers. This makes sense because some breast tenderness is caused by water retention. The diuretic properties of parsley flush excess water from the body. This same action makes this herb useful in helping reduce milk production in preparation for weaning.

• Parsley freshens breath.

• As a diuretic, parsley helps empty the bladder, thus relieving the discomfort of bladder infections. It is also effective in treating kidney disease.

• Bedwetting can be caused by a urinary tract infection; parsley could eliminate this disorder.

• Some people report that repeated applications of crushed parsley leaves will clear up any black-and-blue marks within a day or so.

• Because of its estrogen-like properties, parsley increases the female libido.

Contraindications—None known.

Primrose

Oenothera biennis

Forms—The seeds are used to make an oil and capsules.

Nutritional value—Gamma-linoleic acid (GLA), linoleic acid. Also called evening primrose, this herb is useful in treating a number of disorders.

Medicinal uses—

• Because it is a natural estrogen promoter, primrose is effective in treating hot flashes, menstrual cramps and heavy bleeding, and PMS.

• Although the oil is thought of more as a treatment for the above disorders, medical guides mention it almost as much as flaxseed for treatment of endometriosis. The oil contains GLA and tryptophan, substances that seem to promote general good health in women.

• David Hoffman, author of *The Herbal Handbook,* says evening primrose oil is recommended in the treatment of multiple sclerosis. This is because it contains high levels of GLA.

• The GLA in primrose oil is approved in Great Britain for treating eczema. Research also suggests using the oil in treating dermatitis.

Contraindications—None known.

———————————— **Red Clover** ————————————

Trifolium pratense

Forms—The flowers are used to make dried herb, tea, and tincture.

Nutritional value—Biotin, choline, copper, folic acid, inositol, isoflavonoids, magnesium, manganese, pantothenic acid, selenium, bioflavonoids, zinc, vitamins A, B_1, B_2, B_3, B_6, B_{12}, and C. Red clover is one of the most useful remedies for children with skin problems.

Medicinal uses—

• As mentioned above, red clover is used to treat childhood eczema and psoriasis.

• The expectorant and antispasmodic action make this herb valuable in treating coughs and bronchitis, but especially whooping cough. For the same reasons, it is effective in treating croup and chronic throat conditions.

• Red clover contains the anticancer compound genistein. This compound starves tumors by inhibiting their blood supply.

• This herb contains phytoestrogens that help minimize menstrual cramps by bringing into balance the body's hormone levels.

• Red clover contains 1 to 2.5% isoflavones. Isoflavones are phytoestrogens; they have mild estrogenic activity. Some clovers are so estrogenic that they have been known to cause spontaneous abortion in cattle that overgraze on them. But for humans, this herb can help balance hormones and is used to treat the symptoms of menopause.

• Red clover is good for bacterial infections, HIV and AIDS, inflamed lungs, and inflammatory bowel disorders.

Contraindications—None known.

——————————— **St. John's Wort** ———————————

Hypericum perforatum

Forms—The flowers, leaves, and stem are used to make oil, tinctures, infusions, and extracts.

Nutritional value—Essential oils, glycosides, resins, rutin and other flavonoids, tannins. This herb was named for the plant's blooms, which appear around St. John's Day, June 24. Also, when the buds and flowers are squeezed, they exude a red pigment, which was associated with the blood of St. John the Baptist. The medicinal benefits of St. John's wort have been cited by herbalists for at least 400 years. It is generally used for the treatment of nervous disorders, depression, neuralgia, kidney problems, wounds, and burns. Its ability to treat so many different disorders stems from the number of compounds found in the plant.

Medicinal uses—

• The most prevalent use for this herb is as an antidepressant. Studies have found that it reduces feelings of depression, anxiety, and apathy. Studies show the herb to be comparably effective to many pharmaceutical antidepressants while producing fewer side effects. It is not effective for severe depression, but works very well for mild to moderate depression.

• The herb's pain-relieving ability makes it effective for treating neuralgia, anxiety, and tension. This is useful during menopause, when hormonal imbalance triggers irritability. St. John's wort also eases fibrositis, sciatica, and rheumatic pain.

• As a lotion, the anti-inflammatory herb heals wounds, bruises, varicose veins, and mild burns. The oil works very well for healing sunburn.

• The antiviral compounds found in this herb have been shown to be active against HIV in test-tube studies. Researchers still have a long way to go in determining the effects on humans.

• St. John's wort is useful during childbirth and postpartum healing. The oil is soothing when rubbed on the perineum, the area between the vagina and anus, during labor. After delivery, its anti-inflammatory action eases burning and swelling and speeds the healing of perineal tears.

• Some researchers believe St. John's wort affects the serotonin levels in the brain, decreasing the body's desire for food. A German study found that the herb caused a 50% inhibition of serotonin uptake. This could make the herb useful in treating obesity. More research needs to be done, however.

Contraindications—
• Do not take this herb if you are pregnant.
• Avoid intense sun exposure while using St. John's wort; it can make the skin more sensitive to sunlight.
• This herb contains monoamine oxidase (MAO) inhibitors. If you take an MAO inhibitor on a regular basis, avoid alcoholic beverages and smoked or pickled foods. Also stay away from cold and hay fever remedies, amphetamines, narcotics, tryptophan, and tyrosine.

Sarsaparilla

Smilax officinalis

Forms—The roots are used to make dried herb and tincture.

Nutritional value—Copper, essential oil, fat, glycosides, iron, manganese, resin, saponins, sodium, sugar, sulfur, zinc, vitamins A and D. This herb contains substances similar to testosterone and progesterone. It increases the metabolic rate and balances the glandular system.

Medicinal uses—
• This herb is particularly useful in treating psoriasis and other scaling skin conditions. It is especially effective for these conditions if combined with burdock, yellow dock, and cleavers.
• It can be used for chronic rheumatism, especially rheumatoid arthritis.
• Sarsaparilla is useful for treating frigidity, hives, impotence, infertility, nervous system disorders, PMS, and disorders caused by blood impurities.

Contraindications—None.

———————————— **Saw Palmetto** ————————————

Serenoa serrulata

Forms—The berries are used to make tea, capsules, extracts, and tincture.

Nutritional value—Capric, oleic, palmitic acids, resin. This herb nourishes glandular tissue and has been used to treat the prostate gland.

Medicinal uses—

• This herb is valuable in treating infections of the genitourinary tract.

• Saw palmetto is one of the most popular herbs for treating prostate disorders. It increases urinary flow, reduces residual urine, and decreases the frequency of urination. As a diuretic, it helps flush excess water from the body. The herb also inhibits production of dihydrotestosterone, a hormone that contributes to enlargement of the prostate. It is especially effective when used with horsetail and hydrangea.

• Use this herb to enhance sexual functioning in both men and women.

• A century ago, this herb was best known as a folk approach to breast enlargement. Naturopathic physicians continue to use it for this purpose. Use the capsules or alcohol extract.

• This herb has been used in treating infertility.

Contraindications—None known.

———————————— **Suma** ————————————

Pfaffia paniculata

Forms—The bark, berry, leaves, and roots are used to make capsules, dried herbs, and tablets.

Nutritional value—Albumin, allantoin, germanium, essential oils, pfaffic acid, six saponins, sitosterol, tannins. Suma helps the body adapt to stress and acts as a tonic to the entire system. It enhances the body's immune system, thereby aiding in the prevention of free radical damage.

Medicinal uses—

• Japanese researchers investigated suma in trials against specific types of tumor cells and discovered six saponins called pfaffosides A, B, C, D, E, and F. These are the chemicals present in suma that inhibit tumor cell growth, making this herb valuable in treating and preventing cancer. Because it acts as an immune booster, suma is effective in the fight against AIDS, liver disease, high blood pressure, and weakened immune systems.

• Anemia, fatigue, and stress can be treated with this herb. Research shows that suma may be beneficial in the treatment of diabetes.

Contraindications—None known.

Valerian

Valeriana officinalis

Forms—The roots and rhizomes are used to make tablets, capsules, dried herb, and tinctures.

Nutritional value—Acetic acid, butyric acid, essential oils, formic acid, glycosides, magnesium, pinene, valeric acid, valerine. Valerian root nourishes the nervous system and has soothing properties. It acts as a natural sleeping aid. It provides calming relief to muscles, the nerves, and blood vessels.

Medicinal uses—

• Valerian root promotes sleep. In one study, a combination of 160 mg of valerian and 80 mg of lemon balm extracts brought on sleep as effectively as a standard dose of one of the drugs in the Valium family of pharmaceuticals. Though often believed to be derived from valerian, Valium is not related to the herb in any way.

• Valerian is a safe and powerful muscle relaxant, making it valuable in treating irritable bowel syndrome, menstrual cramps, muscle cramps, and spasms.

• This herb is used throughout the world to treat hypertension and stress-related heart problems. The World Health Organization (WHO) recognizes the research and development of traditional medicine and acknowledges the need to go beyond the test tube for meaningful results. WHO sponsored studies in Bulgaria that researched herbs in the treatment of cardiovascular problems. Valerian is one herb, among garlic, geranium, olive, hawthorn, and European mistletoe, whose use was validated.

Contraindications—

• Thorough investigation has not revealed a single active constituent in this plant, which stresses the importance of depending on the interaction of the constituents as a whole for therapeutic effects.

• Valerian can cause depression if taken in large doses for long periods of time.

Wild Yam

Dioscorea villosa

Forms—The dried underground parts are used to make tea and tinctures.

Nutritional value—Alkaloids, phytosterols, starch, steroidal saponins, tannins. Wild yam is effective in treating many disorders. It relaxes the muscles and promotes glandular balance in women. The phytochemicals help the body balance hormone levels. This herb also nourishes the digestive system and the nerves.

Medicinal uses—
• Because it reduces inflammation, this herb is useful in the treatment of rheumatoid arthritis.
• At one time, wild yam was the sole source of the chemicals that were used for contraceptive hormone manufacture. It is good for treatment of many female disorders, including PMS and menopause-related symptoms.
• Wild yam helps improve gall bladder disorders, hypoglycemia, kidney stones, diverticulitis, and intestinal colic.

Contraindications—Many yam-based products are made from plants treated with fertilizers and pesticides, which may end up in the final product. Try to find organic yam products.

Wintergreen

Gaultheria procumbens

Forms—The leaves, roots, and stem are used to make oil.

Nutritional value—Gaultherin, glycoside, mucilage, tannins, wax. The main activity of this herb is as a pain reliever and anti-inflammatory agent.

Medicinal uses—Wintergreen contains methyl salicylate, a close relative of the salicin found in willow bark. This is a substance similar to aspirin. Because it relieves pain, this herb can be used to

What's in a Label?

With so many herbs and so many herbal combinations available on today's market, it's vitally important to know what to look for on the label.

Take a few extra minutes to read the label before you buy a product. You'll be glad you did.

The product label should include:

• Standardized (% of active ingredient)

• Milligram or microgram dose of each ingredient

• Recommended dosing

• Potential side effects

• Expiration date

• Batch/lot number

• Phone number to call with questions

• Independent lab verification of contents

• Product-specific research

If you've decided to try herbal remedies, you've already taken that first step into the world of "alternative medicine." What you need to remember is that you are still dealing with *medicine*; it's just nature's medicine you're dealing with instead of medicine manufactured by human hands. Give herbs the same respect you would pharmaceuticals; take them responsibly and with caution.

Here are some suggestions to keep in mind when using herbs:

• Pay attention to dosing instructions. These are guidelines that should not be tampered with. They have been determined by experts who are familiar with the herb and its interactions.

• Accept that it usually takes longer to see results when using herbs than synthetic drugs. The upside to this is that you are allowing healing to be the process that it is, which is, for the most part, easier on your body.

• Inform your doctor of your decision to add herbs to a regimen of prescription medication. Although many mainstream physicians don't have expertise in the area of herbal medicine, they should be made aware of what you are putting into your body so that they can make the best and most accurate recommendations.

• Don't self-diagnose the big problems. Granted, you know if you're sunburned, or have been bitten by a bug, or are suffering from PMS; these circumstances are fairly cut-and-dried and easy to treat. But remember that it is important to treat the disorder rather than the symptoms. So if you suspect you may be the victim of a more serious disorder, consult a trained health professional immediately. Then make an informed decision, based on fact rather than speculation, of how to go about treating the condition.

• Listen to your body. Just about any and every drug produces some side effect(s), some more serious than others. It's your responsibility to pay attention to what your body tells you. If you experience dizziness as a result of taking an herb, stop taking it, even if your research tells you this particular herb produces no side effects or may cause something other than dizziness. In the science of herbal therapy, your body is the expert.

• The same goes for allergic reactions. If you experience a reaction after taking an herb, don't take it again. This is especially true if you experience any difficulty breathing within 30 minutes or so of trying a new herb. Play it safe and call 911; some allergic reactions can seem innocuous at first but are, in fact, potentially fatal.

• Be alert to interactions. Herbal medicines sometimes interact badly with certain foods and with each other. Always be especially careful when combining herbs with other herbs or drugs. Regardless of what you've read or been told or heard, adverse interactions are always possible.

• Using herbal remedies can have negative effects during surgery. Experts in the medical field recommend patients to stop taking herbs at least two to three weeks prior to scheduled surgery. Doctors say certain herbs may have dangerous interactions with drugs used to anesthetize patients during surgery, such as problems with blood pressure and bleeding.

treat arthritis, headache, toothache, muscle pain, rheumatic complaints, gout, and sciatica. Sore throat pain can be relieved with a gargle made from wintergreen. The cool, soothing flavor works wonders.

Contraindications—
• This herb is not recommended for children because it works like aspirin. When children take aspirin-like drugs for viral infections, they may come down with Reye's syndrome, a potentially fatal condition that damages the liver and brain.
• Do not take this herb if you are allergic to aspirin.

SECTION II
Diseases, Disorders, and Conditions
from A to Z

In this section, I have compiled information on common ailments, medical conditions, troubling symptoms, diseases, and disorders and arranged them in alphabetical order for you. For each entry, I have given you a brief synopsis of facts about the condition or symptom and then followed that with information about which vitamins, minerals, and herbal remedies help (or may help) the condition and which, if any, may worsen it. You will notice that most of these entries list several vitamins or minerals that current medical research studies, the professional and lay literature, or my own clinical practice experiences have proven beneficial. Let me clarify that by my listing more than one nutrient as having a good effect I don't intend that you should rush out to the nearest health-food store or pharmacy and load up on *all* of the recommended nutrients to try at once. Because there may be various underlying causes for any problem, there may be various remedies; not all of them will work to the same degree for every person. The best and most reasonable approach to altering your nutritional habits—and this includes extra supplementation with a specific vitamin or mineral—is to begin in a systematic fashion.

First, peruse the shelves of your local pharmacy or health and nutrition shop, looking for a complete combined multivitamin and mineral tablet (or group of tablets), with chelated minerals if possible. (I have provided a recommended basic vitamin and mineral intake for various age ranges and specific conditions in this listing.)

Use this combined product as your base of operations upon which to build your nutritional fort. To combat a particular symptom or ailment, you will modify this basic design by adding specific extra fortifications. When you are ready to do so, select one remedy at a time, stick with it long enough to give it a fair trial (in most instances that would be 4 to 6 weeks, at least), and then if you feel you've not benefited from that nutrient, move on to another. I wish I could tell you there is a faster, easier, and surer method of selecting which nutrient of several would be the surefire, magic bullet for what ails you, but that's not possible. Before you begin supplemental use of any specific nutrient, I would also recommend that you carefully reread the discussion about that nutrient in the A-to-Z listings of Section I, so that you will better understand how it works, what might interfere with it, what foods contain it, and the symptoms of taking too much of it.

Also, I would ask that if you currently take prescription medication for any ailment under the direction of your personal physician, you do not alter the dose or discontinue taking the medicine without first consulting your doctor; doing so could be dangerous. That doesn't mean you can't also begin to do a little nutritional rehabilitation in addition to your prescription medication, unless, of course, the recommended vitamin or mineral could interact with your medicine. Remember that sometimes vitamins, minerals, and medications don't mix well; and again, I refer you to the Section I, A-to-Z listings for each nutrient as a cross-check for interactions, side effects, and symptoms of toxicity and deficiency.

And finally, I entreat you to be patient. The symptoms that came about because of nutritional deficiencies didn't arise overnight and, by the same token, won't disappear that way. The first dose or two of any nutrient won't repair the damage and "cure" you; give it time.

Now let's see what the vitamin and mineral shelf has to offer for specific ailments.

Acne Rosacea

What is it?

Acne rosacea, or simply rosacea, as it is sometimes called, afflicts people in middle to older age, who probably inherit a tendency to develop this chronic skin condition. However, the disorder also occurs more often in those people burdened by severe emotional disturbance, chronic alcoholism, and in association with certain gastrointestinal problems that cause a lack of stomach acid. The skin changes seen in rosacea almost always include a pronounced ruddiness or flushed appearance of the face and the formation of facial spider veins. In addition to the redness, the skin may break out with pimple-like blemishes, with scaly, flaky dry patches, or with both. Especially in men, the big increase in oil gland activity in the pores of the nose may cause a growth spurt of the tissues of the end of the nose, leaving it bulbous, lumpy, and misshapen—a condition called *rhinophyma* in medicalese. Only plastic surgery can correct this disfiguring consequence of rosacea.

The similarities of the pimply outbreak to "teenage" acne gave rise to its name; however, when the disorder occurs in middle age, it may strike people who were never troubled by acne vulgaris at puberty. There is sufficient medical evidence (enough, at least, to pique curiosity and further investigation) that the root of the pimply and scaly skin changes may come from inadequate B vitamin absorption. But more on the nutritional aspects in a bit.

It is also interesting to speculate that there may be two components to the skin picture in rosacea: the red flushing and spider veins on one hand, and the pimpled, flaky skin on the other. The reason to so speculate is that oftentimes a nutrient or medical regimen will help the one, but leave the other unchanged. (See "What helps it?" on page 153.)

Some sufferers with rosacea also develop an inflammation of the cornea (the clear covering over the colored part of the eye), called rosacea keratitis, which can be not only irritating but potentially damaging. If your rosacea is associated with eye pain and irritation, you should consult your ophthalmologist for a thorough examination before attempting to treat your eyes yourself.

Severe cases of rosacea may require treatment with potent prescription medications, such as tetracycline antibiotics, metronidazole in pill (Flagyl, Satric, Metronid) or topical gel (Metro-Gel form), or with the vitamin A relative, isotretinoin (Accutane). Before turning to these potent medications, all of which having a potential for unpleasant side effects, let's see what the vitamin and mineral shelf has to offer.

What helps it?

• *Niacin,* given in injectable form into the vein, rapidly improves the pimply red inflamed skin. Injection into the vein, however, is not a very practical mode of administration for home use. And so, try taking it by mouth, in a dose of 100 to 250 mg, one to three times daily to help clear the skin inflammation. Be aware, however, one of the common side effects of niacin in some people is flushing of the skin. If taking the vitamin worsens the flushed appearance, or your blood pressure or pulse increase, discontinue its use. Recommendation: Begin with 100 mg taken once a day. Remain at this dose for 2 to 3 weeks to assess your response. Increase your dose frequency of the 100 mg strength to twice and then three times daily at weekly intervals. If you've still seen no response (and have had no flushing reaction to the medication) move to 250 mg first twice and then, if needed, three times daily.

• *Vitamin B$_6$ (pyridoxine)* is another B vitamin that you might try in doses of 50 mg daily by mouth to improve the pimpling and flaking symptoms. This regimen works well in some people with rosacea. Recommendation: 50 mg daily.

• *Vitamin B$_2$ (riboflavin)* doses of as little as 1 to 4 mg in some studies to as much as 10 mg in others promptly healed the eye disorder rosacea keratitis in 32 of 36 patients studied. In concert with your physician's recommendations for this problem, you might also try that regimen. The effect on your skin symptoms will probably be much less dramatic; however, about half the patients tried on this vitamin did see skin improvement, so riboflavin may help a bit even there. Recommendation: Begin with a dose of 1 to 2 mg taken by mouth each day. Remain at that dose for 2 to 3 weeks to assess your response. Increase every 2 to 3 weeks in 1 to 2 mg increments to a maximum of 10 mg per day.

• *B-complex vitamins by muscular injection* may benefit rosacea sufferers who lack sufficient stomach acid to absorb the B-complex vitamins well by the oral route. If you suffer from chronic indigestion and take frequent doses of antacids or if you have active stomach ulcers and must take daily doses of acid-inhibiting drugs (such as cimetidine or ranitidine, trade names Tagamet and Zantac), these medications may interfere with your ability to absorb the B vitamin group well. In this case, replacement by shots of B-complex may be your only reasonable alternative, and you will most likely have to enlist the aid of your personal physician to either administer the injections periodically, or, depending on how well that physician knows you and your history, he or she might be willing to train you to give your own injections and prescribe a vial of the injectable form of the B-complex for you. Recommendation: A mixture supplying 5 mg riboflavin, 50 mg thiamine, 5 mg pyridoxine, 5 mg pantothenic acid, and 50 mg niacin in each milliliter will suffice. Take $1/4$ to $1/2$ milliliter every 2 to 4 weeks.

• The oral form of the *vitamin A relative isotretinoin (Accutane)* used in severe teenage acne also seems to quiet rosacea flare-ups as well. You can only get this vitamin-like drug by prescription, however. Recommendation: 0.5 to 1 mg for each kg of body weight. (One kg is 2.2 pounds, so a man weighing 150 pounds would be 150/2.2 or about 70 kg. His daily dose would be 35 to 70 mg—i.e., 70×0.5 or 70×1.0.)

Herbal remedies

• *Alfalfa* contains chlorophyll, which has detoxifying properties and supplies many necessary vitamins and minerals. You may also try applying pure *aloe vera gel* to dry skin. Caution: If you experience irritation, discontinue use.

• *Borage seed, dandelion root, dong quai, parsley, sarsaparilla, and yellow dock root* improve skin tone.

• *Burdock root and red clover* are powerful blood cleansers. Calendula, cayenne, fennel seed, ginger, marshmallow root, sage, and slippery elm nourish the skin and promote healing. Caution: Do not use sage if you suffer from any kind of seizure disorder.

• *Milk thistle* aids the liver in cleansing blood.

• *Nettle and rosemary* improve skin tone, nourish the skin, and promote healing.

Dosages may vary, depending on duration and severity of symptoms. Consult a qualified herbal practitioner.

What makes it worse?

• I know of no vitamins or minerals that worsen rosacea; however, its strong association with chronic alcohol abuse would make reduction or elimination of alcohol intake a positive step toward improvement of the skin and eye symptoms.

———————— **Acne Vulgaris** ————————

What is it?

When you were younger, you would have called this breaking out of the skin pimples or blemishes, and in our teenage rite of passage, most of us suffered some degree of heartbreak from these blemishes that always seemed to choose precisely the wrong time to erupt. And although the problem afflicts teenage boys far and away more than girls, neither sex is exempt. And although I hate to be the bearer of bad news to the Boomers among my readers, the trouble doesn't always end at maturity. I recall a 44-year-old patient of mine remarking once that it just didn't seem fair to fight zits and wrinkles at the same time. (Fortunately, however, there are some vitamin-based medical treatments that may actually help both.)

The problem usually begins at puberty when the surging of reproductive hormones (especially the male hormone testosterone, which both sexes have to some degree) stimulates an increase in activity of the oil-producing glands of the skin. The oil gland in the skin has a shape much like a round-bellied flask with a hollow bowl and a skinny neck. Overproduction of oil—or *sebum,* in correct medical parlance—fills the bowl of the gland to overflowing and plugs up the neck. Bacteria on the skin rush into the plugged area, which becomes inflamed and even infected. And voilà, the pimple forms. It may be alone, or it may be one of an army of blemishes across the forehead, nose, cheeks, chin, front of the chest, and the back. The outbreaks may be fairly constant, may wax and wane with the monthly menstrual cycle in women, or may correspond to surges in reproductive/sex hormones in both sexes (i.e., worsening at puberty).

Some people inherit a tendency for severe acne that forms large boil-like cysts, which heal leaving the skin cratered with pocks and scars. While this form of acne, called cystic acne, will benefit from the vitamin and mineral regimens I will describe next, these severe cases may also require more potent vitamin-like medications that only a physician can prescribe and that have enough side effects to warrant close monitoring by that physician during the course of treatment.

What helps (or may help) it?

• Try *folic acid* in a dose of 5 to 10 mg per day. This regimen improved the acne flare-up in over 85% of the patients tested, but remember that the addition of folic acid to your vitamin regimen can hide a B_{12} deficiency that can be damaging to nerve tissues. Be sure to have your physician check your B_{12} level after one month and then every 3 to 4 months during intense folic acid supplementation. Recommendation: Take 5 mg per day for 4 to 6 weeks, and if no response, increase in 1 mg increments monthly to a maximum dose of 10 mg per day. Check blood levels for B_{12} as recommended above.

• *Vitamin A*—although you will recall its being a fat-soluble vitamin and potentially toxic—significantly improved the acne of participants of a large study of men and women. Taken by itself in doses of 150,000 IU, vitamin A proved of little benefit; however, the acne of women on doses of 300,000 IU per day and men on doses of 400,000 to 500,000 IU per day showed clearing of 50 to 75% after 12 to 16 weeks. The downside risks of this high a dose of vitamin A, however, demand that you have very close monitoring by your personal physician or dermatologist for liver and blood fat problems. Side effects typical of hypervitaminosis A (see Vitamin A in Section I, page 39) also appeared in the people involved in this study. The development of vitamin A–like medications and creams with far less toxicity makes the use of these high doses of vitamin A itself unnecessary for the treatment of acne. These newer medications, however, do require prescription by a physician. Recommendation: Women should take 300,000 IU per day (and should use effective contraception to prevent pregnancy), and men should begin with 400,000 IU for 4 to 6 weeks, increasing to 500,000 IU only if they see no results.

• *Beta-carotene* is an effective alternative for those of you who would rather not ingest the high doses required for vitamin A. It is nontoxic and gives excellent results, even in patients with severe acne who were not helped by medication, without exceeding 100,000 IU per day.

• *Isotretinoin,* the vitamin A relative I spoke about on page 154, is available in capsule form under the trade name *Accutane* only by prescription. I mention it here because it indeed is a vitamin derivative captured by the FDA and now controlled in the United States. Use of isotretinoin capsules in doses of 1 mg per kg of body weight per day, however, produces amazing results in severe acne vulgaris and in cystic acne. It is important to note that isotretinoin can cause side effects like dry skin and nosebleeds. Women who are pregnant or who become pregnant while taking the drug run the risk of passing on severe birth defects, such as fetal brain deformities. The cream or gel (topical) forms of the medication, sold under the name *Retin-A,* again only by prescription in the United States, produce substantial clearing of acne flare-ups after twice-daily use for 5 to 8 weeks. (It is here, in fact, where zit and wrinkle treatments coincide, because physicians also prescribe Retin-A to diminish the signs of skin aging—fine-line wrinkling and brown "age spots"). Recommendation: The gel form is more astringent (drying) to the skin than the cream base, so for oily acne, the gel may work better. Wash your face thoroughly with a good cleansing soap and hot water and rinse it very, very well. Allow at least one hour to pass before applying the Retin-A. Begin by sparingly applying 0.5% gel to the involved areas twice daily. If redness develops, increase the wait after washing, or, if necessary, ask your physician to reduce the strength of the medication. If the results are disappointing, you may need a stronger dose of gel. Or you may need to take the Accutane form (by mouth) under the close supervision of your physician. As with Accutane, the drug in Retin-A (tretinoin) should not be taken during pregnancy. In addition, it leaves the skin extremely vulnerable to sun damage.

• *Vitamin E* when taken along with vitamin A can substantially reduce the dose of vitamin A required to reduce acne outbreaks. Recommendation: Try 400 IU of vitamin E along with only 50,000 IU of vitamin A twice a day with meals for 4 to 6 weeks, then reduce the dose of each vitamin by half (taking the combination only once per day) to maintain the clearing.

• *Vitamin B$_6$* taken twice daily improved the premenstrual acne outbreaks in 75% of women between the ages of 16 and 29. Occasionally, B$_6$ and other vitamins in the B group may actually *cause* an acne-like eruption of small uniformly sized blemishes on the forehead, chin, chest, back, and upper arms. This form of B vitamin breakout usually subsides promptly after you quit taking the vitamin. Recommendation: To help combat acne eruptions that follow your menstrual cycle, begin with a dose of 25 mg twice daily and increase to 50 mg three to five times daily if you see no results during the first two monthly cycles.

• *Selenium and vitamin E* may work together to promote clearing of acne breakouts. Try a dose of 200 *micro*grams of selenium plus 10 mg vitamin E (as tocopherol succinate) twice a day for 6 to 12 weeks to improve flare-ups of acne. These nutrients work to clear the inflammation of acne by increasing the antioxidant levels in the

skin. Recommendation: 200 *micro*grams selenium and 200 IU vitamin E twice a day.

• *Zinc* tablets or capsules providing 30 mg of elemental zinc significantly reduces acne flare-ups in some people. In medical studies, zinc sulfate in doses of 90 to 135 mg three times daily (with
meals) over a period of 1 to 3 months resulted in clearing of acne in
some people. Recommendation: Chelated zinc as picolinate or aspartate in a dose of 50 mg per day. Warning: Supplementation of
zinc in ionic form can create deficiencies in other minerals, such as
copper, by competing against them for absorption in the intestinal
tract. Chelation of the zinc prevents this from happening. See pages
30–31, Section I, on chelation of minerals for more information.

• *Essential fat* concentrations, such as the essential fat called
linoleic acid, seem to fall progessively lower in the sebum of people
with acne as their inflammation worsens. Supplementing your diet
with a tablespoon or two of corn oil, canola oil, or cold-pressed virgin olive oil made into a light vinaigrette dressing may prove beneficial. Recommendation: To facilitate the best response from
essential fatty acids, begin with the proper macronutrient framework
(see Section I, eicosinoids, pages 24–25, and macronutrients, page
23). Then to that nutritionally sound base add gamma-linoleic acid to
EPA fish oil in a ratio of 1:4 (GLA:EPA) two to six times daily. The
EicoPro essential fatty acid product manufactured by Eicotec, Inc., of
Marblehead, Massachusetts (1–800–233–EICO) contains ultrapure
sources of linoleic acid and fish oils already combined in the proper
ratio. If you cannot get that product, you can purchase linoleic acid in
a product called evening primrose oil at most health and nutrition
stores, and EPA fish oil as well. Because it is not as pure a form, the
milligram dosing will be different. You can make a reasonable substitute by combining evening primrose oil capsules with fish oil capsules plus vitamin E. Take 500 mg of evening primrose oil (a source
of linoleic acid in capsule form), plus 1000 mg EPA fish oil, plus vitamin E 200 IU one to three times a day. (Warning to diabetics: EPA
fish oil can cause blood sugar fluctuations in some diabetics. Carefully monitor your blood sugar if you use this supplemental oil and
discontinue its use if your blood sugar becomes difficult to control.)

• *Chromium,* which helps you better tolerate carbohydrates, may
prompt rapid clearing of acne outbreaks. Recommendation: 200 *micro*grams chromium picolinate or 1 teaspoon of high-chromium
yeast twice daily.

Herbal remedies

• *Burdock root, milk thistle, and red clover* cleanse the blood.

• *Lavender, red clover, and strawberry leaves* can be used as a steam sauna for the face. Lavender kills germs and stimulates new cell growth. Simmer a total of 2 to 4 tablespoons of dried or fresh herbs in 2 quarts of water. When the pot is steaming, sit with your face at a comfortable distance over the steam for 15 minutes. Splash your face with cold water. Allow your skin to air dry, or pat it dry with a towel. If your acne is severe or badly inflamed, steam treatments may worsen the condition.

• *Tea tree oil* is a natural antibiotic and antiseptic. Dab the oil on blemishes three times daily, or use tea tree oil soap. Other useful herbs are alfalfa, cayenne, dandelion root, echinacea, and yellow dock root.

Dosages may vary, depending on duration and severity of symptoms. Follow package directions, or consult a qualified herbal practitioner.

What may make it worse?

• *Iodine*—which is used medicinally in "contrast" solutions put into the vein for certain kinds of x-ray studies, used as iodinated glycerol in cough control products to thin sinus and bronchial mucus (found in Organidin, Tussi-Organidin, Iophen, and others), in kelp tablets, and in iodized table salt if added in large amounts to food—may worsen or even cause acne outbreaks. Recommendation: Reduce intake of iodized salt, and avoid taking cough medications with iodine when possible.

• *B_{12}*, as well as other members in the B vitamin group, may worsen acne outbreaks. The group hit hardest by this reaction seems to be teenage and adult men who already have an acne problem. Recommendation: Avoid extra supplementation of the vitamin unless you have symptoms of deficiency.

• *Iron* (in its inorganic form) inactivates vitamin E and so may worsen acne. Recommendation: Avoid iron supplementation in doses greater than 10 to 15 mg per day unless you are anemic.

Macronutrient interactions

• Refined *sugar* and dietary *saturated fats* seem to promote acne outbreaks. Eliminating these culprits to as great a degree as is possible from your diet will help decrease acne formation.

• Increased dietary *fiber* (such as a 1-ounce serving of an all-bran cereal each day, 1 to 2 FiberCon tablets taken with daily meals, or bulk vegetable psyllium powders such as Metamucil, Konsyl, and Citrucel) helps to clear acne eruptions. Studies have so far not uncovered precisely how the bran exerts this beneficial effect on the complexion, although it may be through improving bowel elimination and limiting the absorption of saturated fats, acne-aggravating nutrients, and toxic substances. Recommended dose: Gradually work up to a total daily fiber intake of 30 to 40 grams per day.

Age Spots

What are they?

These brown, freckle-like spots appear usually first on the backs of the hands, the face, and upper chest, in areas chronically exposed to sun. The medical name for them is *lentigines,* and they, like the freckles of childhood, are nothing more than an area where the skin cells contain an excess of coloring pigments. If you run your fingertip over an age freckle with your eyes closed, you will feel nothing. They are totally flat and different in that regard from the rough, raised spots caused by sun damage, called solar keratoses, that can become skin cancers. The lentigines pose no health threat, but I can attest that they can precipitate an emotional crisis when at 30-something you first find them on your hands.

What helps them?

• Some evidence suggests that *vitamin E oil* applied daily to the areas involved may help slow down the aging process in the skin, and the natural leap of intellect would be to assume this would reduce age spotting. I have found the application of vitamin E helps lessen various kinds of pigmented skin spots in my own patients, and this effect makes excellent medical sense. However, there is not much in the way of hard science to prove a role for vitamin E in age spot treatment. Still, topically, it's quite harmless, and it does have a generally beneficial effect on skin, keeping it soft and supple.

I would recommend that you purchase either vitamin E oil to apply nightly to the spotted areas, or purchase vitamin E 200 to 400 IU capsules, which you can pierce or snip the end from and squeeze the contents out of. I prefer the latter form, because the capsules are a "two-fer," meaning that you get two modes of treatment for the price of one: you can take them by mouth as a vitamin supplement or you can rub the contents onto your skin.

To cover larger areas of skin, mix the contents of one or two capsules in the palm of your hand with a puddle of any richly moisturizing body lotion you like. Recommended dose: 200 IU to 400 IU applied to spotted areas twice daily mixed with moisturizing lotion.

• *Vitamin A,* or at least its prescription cousin, isotretinoin (Retin-A), applied sparingly to the age-spotted areas of the backs of the hands and arms or on the face, markedly improved the condition in clinical trials. In some countries, pharmacies sell Retin-A over the counter, but in the United States it still requires a prescription. If you use this vitamin relative, whether purchased in this country or elsewhere, discipline yourself to apply only the tiniest amount in a very thin film and never on freshly scrubbed skin. Even the lowest-dose cream (0.25% cream) is potent enough to cause redness and drying of the skin if you use or absorb too much. Recommended dose: Apply a very light film of cream or gel to skin once or twice daily no sooner than 1 to 2 hours after washing your skin. Follow in one hour with a good moisturizing lotion.

• *Essential fatty acids*—in a form suitable for applying to your skin—are available, to my knowledge, only in a nonprescription product called EicoDerm (produced by Eicotec, Inc., of Marblehead, Massachusetts). The essential fatty acids produce much the same benefit of the vitamin A–related creams, but with virtually zero side effects or potential for skin irritation. You can add a few drops of this formulation of essential fatty acids to your facial rinse water twice daily, or apply the oil directly to the skin's spotted areas morning and night; the formula absorbs readily into the skin used either way. If it's going to do the job, you should see some visible lightening of the spots after 3 to 4 weeks of twice-daily use. Recommended dose: Apply a light film to the damaged skin areas twice daily.

Herbal remedies

• *Burdock, milk thistle, and red clover* cleanse the bloodstream.
• *Ginkgo biloba* improves circulation and has potential antioxidant properties.
• *Ginseng and licorice* are beneficial for age spots. Caution: Do not use either of these herbs if you have high blood pressure.

Dosages may vary, depending on the duration and severity of your symptoms. Follow package directions, or consult a qualified herbal practitioner.

What makes them worse?

• *Sun exposure,* natural sun or sunbed use, because of its aging effect on skin, may promote an increase in age spotting. No nutrients, to my knowledge, directly worsen this problem.

AIDS/ARC

What is it?

In this day and age, I would expect that acquired immunodeficiency syndrome (AIDS) and AIDS-related complex (ARC) probably need no introduction. Laymen and scientists have written entire volumes about AIDS since it was first recognized in 1981, and rare would be the talk show, magazine, soap opera, TV drama, or movie company that has not devoted some time to discussing this tragic disease. There really isn't space enough for me to go into great detail about them in a book of this nature, so let me simply give you an abbreviated nutshell description.

The underlying process in AIDS occurs because of infection by HIV (the human immunodeficiency virus), which attacks parts of the body's immune defense system. The weak defense leaves people with the virus vulnerable to attack by a variety of infections that a healthy immune system could defend us from easily, and so HIV-infected people contract and sometimes succumb to unusual infections and unusual cancers. And it is these culprits, not the HIV per se, that cause the disability and death from AIDS. They could not do so, however, without the initial assault by the virus to weaken the defenses arrayed against them.

Statistics from 1993 estimated that about 85% of the reported AIDS cases in America have been men who got the virus through sex with an infected man, or men and women who were infected through intravenous drug use. The remaining 15% is made up of infants and heterosexual partners of infected people and those who contracted the virus from blood transfusions before screening techniques made the American blood supply safe. However, in Africa, India, and other third world areas, the disease knows no gender, and heterosexual transmission of the virus occurs widely. There is no one of any gender or age group not potentially at risk for this disease.

In that broad gray area between those people who merely test positive for exposure to HIV but are in no way ill and those who suffer calamitous assault by a host of unusual infections or cancers and develop the disease we call AIDS lies what scientists term ARC: people with the virus and with some early signs of immune system weakness, but without active illness. What makes the difference between the ends of this spectrum of disease? Why do some people acquire the disease after coming in contact with the virus and others do not? What caused the explosive degree of heterosexual spread of the virus in African nations? Certainly that is the $64,000 question with a Nobel Prize attached to its correct answer, but a good deal of recent research suggests that at least part of the explanation may lie in the nutritional status of the person under viral attack.

Worldwide, the disease claims far more victims among the poor, the sickly, the very young: groups with inadequate intake of essential nutrients, of good-quality protein, vitamins, minerals, and fats. That is not to say that those of us who strive for nutritional excellence would be immune from attack by the virus—that simply is not the case; however, a strong immune system, which sound nutrition provides, probably makes a difference not merely in resistance to the viral attack upon exposure, but in the course of the illness if it does strike. Let's see what kind of nutrients offer some benefit in strengthening our defenses.

What helps it?

• A number of studies have shown the blood of HIV-positive patients to be low in *folic acid*. The decrease may arise in part from the fact that many of the drugs used to treat the unusual infections that befall AIDS patients can deplete folic acid. Because of its role in building new body proteins, genetic material, and blood cells, a deficiency of folic acid would contribute to weakening the immune system. Recommendation: 1 to 2 mg per day is an adequate beginning point. The maximum dose available without prescription is less than $1/2$ mg, so you must double, triple, or quadruple the over-the-counter dose or obtain a prescription from your physician for 1 mg folic acid. In either event, to assess your response, ask your physician to draw blood to check a red blood cell folate level. If it is still low, increase your dose to 3 to 4 mg per day and have your physician recheck the response with a red blood cell folate level in 6 weeks and at this time perhaps also check your B_{12} level. It is important to keep the balance of folic acid and B_{12}. If folic acid is given to someone already deficient in B_{12}, that deficiency will become severe, and vice versa.

• A number of studies on both patients with AIDS (as well as people who only test positive for HIV) documented B_{12} deficiency. You should ask your physician to perform a blood test to check for deficiency of B_{12}, and if present, begin to supplement by injection. Recommendations: 1000 *micro*grams by injection into the muscle, weekly for about 4 to 6 weeks, then monthly indefinitely.

• Several research studies have documented thiamine deficiency in patients with AIDS, and others have implicated the low blood levels of *thiamine* as a possible cause of the nerve damage and dysfunction seen in some AIDS patients. Supplementing thiamine, therefore, should correct the deficiency and lessen the likelihood of developing nerve problems. I could find no hard science to verify a clear role for thiamine in this regard, but the trail certainly leads that way. Since the vitamin has virtually no toxicity, even at large doses, I would recommend supplementation. Recommendation: Begin with a minimum dose of 10 to 25 mg per day. You can gradually increase to as much as 100 mg to 200 mg without danger. Your kidneys will excrete any excess that your body doesn't need. Illness and especially fever increases your thiamine requirement; therefore, at such times, you should increase your dose to the 100 mg to 200 mg level.

• In studies on laboratory mice that serve as AIDS models (those being certain types of mice specifically bred to be able to develop an AIDS-like syndrome), supplementation with *vitamin A* reduced the risk of their developing cancers. Early human studies with vitamin A seem to point the same way. Recommendation: Try doses of vitamin A at doses of no greater than 10,000 to 20,000 IU to begin. With great caution, or under the care of your personal physician, you may increase the dosage to 50,000 IU if symptoms of deficiency (see page 39) of the vitamin persist. Remember, however, that vitamin A levels can build up and in some cases may cause severe symptoms of too much of the vitamin. Refer to the listing of vitamin A for toxic side effects and reduce your dose if you develop these kinds of symptoms.

• Very recent studies have shown that large doses of *vitamin C (ascorbic acid)* not only inhibited the ability of HIV to duplicate itself in patients with AIDS, but improved the function of the crippled immune cells, markedly reduced the number of people developing unusual infection, and shrank the size of the unusual cancer, Kaposi's sarcoma (the purple-pink skin tumors that afflict some AIDS patients). Recommendation: Using crystalline (powdered) vitamin C with a strength of 4 grams per teaspoon, begin with $\frac{1}{2}$ teaspoon (2 grams) twice daily for one week. Increase to 1 teaspoon (4 grams) twice daily for one week. Gradually increase the daily dose by $\frac{1}{2}$ teaspoon daily until you develop loose stools. This effect, called bowel tolerance, lets you know that you've reached the maximum dose you will be able to take at this time. Your ability to tolerate more vitamin C will increase if you become ill, run a fever, or are under added emotional or physical stress, and you can sneak the dose up in 2 gram increments at these times. Some people tolerate doses as high as 250 grams (given by vein) in a single day without problems; however, because your own ability to tolerate vitamin C may not permit a dose of this magnitude no matter what physical assault you may be under, begin at 2 to 4 grams per day and slowly work up until your bowels tell you "enough!"

• *Vitamin E,* because of its role in maintaining a healthy cell membrane,* has also begun to receive attention in AIDS research. It indeed appears that supplementation may be beneficial, but the final data simply are not in yet. Recommendation: At this point, I would recommend a conservative 800 IU to 1200 IU per day. Recommendation: While the jury is still out on any specific application for HIV, I would recommend that you ask your physician to check to see if your level of calcium or magnesium is low or "low normal" (still technically normal but on the lowest edge of the normal range). In either of these events, I would recommend an intake of these minerals sufficient to bring the level in your blood up to normal. In the case of "low normal," that may mean simply eating more foods rich in calcium and magnesium, whereas if your level lies truly below the normal level in blood, correction would likely require supplements of calcium of 500 to 1500 mg per day or of magnesium (Slo-Mag)

---

*Some studies document lower than normal blood levels of *calcium and magnesium* in people infected with HIV. As yet, I could not find any published data that addresses whether these deficiencies contributed to specific health risks for HIV-positive people. However, both calcium and magnesium are critically important minerals for muscle, bone, and heart health, as well as for proper nerve transmission, and so for reasons of good health you would not want to be deficient in either of them.

of 200 to 400 mg per day. Low levels may occur for many reasons besides inadequate intake (such as low vitamin D intake or inadequate exposure to sunlight), so I refer you to the specific listings for calcium (page 54) and magnesium (page 82).

• *Germanium* is a trace mineral that improves cellular oxygenation. It fights pain, enhances the functioning of the immune system, and rids the body of toxins and poisons. Because it carries oxygen to the cells, germanium, when obtained through foods, is an effective way to increase tissue oxygenation. Foods containing germanium include garlic, shiitake mushrooms, and onions. Japanese scientist Kazuhiko Asai found that an intake of 100 to 300 mg of germanium per day improved many illnesses, including AIDS.

• Attention has focused on *zinc* deficiency as a contributor to furthering the immune system problems in AIDS patients. Zinc deficiency causes the tissues that produce immune-fighting cells to shrink, weakening the defense system and leaving the person more vulnerable to disease. Recent studies demonstrate that many AIDS patients are zinc deficient, which may be one of the nutritional factors leaving them vulnerable to infection by the virus upon exposure. Zinc deficiency may also hasten the progression from symptom-free HIV-positivity to a worsening of their disease and the development of AIDS. Recommendation: 150 mg chelated zinc daily for 3 to 6 months. Warning: Supplementation of zinc in its ionic form can create deficiencies of other minerals, such as copper, by competing with them for absorption from the intestine. Chelation of the minerals (see pages 30–31 on chelation) prevents this competition to get into the body, allowing you to fully absorb each of them.

• Certain of the *amino acids,* which are the basic subunits for building protein, appear to bolster immune function. Let me first underscore the importance of avoiding general protein deficiency in any debilitating disease and the value of eating a diet rich in complete protein (containing all the essential amino acids) sufficient to provide for the lean tissues. (See "Leveling the Playing Field," pages 23–24.) Providing your body with extra amounts of specific amino acids in supplemental form over and above your basic protein requirement, however, also appears to benefit the immune system in HIV, so let me discuss these amino acids in greater detail.

Arginine taken in doses of 30 grams per day for 3 days increases the activity of natural killer cells (a certain type of immune fighter cell crippled by HIV infection). Because one of the ways in which the virus takes control of the immune system is by silencing these killing immune fighters, enhancing their ability to keep on killing would logically be a benefit to you.

Cysteine has a twofold role in HIV. It has been shown to slow down the reproduction of immunodeficiency viruses in the laboratory and is necessary in staving off attack by free radicals. The latter effect occurs because cysteine is made into glutathione, one of the body's potent antioxidant scavengers of free radicals, and therefore, a deficiency in dietary cysteine results in your body's not being able to make as much glutathione as it needs to protect your tissues from free radical attack. I refer you to pages 19–23, where I discuss free radicals and their role in damaging the body's tissues. The recommended dosage is a total dose of 1600 to 1800 mg daily, as a single 600 mg tablet three times daily, or in powder form, a 400 mg dose taken four times daily. Please see the entry for glutathione (page 168) for other supplementation suggestions.

• Another nutritional substance made from egg yolk, called *egg lipid extract, or AL 721,* appears in research studies to render HIV less able to infect—in effect, to cripple it. Let me interject that none of the studies done so far on this very innocuous substance has been a "controlled" study, but the work on AL 721 is at least promising and deserving of more intense scrutiny, which I feel sure it will get. Recommendation: Again, for now, you will only have access to the whole-food source—eggs—which I would encourage you to eat. Make an egg or two a part of your daily dietary intake. One additional note: Some of you may become concerned about your cholesterol going up if you eat eggs daily. Please rest easily on that score. Most patients with AIDS (or any severe debilitating disease) suffer from too low a cholesterol level, not from an elevated one. And too low a level carries its own health risks in the form of susceptibility to infection and cancer—an added burden you don't need. However, you might ask your personal physician to check your cholesterol level periodically if the specter of rising blood levels alarms you. The number you are seeking for good health purposes is a total cholesterol reading between about 180 mg/dl and 220 mg/dl, but the most important aspect of normalcy in cholesterol is a number representing the ratio between the HDL "good" cholesterol number and the total cholesterol. To calculate this ratio, take your total cholesterol reading and divide it by your

HDL cholesterol reading; if that ratio is 4 or less, you're in good shape.

• *Glutathione* itself comes in tablet or capsule form for supplementary use. It is expensive, however, and the effectiveness of oral formulas is questionable. You would be better off supplying your body with the raw materials it uses to make glutathione: cysteine, glutamic acid, and glycine. NAC is particularly effective for this purpose. What *does* seem to work well is the combination of supplements of NAC, glutathione, and vitamin C. Studies show that when taken together, the results are more effective than when taken alone. NAC and glutathione have been shown to work together to extend the latency period of HIV. Researchers also suggest that the two inhibit expression of HIV. This means that although a person may test positive for HIV, there is no physical evidence of the infection. Both NAC and glutathione are natural and nontoxic. Recommendation: Begin with a dose of 150 mg per day and increase to 300 mg per day.

• Some recent research shows that AIDS patients develop deficiency in *coenzyme Q_{10}* and that supplementation improves their resistance to infections. Recommendation: 200 mg coenzyme Q_{10} daily and continued indefinitely.

• The *essential fatty acids* (see the discussion of eicosinoids, pages 24–27) linoleic acid (GLA) and EPA (fish oil) appear to be able to destroy the envelope or protective coat of the HIV and may therefore help in slowing progression of the disease. These fats when taken in the proper ratio also improve immune function. Recommendation: To facilitate the best response from essential fatty acids, begin with the proper macronutrient framework (see Section I, Macronutrients, page 23). Then to that nutritionally sound base add gamma-linoleic acid to EPA fish oil in a ratio of 1:4 (GLA:EPA) one to three times daily. The EicoPro essential fatty acid product manufactured by Eicotec, Inc., of Marblehead, Massachusetts, contains ultrapure sources of linoleic acid and fish oils already combined in the proper ratio. If you cannot get that product, you can purchase linoleic acid in a product called evening primrose oil at most health and nutrition stores, and EPA fish oil as well. Because it is not as pure a form, the milligram dosing will be different. You can make a reasonable substitute by combining evening primrose oil capsules with fish oil capsules plus vitamin E. Take 500 mg of evening primrose oil (a source of linoleic acid in capsule form), plus 1000 mg EPA fish oil, plus vitamin E 200 IU one to three times a day. (Warning to diabetics: EPA fish oil can cause blood sugar fluctuations in some diabetics. Carefully monitor your blood sugar if you use this supplemental oil and discontinue its use if your blood sugar becomes difficult to control.)

Herbal remedies

• *Licorice* tea contains a constituent called glycyrrhizin, which inhibits a number of processes involved in viral replication. Studies indicate that glycyrrhizin inhibits the growth of HIV in test tubes. Clinical trials have also produced positive results.

• *Oregano* and *self-heal* contain antioxidants that can help maintain immune function in those who are HIV-positive.

• *St. John's wort* contains two antiviral compounds: hypericin and pseudohypericin. Much research still needs to be done to determine the full therapeutic value of these two compounds in treating HIV. The results of test-tube and animal studies have been positive. A mixture of hypericin and several derivatives has been patented as a treatment for cytomegalovirus infection, one of the many infections that strike people with AIDS. Caution: This herb contains MAO (monoamine oxidase) inhibitors. Do not take if you're pregnant. Avoid prolonged sun exposure while using St. John's wort; it can make skin more sensitive to sunlight.

• There is some evidence that acemannan, a compound found in *aloe,* may be beneficial in treating AIDS. Test-tube studies show it to be active against HIV.

• *Astragalus,* while not having demonstrated any anti-HIV effect, is an immune booster. Caution: Do not use if you have a fever.

• A research report claimed that the root extract of *black-eyed Susan* stimulates the immune system better than echinacea extracts.

• *Blessed thistle* contains compounds with anti-HIV activity.

• *Burdock* juice or extracts have shown test-tube activity against HIV.

• One of the most powerful and popular immune-boosting herbs is *echinacea.* It has antiviral properties and increases the efficiency of white blood cells.

• *Garlic* contains a compound called ajoene, which may inhibit the spread of HIV within the body. Garlic is also effective against a number of the opportunistic infections of AIDS.

• One of the best sources of the antioxidant compound quercetin is the *onion*. It has many of the same antiviral effects as garlic. Cook with onion and leave the skin on; that's where the majority of the quercetin is.

• *Pears* contain caffeic and chlorogenic acids. The former is an immune stimulant, the latter has been studied and shown to have activity against HIV.

• The life expectancies of people who were HIV-positive more than doubled by adding gamma-linoleic acid (GLA) and omega-3 fatty acids found in fish such as salmon and swordfish to their diets.

• *Evening primrose* is an excellent source of GLA.

• *Iceland moss* contains compounds that inhibit an enzyme essential to replication of HIV. AZT and other AIDS drugs do the same thing, but with toxicity and the inability to completely inhibit the virus. The moss, however, is nontoxic to cells.

• *Cat's claw* boosts immune function, and has been helpful for people with AIDS and AIDS-related cancers. Caution: Do not use if you are pregnant.

Dosages may vary, depending on the severity of your symptoms. Consult a qualified herbal practitioner. Be sure to let your physician know of your decision to use herbs; not all herbal remedies are useful or safe when used in conjunction with conventional pharmaceuticals.

What makes it worse?

• Diets composed primarily of *whole cereal grains and green vegetables* can interfere with adequate absorption of zinc, creating deficiency, and weakening your immune function.

• Diets *inadequate in regular intake of complete protein* can also increase susceptibility to infections.

• A diet high in *sugar* debilitates your immune system by reducing your ability to produce antibodies against disease as well as by reducing the killing power of certain immune defenders. Recommendation: Eliminate or sharply curtail your intake of refined sugar, corn syrup, high-fructose corn syrup, molasses, and all products made with these substances.

——————————— **Alcoholism** ———————————

What is it?

Abuse of alcohol takes two basic forms: problem drinking and true addiction, the first often progressing to the second. In susceptible people (and medical studies do indicate that some people inherit a tendency to develop the addiction), frequent and repeated use of alcohol can lead to dependency. Dependency means that your body suffers physical and emotional discomfort with "withdrawal" of your access to liquor, wine, or beer. Once dependent, an alcoholic will continue to drink even when doing so threatens his/her job, home life, and health. Prolonged heavy drinking can cause damage and destruction of the liver and brain tissues and nerves, may contribute to the development of depression, and may promote nutritional deficiencies. Many of the severe symptoms associated with chronic alcoholism arise because of these nutritional deficiencies. Let's take a look now at the nutrients that help to decrease the toxicity of alcohol to the body and may also curb the craving for alcohol.

What helps it?

• Deficiencies in *vitamin A* and *zinc* cause a wide range of problems associated with alcohol abuse, among which are night blindness, reduced sexual function, loss of taste, and decreased sense of smell. Correction of these deficiencies will alleviate these problems. Recommendation: Begin first by eating a diet rich in foods containing vitamin A (or beta-carotene) and zinc. In addition, you may wish to add 5,000 to 10,000 IU of vitamin A or 15,000 to 20,000 IU beta-carotene along with zinc in a dose of 100 to 150 mg per day. You should see improvement of these symptoms after using the combined regimen for at least 4 weeks. You may continue the regimen indefinitely as long as you do not develop any of the symptoms of taking too much vitamin A (see page 37).

• Alcohol abuse often leads to deficiencies in the *vitamin B-complex* (especially thiamine, pyridoxine, folic acid, and B_{12}). Deficiency of the B vitamins leads to a host of maladies of skin, blood cells, and energy level but, more important to this discussion, may increase your craving for alcohol. Recommendation: Begin with 100 mg B-complex daily. An injection of 1 milliliter B_{12} (cyanocobalamin 1000 *micro*grams per milliliter) with $1/4$ to $1/2$ milliliter B-complex (containing 5 mg riboflavin, 50 mg thiamine, 5 mg pyridoxine, and 50 mg niacin) added to it bypasses your stomach and ensures that your body will absorb the vitamins. Specific members of the B vitamin family also have more direct effects on lessening alcohol damage and in helping to curb the addictive cravings. Let's look at these now.

• *Vitamin B₃ (niacin)* may also become depleted in chronic alcohol abuse and may contribute to the agitation, confusion, mental cloudiness, and disorientation sometimes seen in this condition. Correcting the deficiency by eating a diet rich in food sources for niacin and by supplementation may reduce both your craving for alcohol and its toxicity to your body. Niacin also seems to reduce the physical pain associated with alcohol "withdrawal" in people trying to stop drinking. Recommendation: Take 250 mg niacin twice a day for 4 to 6 weeks. If you have seen no improvement in the symptoms, increase your supplemental intake to 500 to 1000 mg daily of time-release niacin for another 4 to 6 weeks. If at that time mental cloudiness and alcohol cravings have still not diminished, you may increase the dose to 2 grams (2000 mg) or even 3 grams (3000 mg). Because niacin can cause uncomfortable side effects, such as flushing, in some people (see page 88), I would recommend that you increase slowly and that you stick with the lowest dose at which you see a response.

• *Vitamin B₁ (thiamine)* deficiency may arise not only because of poor dietary habits in alcohol abuse, but also because alcohol prevents absorption and efficient use of thiamine by the body. Some of the damage to the brain and nervous system that medical research attributes to the toxic effects of alcohol may actually be caused by thiamine deficiency. Mental symptoms ranging from mild agitation to hallucinations (the "pink elephants" that pop culture associates with inebriation) appear to respond to thiamine supplementation. In the research laboratory, rats "trained" to drink alcohol, then given the choice of water or alcohol, picked alcohol less often when they ate a diet containing adequate thiamine. Their thiamine-deficient friends, however, chose alcohol over water five times more often. What that means in human terms is that thiamine may actually reduce the desire to drink alcohol. Recommendation: Take thiamine 200 mg per day, 3 times a day (along with the entire B-complex as described above).

• *Vitamin C (ascorbic acid)* may improve the body's ability to detoxify and "clear" alcohol from your system as well as prevent some of the liver damage brought on by alcohol use. The two effects go hand in hand, because the liver is the primary organ in the body responsible for handling toxic substances, altering them in such a way as to make them less harmful (a process called detoxification) and then getting rid of them (the clearing process). The healthier your liver, the better able it will be to protect you from toxins, such as alcohol. Recommendation: 3 to 5 grams of time-release vitamin C daily. Another ½ to 2 grams taken 1 hour before alcohol consumption may also help to blunt the immediately toxic effects of alcohol on the liver.

• Chronic use of alcohol can also lead to low levels of another important antioxidant and tissue protector: *vitamin E.* Deficiency in vitamin E may also worsen the risk of alcoholic damage to the muscles, including the heart muscle, and the liver. Recommendation: Supplement daily with at least 800 IU (but safe in doses up to 1200 IU) to help protect against damage to vital organs. Begin slowly at a dose of 100 IU per day. After one week, check your blood pressure, because vitamin E can cause an elevation of pressure in some people. If the average of 4 or 5 readings on different days does not exceed 140/90, you may increase your dose weekly, checking pressures between dose changes, to 200 IU, then 400 IU, then 600 IU, then finally 800 IU, where most people will stop.

• *Zinc* deficiency in alcohol abuse is common and may arise not only because of insufficient dietary intake but because the body requires zinc to metabolize and detoxify alcohol. Increased demand for zinc leaves even an "adequate" dietary intake lacking. In laboratory research, rats low in zinc voluntarily drank more alcohol than their study mates with adequate zinc. In human terms, that means that alcoholic cravings may be worse in a state of zinc deficiency or, conversely, that your ability to abstain from alcohol may improve with adequate zinc in your diet. Recommendation: Take 50 to 60 mg of chelated zinc three times a day. Warning: Ionic zinc supplementation can cause deficiency of other minerals, notably copper, which you can avoid by taking the mineral in chelated form (such as zinc picolinate, zinc aspartate, or other zinc chelates).

• *Selenium* is essential for your body to produce the free radical scavenger glutathione, which protects your liver from alcohol damage. Selenium, often deficient in alcohol abusers, also works with vitamin E in protecting the liver. Recommendation: Take 100 to 200 *micro*grams daily. Alternatively, you can take *glutathione* itself in a dose of 3000 mg daily.

• *Magnesium* depletion can occur in alcohol use, even at moderate (1 ounce) daily intake. And reduced levels of magnesium contribute to muscle weakness and damage—including the heart muscle. Because of the complex interplay of magnesium, calcium, and phosphorus, you might want to review the discussions of these nutrients in Section I. Recommendation: You can supplement with a combined calcium and magnesium product, such as dolomite powder, in a dose of ¹/₂ teaspoon 3 times daily. Or if your calcium intake is sufficient from other sources, take only magnesium glycinate 200 to 400 mg daily. The proper ratio of calcium and magnesium is 2:1—that is, take twice as much calcium as magnesium.

• The amino acid (protein building block) *glutamine* appears to blunt the craving for alcohol in human research studies. Recommendation: Take 200 mg glutamine in tablet or capsule form 5 times daily for 6 weeks. If effective, your response should be improved sleep, lessened anxiety, and a reduced desire to drink. Once you achieve a good response, you may reduce your dose to 2 or 3 times a day (sometimes even discontinue entirely), unless symptoms return when you attempt to do so.

• Deficiency of *tryptophan,* another of the amino acids, may contribute to depression, memory difficulties, blackout spells, aggressive behavior, and suicidal tendencies in alcohol abuse. Dietary tryptophan seems to reduce these symptoms and may also reduce continued craving for alcohol. Recommendation: Take a 300 mg dose of L-tryptophan 1 to 4 times daily. (Note: Years ago, a number of people developed a severe muscular disorder [called EMS] from taking tryptophan supplements. At the time, the FDA ordered all supplemental forms of this amino acid removed from the shelves until the cause of the disorder surfaced. Ultimately, the culprit proved to be a contaminant in supplements made by a single large manufacturing source and not the tryptophan itself; however, the FDA has still not approved return of this harmless amino acid to the market. If it should ever do so, you may follow the recommended doses in this listing.)

• *Carnitine* is a "pseudovitamin" nutrient that improves the metabolism of fats in the liver and may protect the liver from alcoholic damage. Recommendations: Use only l-carnitine (not d- or dl- mixtures) in a dose of 250 mg once or twice daily.

• *Choline* is another of the pseudovitamins not classified as a vitamin by the FDA, and without a clearly identifiable deficiency disease when we lack it. Though not an essential vitamin, it is still important to good health. Studies show that it alleviates the accumulation of abnormal quantities of fat in the liver. In addition, choline transports and metabolizes fats that *may* play a role in reducing the toxic effect of alcohol on your liver. I have to say *may* do so, because animal studies have shown both that it helps and that it doesn't. In some studies, choline helped stop fatty liver damage, and in others, not only did it not stop damage, massive doses of choline actually proved toxic to the liver. This conflict may be an example of the need for an adequate macronutrient framework onto which we add the micronutrient (see Macronutrients, Section I, page 23), because when researchers increased dietary protein in the animal subjects and then added choline, they were able to prevent or lessen the liver damage caused by alcohol and even promote healing of damage. However, be aware that the protective and healing effect of choline fails if you continue the insult to your liver by continuing to drink alcohol. Recommendation: I recommend using lecithin, a natural substance high in choline. It is more easily assimilated and less irritating at higher doses than other forms. Take 1200 mg 3 times daily, before meals.

• The *essential fatty acids* linoleic acid (GLA) and fish oils (EPA) may lessen the physical pain of alcohol withdrawal as well as help to prevent liver damage from alcohol. Refer again to the discussion of essential fats in Section I (eicosinoids, pages 24–27) for an overview of these important macronutrients. Recommendation: Your optimal benefit will come from essential fats in the proper ratio of 1 part pure GLA to 4 parts pure EPA. EicoPro (from Eicotec, Inc., Marblehead, Massachusetts) provides the proper premixed ratio of ultrapure oils that you may take in doses of 2 capsules 1 to 3 times daily. If you are unable to get this product, you can achieve much the same end by taking 500 mg of evening primrose oil (a source of linoleic acid in capsule form) with 1000 mg EPA fish oil 3 times a day. (Warning to diabetics: EPA fish oil can cause blood sugar fluctuations in some diabetics. Carefully monitor your blood sugar if you use this supplemental oil and discontinue its use if your blood sugar becomes difficult to control.)

Herbal remedies

• *Alfalfa* is a good source of necessary minerals.
• *Burdock root and red clover* cleanse the bloodstream.
• *Dandelion root and milk thistle* repair damage done to the liver.
• To calm you down and help you sleep, take *valerian root* at bedtime.
• *Siberian ginseng* supports the liver and has been shown to reduce the chances of the patient's reverting back to alcohol use after rehabilitation.

Dosages may vary, depending on the severity and duration of your symptoms. Consult a qualified herbal practitioner. Let your physician know of your decision to treat herbally; not all herbal regimens can be used in combination with conventional pharmaceuticals.

What makes it worse?

• Paradoxically, although alcohol abuse often leads to a deficiency of vitamin A and to the development of symptoms from its lack, supplemental *vitamin A* may sometimes worsen the liver damage brought on by chronic alcohol abuse; therefore, I urge you to take care in supplementing this vitamin at a level above 5,000 IU to 10,000 IU per day if your physician has told you that your blood chemistry profile shows any indication of liver damage.

• A diet high in *sugar and refined starch*—dietary substances that cause the body to produce large amounts of insulin and make the blood sugar erratic—may stimulate your desire to drink. Read again the discussion of macronutrient effects, page 23, for basic dietary recommendations.

• One very obvious point, but so important to your good health that I will include it: continuing to drink *alcohol* worsens the damage already wrought.

—————————— **Allergies** ——————————

What are they?

About 10% of the population of the United States suffers from what we physicians term *atopic allergy*. This broad category includes hay fever (the runny nose, itchy eyes, and sneezing that come from exposure to pollens and molds), allergic eczema (the inflamed, red, scaling skin condition that accompanies food and pollen allergies), allergic asthma (restriction of the breathing passages in the lungs as a consequence of inhaling substances to which you are sensitive), and anaphylaxis (the life-threatening condition of immediate and extreme reaction to an allergic substance complete with hives, swelling, restricted breathing, and finally "shock," which in the true medical sense means not emotional crisis but circulatory collapse: a state in which you cannot maintain a blood pressure sufficient to support life).

Allergic symptoms occur because of a misidentification on the part of your immune defenses. Those defense systems function normally by protecting us from anything that is *not us*. By that I mean anything foreign, whether it be a bacterium, virus, or fungus trying to infect us, one of our own cells gone haywire and trying to become cancerous, or a substance of truly foreign origin, such as a medication, pollen grain, or mold spore. Most of us have an immune system that has in a sense "made peace" with our environment, and we, therefore, do not react to the things around us with weepy eyes, runny noses, or hives when the pollen flies or the cat hair floats. Some of us, however, have an immune defense that does raise up and fight when these "foreign" substances invade. And in the wake of the battle, the allergy sufferer—the battleground—pays the price in symptoms. The main culprit in initiating the symptoms is a substance released by a certain type of immune fighter—the mast cell—called histamine. That is why *anti*histamines—or other substances that prevent the mast cells from releasing their histamines—help to curb allergy symptoms. There are also nutrients that help to decrease your sensitivities to the world around you. Let's take a look at these.

What helps them?

• *Niacin* in laboratory studies prevents the release of histamine by the mast cells. That being the case, in human allergy, niacin ought to reduce the severity of allergic response. Indeed, in human studies, seasonal allergy sufferers showed rapid improvement of hay fever symptoms when given niacinamide injections in the muscle or into the vein. While these routes of administration are not handy for home use, you can take niacin (in the form called niacinamide) by mouth. Recommendation: Niacinamide in a dose of 200 to 300 mg per day should help to reduce seasonal allergy symptoms.

• *Pantothenic acid* has proven to reduce allergic drainage and nasal stuffiness in a number of clinical reports. Recommendation: Begin with a 100 mg dose at bedtime. Earliest signs of relief of symptoms may occur in 15 to 30 minutes. If your symptoms fail to respond sufficiently, you may have to increase your dose to 250 mg once or even twice daily.

• In people who suffer symptoms from MSG sensitivity (and cannot tolerate Chinese food prepared with monosodium glutamate, MSG, as a result), *vitamin B_6 (pyridoxine)* has proven to be of some use. I know of no information, nor could I find reports of any, that suggested that this vitamin might be beneficial in allergy to other substances. Recommendation: Take 50 mg of vitamin B_6 daily for at least 12 weeks.

• *Vitamin B$_{12}$ (cyanocobalamin)* supplementation has shown benefit in allergic asthma, chronic hives (urticaria), chronic allergic dermatitis, and sensitivity to sulfites (found, for example, in egg yolk and some wines). Recommendation: B$_{12}$ taken orally or by injection in a dose of 500 *micro*grams weekly for 4 weeks should result in improvement to these allergic symptoms. Several medical studies reported the use of 2000 to 4000 *micro*grams of B$_{12}$ in a sublingual (one that dissolves under the tongue) form that absorbs rapidly—in 15 minutes—and hangs around for a 24-hour period, making it ideal to combat sporadic but predictable exposures to allergens. (Such exposures would be cleaning out the attic, visiting a relative who has cats, or drinking an unknown wine that might contain sulfites.)

• A whole host of clinical research indicates that *vitamin C (ascorbic acid)* helps to reduce seasonal allergy symptoms, probably by reducing the release of histamine by the mast cells, and may protect against life-threatening anaphylactic reactions. Recommendation: Take 1 to 4 grams of vitamin C daily. Unless you already take vitamin C for other reasons, begin slowly, at 500 mg a day, and work up to a dose of 4 grams per day over a period of a week or two. I recommend that you use the crystalline (powdered) form of ascorbic acid instead of tablets or capsules, because it's easier to inch the dose upward. The usual strength of the powder is 1 teaspoon equals 4 grams. Mix your dose into a citrus-flavored beverage (lemon-lime, orange, grapefruit) to blunt its sourness. It will not go into solution unless the beverage is carbonated, which I also heartily recommend for this purpose.

• *Vitamin E,* at least in clinical study, has also shown some antihistaminic properties, but the hard science is sketchy so far. There are so many other reasons to take vitamin E, however, that those of us interested in health and longevity will already be supplementing it. Recommendation: Take 600 IU vitamin E daily. Begin with a 100 IU dose and check your blood pressure. Some people will suffer an elevation of blood pressure on supplemental vitamin E. If your pressure remains at or below an average of 140/90 on 4 or 5 readings, you may increase to 200 IU. Check again. If your pressure is still normal, increase to 400 IU, and so on, to 600 IU.

• *Calcium* and *magnesium,* if deficient, may worsen allergic asthmatic symptoms. While I could find no specific dosage recommendations for treatment in the literature, the connection of deficiency and symptoms seems valid. Recommendation: Prevent deficiency of these two minerals by consuming at least a baseline intake of 500 mg calcium and 200 mg magnesium.

• *Molybdenum* is a trace element necessary to detoxify sulfites and is found to be low or lacking in the majority of people sensitive to sulfites (in egg yolks or wine). Cases of severe sulfite allergy with asthma have responded to molybdenum treatment by administration into the vein twice weekly (doses of 250, 500, then 750 *micro*grams). Although the intravenous route won't work for general home use, you can take the element by mouth. Recommendation: Begin with about 100 *micro*grams daily and, after 2 to 3 weeks, increase to 200 *micro*grams, then 400 *micro*grams if needed.

• In people with chemical sensitivities, deficiency in *zinc* seems to worsen the problem. Supplementation to correct the deficiency seems to help, and may do so by inhibiting the release of histamine from the mast cells. Recommendation: Begin with 50 to 60 mg chelated zinc (the picolinate, aspartate forms) daily. Increase the dose to twice daily. Warning: Zinc supplementation with an ionic (not chelated) form of the mineral, such as zinc sulfate, can cause you to become deficient in copper, leading to anemia.

• Research has shown that *quercetin,* one of the bioflavonoids, reduces allergic symptoms by preventing histamine release from the mast cells and by inhibiting inflammation. Recommendation: Take a total daily dose of 1 to 2 grams of bioflavinoid complex (containing quercetin) divided throughout the day (for example, 500 mg 3 times daily) for no longer than 2 to 3 weeks.

Essential Fats

• *Oleic acid,* a fat found in olive oil, has been shown to inhibit histamine release. Recommendation: Use this oil where possible in cooking.

• *Linoleic acid (GLA) and fish oils (EPA)* also inhibit the inflammation that causes swelling and irritation from allergies. If you suffer with allergies, you feel this inflammation in your stuffy nose, weeping red eyes, and wheezy breathing, as well as the itch and redness of your skin if you break out in rashes from allergy. Refer to the eicosinoids, (Section I, pages 24–27) for more information about these fats. Recommendation: EicoPro, 2 capsules, 1 to 3 times daily. You can construct a reasonable substitute for this combined product with a daily intake of 500 mg of evening primrose oil (a source of linoleic acid in capsule form), plus 1000 mg EPA fish oil, plus 200

IU vitamin E. Take the combination 1 to 3 times a day. (Warning to diabetics: EPA fish oil can cause blood sugar fluctuations in some diabetics. Carefully monitor your blood sugar if you use this supplemental oil and discontinue its use if your blood sugar becomes difficult to control.)

Herbal remedies

• *Garlic and onion* contain quercetin, which retards inflammatory reactions.

• The leaf extract of the *ginkgo* tree contains substances that interfere with the platelet-activating factor, or PAF. This PAF has a starring role in triggering allergies, asthma, and inflammation. Caution: In large amounts, this herb can cause diarrhea, irritability, and restlessness.

• Dr. Andrew Weil has said he knows of nothing so dramatic as the hay fever relief afforded by freeze-dried *stinging nettle* leaves.

Dosages may vary, depending on the duration and severity of your symptoms. Consult a qualified herbal practitioner. Let your physician know of your decision to treat herbally; not all herbal remedies can be used in combination with conventional pharmaceuticals.

What makes them worse?

• Continued exposure to the offending substance naturally worsens the problem. Although this statement sounds trite, I think it's important that I address it. If you are an "allergic" or "sensitive" person and have not been tested by an allergist for environmental allergens, as well as food and food additive allergies, you would be wise to do so. The best remedy for your symptoms, when it's feasible, is to remove the cause. Sometimes, however, it seems like everything you enjoy offends your immune defenses, and unless you plan to live in a plastic bubble, you have to find some way to deal with the problem. In addition to nutritional treatment, allergy desensitization (by taking allergy shots) may give you some peace from your body's overactive allergy alert system.

—————————— **Anemia** ——————————

What is it?

When your body's supply of red blood cells falls below normal, you are said to be anemic, and you might complain that you tire easily, or that your heart beats rapidly or skips beats, and that you become out of breath and puff and pant when you climb stairs, walk, or otherwise exert yourself. The cause of the falling number of red blood cells can be because they are being lost through bleeding, because they are damaged or destroyed, or because your body is not producing enough of them. Although there are many types of anemia, the kinds with a nutritional basis involve specific dietary deficiencies in iron, folic acid, or vitamin B_{12}, and in cases of general overall malnourishment. Let's take a look at how nutritional supplementation can help in various anemias.

What helps it?

• *Folic acid* deficiency clearly causes an anemia in which the red blood cells produced are few in number but quite large (called a megaloblastic anemia). Supplementation restores the cells to a normal size and number. Addition of folic acid to the diet may also benefit people who suffer from sickle cell anemia (an inherited anemia seen primarily among blacks) and even aplastic anemia (a life-threatening condition in which the red blood cell–producing tissue the bone marrow shuts down production). Recommendation: Take 2 to 5 mg daily. Refer to the listing for this vitamin in Section I and note that when you supplement folic acid, you must be certain to ask your physician to check your blood level of vitamin B_{12}. Since they both cause the same kinds of anemic problems, deficiency of one can mask deficiency of the other.

• *Riboflavin* deficiency may cause an anemia in which the cells are few in number but normal in size, shape, and color. Recommendation: Begin with a dose of 20 to 30 mg per day. After 3 to 6 weeks, ask your physician to recheck your red blood count. If you have had no response by 6 weeks, another cause of anemia may be at work.

• *Thiamine* deficiency may cause anemia with few, large red blood cells. Supplementation to correct the deficiency corrects the anemia as well. If an anemia with large red blood cells fails to respond to B_{12} or folic acid, thiamine may be the culprit.

Recommendation: Take 20 mg of thiamine per day for 3 to 6 weeks and then recheck your blood count.

• Among the many other physical ailments that occur in *vitamin A* deficiency, one of the early changes involves problems in producing hemoglobin (the iron-containing, oxygen-carrying pigment of red blood cells). Without enough hemoglobin, your body cannot produce normal-sized red blood cells in normal numbers, and voilà, anemia results. However, because vitamin A can build up and cause problems, I would ask that you reread the discussion of this vitamin in Section I to become familiar with the symptoms of taking too much. Recommendation: Take 10,000 IU vitamin A or 25,000 IU beta-carotene daily for 3 to 6 weeks. At that time, ask your physician to repeat your blood count to see if it has improved.

• *Vitamin B_6* deficiency can occasionally cause an anemia with small, pale red blood cells much like we see in people deficient in iron, and supplementation with B_6 improves the anemia. Some patients with sickle cell anemia have also responded (with fewer pain crises and better blood counts) from supplementation with vitamin B_6 daily. Recommendation: 50 to 100 mg B_6 daily.

• *Vitamin B_{12}* deficiency causes a quite well-known anemia, called *pernicious anemia,* in which the red blood cells produced are few in number but large in size. Symptoms of severe weakness, fatigue, and mental cloudiness accompany the low blood count. Recommendation: To be certain your body absorbs this vitamin, I would recommend that you take it in shot form in a dose of 1000 *micro*grams of cyanocobalamin or hydroxocobalamin weekly for 4 to 6 weeks, then monthly for at least a year and possibly indefinitely. After you've restored your body's levels of the vitamin to normal, you may be able to take the vitamin by mouth or under the tongue.

• *Vitamin C* improves your ability to absorb iron, and failure to take in enough vitamin C may contribute to the development of an anemia of small pale red blood cells. Recommendation: At the barest minimum, take 500 mg vitamin C per day. Most adults will tolerate (and if Dr. Linus Pauling is correct, should make every effort to take) a daily dose ranging from 3 or 4 grams (3000 to 4000 mg) up to 8 or 10 grams with ease. Refer to Section I and the discussion of the history of vitamin C for additional information about this important vitamin.

• *Vitamin E* supplementation appears to make the red blood cells less fragile (less prone to easy bursting, which is often their fate) in some of the inherited anemias, such as sickle cell anemia, Mediterranean-type G_6PD deficiency, thalassemia, and the anemia that patients with cystic fibrosis develop. (I won't go into detail about exactly what these anemias are, because if you have them or if they run in your family, you will know about it. If they do not, you are not at any risk to develop them.) The reason the vitamin helps make the red blood cells stronger, if you will, probably lies in its antioxidant properties. Recommendation: Take 400 to 800 IU per day.

• In the medical literature, cases of anemia with production of small, pale red blood cells (a picture identical to iron-deficiency anemia) occurs with *copper* deficiency. That the two minerals should cause such similar kinds of anemia makes perfect scientific sense, because to make hemoglobin (the red, oxygen-carrying pigment) the body requires both copper and iron. The red blood cells are small and pale precisely because there isn't enough hemoglobin to fill them up and make them full size and ruddy-red in color.

Copper deficiency rarely occurs under "normal" dietary conditions; however, ailments causing chronic diarrhea or poor absorption of food can cause low levels of copper, as can supplementation with other minerals that compete with the copper and hinder its absorption. Supplementation with zinc in its ionic form can create this kind of competition deficiency in copper; however, chelated zinc does not. Please refer to the discussion in Section I on the importance of chelation of minerals to their absorption.

On the other side of the coin, however, oversupplementation of copper can also cause problems for some people who suffer from a disorder called Wilson's disease, which causes them to store copper too easily. The buildup of copper in their brain and liver tissues causes severe symptoms, such as poor coordination, shaking tremors, difficulty speaking, drooling, and emotional disturbances. Recommendation: Unless your physician has tested and proven you to be low in copper, I would recommend you not supplement with extra tablets or capsules, but rather eat more of foods rich in copper (shellfish and other seafood, liver and kidney, and lamb) to prevent deficiency. However, if you are taking ionic zinc supplements (zinc sulfate, for example), you may also require the addition of 2 mg to 4 mg chelated copper per day.

• *Iron,* the commonest mineral deficiency cause for anemia, occurs more often in women of reproductive age still having monthly menstrual periods than in men. The cause is that of monthly loss of blood (and therefore, iron loss) exceeding the amount they replace in their diets. The anemia caused by lack of iron is one in which the red blood cells are small and pale. Recommendation: 20 to 30 mg iron glycinate daily (along with vitamins A, C, and E and adequate copper—see the specific listings for each of these nutrients). Before using an iron supplement, check with your doctor to be sure you have a deficiency. Excess iron can damage the liver, pancreas, heart, and immune cell activity. It has also been linked to cancer. Supplement only under qualified supervision.

• People who suffer from sickle cell anemia often have low levels of *zinc,* and studies have shown that supplementation with this mineral alleviates some of their symptoms (especially the number of pain crises they suffer). Recommendation: Take 40 to 50 mg of chelated zinc daily. Warning: Taking ionic zinc (such as the sulfate form) may cause deficiency of other minerals, notably copper, which may worsen anemic symptoms.

Herbal remedies

• *Alfalfa, bilberry, cherry, dandelion, goldenseal, grape skins, hawthorn, mullein, nettle, red raspberry, shepherd's purse, and yellow dock* are good for anemia. Caution: Do not take goldenseal during pregnancy, or for more than one week at a time if you have a history of cardiovascular disease, diabetes, or glaucoma.

Dosages may vary, depending on the duration and severity of your symptoms. Consult a qualified herbal practitioner. Alert your physician to your decision to use herbs. Not all herbal remedies can be used in conjunction with conventional pharmaceuticals.

What makes it worse?

• *Milk,* wholesome as it is, can cause some problems in certain people. At least in infants, gastrointestinal intolerance to nonhuman milk may cause worsening of anemia through loss of small but steady amounts of blood in the bowel movement. Breast milk usually does not cause this kind of intolerance. When babies develop anemia, this source of blood loss has to be considered. The amount lost would not necessarily be visible to the naked eye, but you could find it chemically with cards or strips designed to detect occult (hidden) blood. You can purchase these test cards at the pharmacy or from your physician. If you detect blood, you should consult your personal physician, pediatrician, or allergist.

• Overzealous use of *stomach acid–inhibiting drugs,* such as Tagamet (cimetidine) or Zantac (ranitidine), used in treating stomach ulcers or gastritis, could create a lack of stomach acid. Without at least some stomach acid, you cannot properly absorb iron.

— Aphthous Stomatitis (Canker Sores) —
What is it?

You may have called them by other names—canker sores or mouth ulcers—but whatever name you care to apply to these repeated outbreaks of sores inside the mouth, one thing is certain: they hurt. The ulcers themselves are usually creamy white or yellowish craters with a red rim. They may be single or many, and usually form on the lining inside the cheeks or lips, and less often on the gums or roof of the mouth. The ulcers can vary in size from 1 to 2 mm (about like the head of a pin) to 10 or 12 mm (about the size of a dime). Even a small one can make your entire mouth and that side of your face tender and talking and chewing a misery, and may last for a week or two. When you're the victim and your misery index is high, you just want relief of the discomfort. Between outbreaks, however, you might wish to know what causes them.

Unfortunately, medical science has yet to settle the ongoing debate on their precise cause, although theories abound. They can be triggered by poor dental hygiene, irritation from dental work, food allergies, nutritional deficiencies, hormonal imbalances, viral infection, an underlying immunologic disease, trauma, stress, and/or fatigue. Sometimes they are associated with Crohn's disease. I favor the multiple-cause hypothesis, that they arise from various causes in different people, such that in a particular person any one of these explanations might be accurate. I suffered with these myself during my teens, and occasionally will still have the beginnings of one; however, I have become firmly convinced that mine at least are viral, and I treat them accordingly with antiviral prescription medications and nutrients that help to stimulate solid immune function (see Immune System Health listing). I am just as convinced, however, that other causes exist, but whatever those may be, what role, if any, do nutrients play in treating them?

What helps it?

• *Zinc* supplementation as well as application of a topical paste containing zinc seems to help (possibly through its immune system–

stimulating effects). Recommendation: Take 50 to 60 mg of chelated zinc (picolinate, aspartate) by mouth 1 to 3 times daily. Alternatively, apply 1% zinc sulfate in Orabase (dental paste) to the ulcer. To get the best results, place a small dot of the paste on your finger and apply it to the ulcer without rubbing. Hold it in place for a few seconds, then gently lift your finger away. Reapply 2 to 3 times daily. Warning: Zinc sulfate (ionic zinc) can compete with copper and other minerals for absorption from the gastrointestinal tract, creating deficiencies in the other minerals, and although you will only be using this preparation on the surface, don't overuse the paste. With regard to the zinc tablets, be certain the zinc is in the chelated and not ionic form to prevent creating deficiencies of other minerals (see discussion of chelation of minerals, Section I, pages 30–31).

• Some people with aphthous ulcers respond to a combination of blood-building vitamins and minerals: *folic acid,* vitamin B_{12}, and *iron.* This good response happens especially when the mouth ulcers occur along with other symptoms, such as anemia, painful tongue, and cracking of the corners of the mouth. Recommendation: Try a combination of 5 mg folic acid 3 times daily, 1000 *micro*grams B_{12} by injection every 2 months, and 10 mg chelated iron (iron glycinate) per day for 4 to 6 months. You should consider a good response to be fewer outbreaks, shorter length of outbreaks, and/or reduced pain with outbreaks.

• *Lactobacillus acidophilus or bulgaricus,* the "friendly" bacteria used to culture yogurt and buttermilk, also seems to help lessen the pain of aphthous ulcers, to decrease the formation of the ulcers themselves, and to speed clearing of the sores. Recommendation: Drinking bulgarian cultured buttermilk or eating cultured yogurt may help. Or, you can dissolve 2 tablets containing these bacteria in your mouth 4 times daily. You should be able to find the tablets at pharmacies and health and nutrition shops.

Herbal remedies

• *Myrrh* contains high amounts of tannins, an antiseptic that also has antibacterial and antiviral action. It is especially helpful in the treatment of mouth sores caused by bacteria, fungus, a virus, or an allergy.

• *Cankerroot* got its name because of its traditional use as a treatment for canker sores. It shares many of the same active ingredients as goldenseal.

• *Goldenseal* or *tea tree oil* can be applied on the sore twice during the day and again at bedtime.

• *Red raspberry tea* contains those valuable flavonoids and is very helpful in treating canker sores.

• American Indians and early settlers used the root of *wild geranium* to treat and wash canker sores.

Dosages may vary, depending on the duration and severity of your symptoms. Follow package directions, or consult a qualified herbal practitioner.

What makes it worse?

Any *foods* to which you might be allergic. An allergy specialist can test you for skin or blood evidence of specific food allergies. Armed with that knowledge, you can then set about to discover which of these foods might actually stimulate eruptions with an elimination trial—that is, select a suspected culprit food and cut it out of your diet entirely for 3 to 4 weeks to see if symptoms disappear. If the ulcers clear, you're halfway there. To be certain that food causes the outbreak, you must eat that food again to see if ulcers reappear. If they do, to continue to eat that food is to risk breaking out in mouth ulcers. If ulcers do not break out when you next eat the food, it's "off the hook" and safe to eat, and you're ready to move on to test another food. Check only one food at a time or you won't know which of several foods might have been responsible. Recommendation: If you have no allergy test results to guide you, you can begin by eliminating foods that frequently cause allergic reactions in others—chocolate, citrus, strawberries, nuts, tomatoes, wheat—but recognize that any food, beverage, or chemical *could* be the culprit.

Arrhythmias

(see Cardiac Arrhythmias)

Atherosclerosis

What is it?

The term *atherosclerosis* derives from the Greek words for gruel *(athere)* and hard *(skleros)*. We use this word to describe the hardened deposits of fatty cholesterol droplets into the walls of arteries. The process of atherosclerosis, or hardening of the arteries, can occur in any artery anywhere in the body. When it occurs in the arteries supplying blood to the heart, we speak of coronary artery disease, a condition that leads to heart attacks. In the arteries of the brain, we call it cerebral vascular disease, but this is the place most Americans probably think of in connection with the phrase *hardening of the arteries*. Atherosclerosis in the brain arteries leads to senility and to stroke. In the big arteries leading into the legs, hardened cholesterol deposits can cause painful cramping in the calves of the legs (called claudication) with walking even short distances. But wherever it occurs, atherosclerosis is the same process, and basically, the same factors influence its development.

The major cause of atherosclerosis in Western civilization, in my opinion and in that of a growing number of experts in this field, comes from a tendency to overproduce the hormone insulin when we eat, a tendency that becomes increasingly worse as we age. When insulin levels remain high in your blood a majority of the time, a number of unpleasant processes occur: fluid retention, elevation of blood pressure, increased storage of fat, and a tendency to develop diabetes. (You may be interested in the related discussions under Obesity and Hypertension for more information.) But aside from these other problems, high insulin also stimulates your liver to produce more cholesterol and triglycerides, the major blood fats associated with atherosclerosis. Chronically high insulin causes you to produce less of the HDL cholesterol (the "good" cholesterol) and significantly more of the LDL, or low-density cholesterol, that worsens heart disease risk. And then, by a means not yet clear, high insulin promotes the changes in the cholesterol molecules that makes them more likely to deposit in the artery walls, setting the stage for atherosclerosis. If you add other stimuli to atherosclerosis, such as smoking, on top of that picture, you accelerate the rate at which your arteries harden.

Even though surgery to remove and replace seriously damaged arteries may be necessary in the later stages of atherosclerosis, nutrition can help to prevent its progression before that time and can certainly help to discourage its development in the first place. Let's see how.

What helps it?

• *Proper dietary construction* plays a clear role in reducing your risk of developing atherosclerosis. Eating a diet that provides plenty of lean protein, is high in dietary fiber and rich in low-starch vegetables, with the proper amount of fats and oils, and virtually devoid of refined sugars and starches will do more to curb your tendency to harden your arteries than any one single nutrient will do by limiting the foods that make your body produce the most insulin. Recommendation: Refer to Macronutrients on page 23. Using the basic guidelines provided there, construct a diet for yourself that provides at least ½ gram of complete protein for each pound of your lean body mass. (You will find the information you need to calculate your lean weight in the discussion.) Vary your protein choices, relying heavily on all types of poultry, regularly adding seafood and fresh-water fish, low-fat dairy products, leanest cuts of beef or pork, and egg whites to make up about 30% of your day's total caloric intake. Then choose from a wide variety of green, yellow-orange, and dark green leafy vegetables, rice, and oats to make up another 40% of your day's calories. Although you need not avoid them entirely, you should limit your intake of wheat, corn, and potato, since these starches, like sugars, strongly stimulate insulin release. The final 30% of your day's calories should come from fats and oils, but specifically from cold-pressed oils such as olive oil and canola oil, with a little animal fat (about 10% of your calories) thrown in. Do not use hydrogenated vegetable oils, such as margarine or solid vegetable shortening, because these oils may actually promote atherosclerosis. And absolutely don't deep-fry anything! Even a high-quality, healthful oil will change chemically when you burn it repeatedly at 400 to 500 degrees.

• A diet high in *fiber* also helps to keep a cap on cholesterol levels, by binding up the cholesterol in your intestine and slowing down its absorption. Recommendation: Eating the kind of diet outlined above will already have you well on your way to eating more dietary fiber, but in addition, you should add a supplemental vegetable fiber bulking powder (such as Metamucil, Konsyl, or Citrucel) to increase your daily fiber intake to 50 or more grams per day. I caution you not to rush from the current American average intake of 10 to 15 grams to 50 grams overnight, because if you do, you will suffer abdominal bloating, cramping, and gas. Increase slowly. Use the regimen I describe under the heading Colon, Spastic to get there gradually.

• Your body uses *essential fatty acids* as raw materials from which to make a family of potent chemical messengers called the eicosinoids. Refer to the Yin and Yang of Human Health on pages

24–27 for more information about how these messengers work. Like all families, the eicosinoids have some "good" members and some "bad" ones. The good eicosinoids help, among other benefits, to reduce cardiovascular risk (heart disease and hardening of the arteries) and lower blood pressure. Recommendation: Begin with the proper basic dietary framework as just outlined to pave the way for best results. To that sound base, add gamma-linoleic acid (GLA) and EPA fish oil in a ratio of 1:4 (GLA:EPA) 1 to 3 times daily. The EicoPro essential fatty acid product manufactured by Eicotec, Inc., of Marblehead, Massachusetts, contains ultrapure sources of linoleic acid and fish oils already combined in the proper ratio. If you cannot get that product, you can purchase linoleic acid in a product called evening primrose oil at most health and nutrition stores, and EPA fish oil as well. Because it is not as pure a form, the milligram dosing will be different. You can make a reasonable substitute by combining evening primrose oil capsules with fish oil capsules plus vitamin E. Take 500 mg of evening primrose oil (a source of linoleic acid in capsule form), plus 1000 mg EPA fish oil, plus 200 IU vitamin E 1 to 3 times a day. (Warning to diabetics: EPA fish oil can cause blood sugar fluctuations in some diabetics. Carefully monitor your blood sugar if you use this supplemental oil and discontinue its use if your blood sugar becomes difficult to control.)

• A deficiency of *folic acid* can increase your risk of atherosclerosis, because your body needs this vitamin to convert one of the amino acid protein building blocks (homocysteine) that may increase your arteries' tendency to harden into another amino acid (methionine) that does not. Recommendation: Take 5 mg of folic acid per day for 14 days, then reduce your dose to 1 gram per day. Take a 100 mg dose of vitamin B-complex along with the folic acid; the B vitamins work best together. Warning: Supplementing folic acid can hide a deficiency of vitamin B_{12}. You should ask your physician to check the level of B_{12} in your blood; if deficient, you should supplement B_{12} as well.

• Deficiency of *vitamin B_6* (pyridoxine) can also contribute to the development of atherosclerosis for generally the same reasons as its fellow B vitamin folic acid; it is necessary to convert homocysteine into another harmless amino acid, cystathionine. Without B_6, the damaging homocysteine builds up in artery walls, and this accumulation may increase the tendency of cholesterol to deposit there.

Recommendation: Take vitamin B_6 in a dose of 40 to 50 mg per day along with 50 mg of B-complex.

• Deficiency of *vitamin B_{12}* also causes the homocysteine buildup, because your body must also have this vitamin to convert the homocysteine to the harmless cystathionine. Recommendation: Take 500 to 1000 *micro*grams of sublingual (under the tongue) vitamin B_{12} weekly for 4 to 6 weeks, then at least monthly. Take a 50 to 100 mg dose of B-complex daily.

• The most recent work of Dr. Linus Pauling into the many benefits of *vitamin C* centered on its role in preventing atherosclerosis. He felt quite strongly, and his research bears him out, that a deficiency in vitamin C results in your body's making poorly formed, weak fibrous framework for the arteries. In the absence of enough vitamin C, your body increases its production of certain blood fats that "patch" the tiny damaged areas in the walls of the arteries. These patches may then be the beginnings of cholesterol plaques, which plug up and harden the arteries. Recommendation: Take vitamin C in a dose of at least 1 gram (1000 mg) 3 times a day. Please refer to the listing for this important vitamin for other information about its role in human health.

• The Harvard Nurses Study has shown that daily intake of *vitamin E* can help to reduce your risk of heart disease (and, by extension, probably atherosclerosis in other locations as well). Recommendation: Take a minimum dose of 200 IU of vitamin E, as d-alpha-tocopherol succinate, per day. Vitamin E can cause elevation of blood pressure in some people. If a 200 IU dose does not elevate your pressure, you can increase it to a daily intake of 600 IU.

• Deficiency of *calcium* may contribute to the development of atherosclerosis by several means: it may contribute to an increase in your levels of cholesterol and triglycerides, and it may increase the tendency of your platelets (blood cells that congregate in an area of blood vessel damage to patch a tear and begin the process of forming a clot) to stick together and therefore increase the risk of blood clots. Supplementing calcium in your diet can help to offset some of these problems, but take care not to overdo it. High levels of calcium can promote hardening. Recommendation: Keep your daily intake of calcium (from food and supplements) around 1500 mg per day. Calcium and magnesium work together, and you should take them both, if you take one of them (see Magnesium on page 192).

• Deficiency of *chromium* may contribute to atherosclerosis, and supplementation can help to "normalize" blood fats—that is, increase the good kind of cholesterol and lower the bad. Recommendation: Take 200 *micro*grams chromium picolinate per day.

• Deficiency of *magnesium* increases risk of atherosclerosis of heart arteries, heart attack, and dangerous heart rhythm changes. Supplementation with magnesium may help to prevent calcification (hardening) of blood vessels throughout the body. Recommendation: Take magnesium aspartate in a dose of 250 to 500 mg per day. Calcium and magnesium work together, and you should take them both, if you take one of them.

• Because your body must have *selenium* to make its own natural free radical scavenger, glutathione peroxidase, a deficiency in selenium can increase your risk of free radical damage to tissues. Oxidation (free radical damage) of the LDL cholesterol molecules may also contribute to their becoming more easily embedded in the walls of the arteries. Recommendation: Take selenium aspartate in a dose of 100 to 200 *micro*grams per day.

• The recent study of Harvard physicians showed that daily intake of *beta-carotene* helped to reduce heart disease. Recommendation: Increase your intake of foods rich in beta-carotene, such as green, yellow-orange, and dark green leafy vegetables. You should also take 25,000 IU supplemental beta-carotene daily.

• Some studies show that *coenzyme Q_{10}* helps to protect against atherosclerosis and may help to reduce the tendency of blood to form clots readily. (When the hardened arteries become narrowed by cholesterol plaques, even a small clot can occlude the artery and stop blood flow, causing a heart attack or stroke.) Recommendation: Take 30 mg of coenzyme Q_{10} 1 to 3 times daily.

What makes it worse?

A diet high in *refined starches and sugars* promotes the development of atherosclerosis by increasing insulin levels in your blood. Recommendation: Eliminate or sharply reduce your intake of all refined starches, including white flour and highly milled corn meal and all products made with these substances, and sugars, including table sugar, corn syrup, high-fructose corn syrup, molasses, and all products made with these substances. Heavy consumption of *alcohol* may increase your risk for atherosclerosis; however, a modest intake of alcohol may actually be of benefit. Recommendation: You should limit your alcohol intake to no more than a single glass of wine, a single "lite" beer, or a single ounce of distilled spirits per day.

Arthralgia (Joint Pain)

What is it?

The term *arthralgia* means joint pain, but tells us nothing about a reason for the pain. It could come, for example, from overuse of the joint: bursitis in a golfer's shoulder or tennis elbow; from joint irritation caused by a viral infection: the severe aching in the back that accompanies influenza; or from arthritis: the true inflammation that reddens, swells, and sometimes gnarls the joints.

What helps it?

• Because the kind of nutritional supplement that will help joint pain is going to depend on what causes the problem, I would refer you to the listings of specific causes for joint pain: arthritis or osteoarthritis (the wear-and-tear, old-age kind), rheumatoid arthritis (the destructive kind that strikes younger age groups, even children), carpal tunnel syndrome, lupus erythematosus.

What makes it worse?

• Again, see specific conditions.

Arthritis

What is it?

Arthritis means inflammation of a joint and is a generic, nonspecific term that people often use to describe anything that hurts a joint. Pain, however, is not the only criterion; there must also be some visible sign of inflammation—that is, the joint must be red, warm to touch, swollen somewhat, *as well as* painful. Although there are many types of arthritis (over 100, really) for the purposes of this discussion, I will use "arthritis" to mean *osteoarthritis,* the wear-and-tear type of joint inflammation that comes with age. The other major conditions causing arthritic symptoms or pain around the joints I will list and discuss under their specific names: rheumatoid arthritis, lupus erythematosus arthritis, psoriatic arthritis, gout, bursitis, etc.

Osteoarthritis, also called degenerative joint disease, or DJD, usually strikes the most frequently used (or overused) joints of women in their 50s and 60s and men in their 40s and 50s. Although either gender can develop this kind of arthritis in any joint, women more often tend to suffer from osteoarthritis in the small joints of hands and fingers and in their necks and backs, whereas this so-called wear-and-tear kind of arthritis usually afflicts men in the larger weight-bearing joints: the hips, knees, ankles, feet, and backs. Once thought to strictly be a consequence of years of use, recent medical study has uncovered a genetic link for osteoarthritis—meaning the tendency to develop it runs in the family, and it's more than just wearing out the joint surfaces. If your joints have begun to ache and this kind of arthritic problem runs in your family, does nutrition offer you any help? Sure. Let's take a look.

What helps it?

• A recent and widely accepted treatment for osteoarthritis combines *glucosamine* with *chondroitin*. This duo can actually repair damaged or eroded cartilage. Glucosamine is made up of glucose and an amino acid called glutamine. It provides structure to the bone and cartilage. It is available in four forms in the United States, *glucosamine sulfate* being the most popular. Although it relieves symptoms when used alone, its healing and restorative qualities are greatly enhanced when paired with the chondroitin sulfates. These sulfates act as liquid magnets, attracting proteoglycan molecules, which fill in the spaces within the cartilage "netting." The fluid is important because it acts as a shock absorber while it sweeps nutrients into the cartilage. Without this fluid, cartilage becomes malnourished and fragile. Daily dosage depends on your weight. Recommendation: If you weigh less than 120 pounds, take 1000 mg glucosamine plus 800 mg chondroitin sulfates. If your weight falls between 120 and 200 pounds, take 1500 mg glucosamine plus 1200 mg chondroitin sulfates. Anyone over 200 pounds should take 2000 mg glucosamine and 1600 mg chondroitin sulfates. Everyone's needs vary, so be sure to have a thorough consultation with a physician and make clear your intent to follow this treatment.

• *Niacin* appears to decrease pain and increase mobility of painful joints after as little as 2 to 6 weeks of supplementation. Case reports show the effect to be especially beneficial for osteoarthritis of the knees. Recommendation: Begin with 500 mg of niacin (as niacinamide) and 100 mg B-complex twice a day for a week. Increase your niacinamide dose to 500 mg 3 times daily for a week. Then increase your first morning dose of niacinamide to 1000 mg, then both the morning and noon doses to 1000 mg, and then increase all 3 doses to 1000 mg. Continue the B-complex at 100 mg twice daily throughout. Once you have seen a good response in relief of pain or increase in joint mobility, you may taper the dose back down to a single 500 mg dose of niacinamide plus 100 mg B-complex and remain there. Warning: Read the listings for niacin supplementation. Some people cannot tolerate increased amounts of niacin without symptoms of severe flushing, blood pressure increases, and racing pulse. Begin slowly and increase only if you tolerate the niacin without side effects. Stop the medication if you develop flushing.

• *Pantothenic acid* seems to help some people with arthritic joint pain and not to benefit others, but the same can be said for almost any arthritis treatment, prescription or otherwise. In studies that used pantothenic acid in conjunction with the other members of the *vitamin B-complex,* over three-quarters of the participants reported significant improvement of symptoms after 2 weeks, suffered relapse of discomfort when taken off the vitamin, and improved again upon resuming the therapy. Recommendation: Take 100 mg pantothenic acid along with 100 mg vitamin B-complex twice daily for 2 to 4 weeks.

• *Vitamin C* plays a crucial role in the formation of collagen, the chief protein component of cartilage and bone, and should always be a part of the vitamin and mineral regimen in the treatment of arthritic conditions. Your body needs vitamin C not only to be able to build and repair the smooth cartilage surfaces that cover the bone ends and build the framework for bones themselves, but also to build and maintain the tendons and ligaments that attach to the bones. Arthritis does run in the family, and for that reason, young people who carry an increased family risk for developing arthritis should begin to supplement extra vitamin C *before* they begin to develop joint wear and tear and pain. Vitamin C's powerful antioxidant capabilities also make it important in slowing down the aging of tissues, a process that would hasten the development of osteoarthritis. Recommendation: Based on weight, I recommend a starting dose of 10 to 20 mg per pound of body weight per day. Divide the dose into 2 or more doses throughout the day. By that calculation, a 50-pound child at risk for arthritis would take 500 to 1000 mg of vitamin C per day in divided doses, a 100-pound adult would take 1000 to 2000 mg per day in divided doses, and a 200-pound adult would take

2000 to 4000 mg per day in divided doses. If you currently suffer with osteoarthritis symptoms, begin and hold at this starting dose for 3 to 4 weeks, then increase in 500 mg per dose increments until you reach your bowel tolerance level. (See discussion of vitamin C in Section I, pages 50–54.)

• *Vitamin E,* because of its antioxidant protection of essential fats (see Section I, eicosinoids, pages 24–27, for more in-depth discussion) reduces pain both at rest and with movement, in osteoarthritic joints, as well as decreasing the need for pain and anti-inflammatory medications. Recommendation: 400 to 600 IU of vitamin E daily. Children old enough to swallow capsules can take 100 IU per day. Younger children can at least increase their intake of vitamin E by regularly eating seeds and nuts (sunflower seeds are a favorite for most kids).

• *Selenium,* which is necessary for the body to produce the natural antioxidant and free radical scavenger glutathione peroxidase, works well in conjunction with vitamin E toward reducing the symptoms of pain and stiffness in arthritic joints. By taking the two together, you can see good results on a lower dose of vitamin E per day. Recommendation: As an adult, you should take 100 to 200 *micrograms* of selenium (as sodium selenite or selenium aspartate) plus 100 to 200 mg vitamin E daily.

• A number of studies done in various countries have shown that in areas where the soil is deficient in *boron,* more people seem to develop osteoarthritis. By the same token, supplementation with boron also seems to alleviate the pain and stiffness of arthritis once it does develop. Recommendation: Begin by taking 6 to 9 mg of elemental boron (50 to 75 mg borax) daily until your symptoms improve. Then you may drop your daily dose to 3 mg (25 mg borax) and maintain there. Note: Borax is a boron-containing compound available at health and nutrition stores, not the laundry detergent by the same name.

• *Essential fatty acids* linoleic acid (GLA) and fish oils (EPA) are the basic nutrients from which your body makes potent natural anti-inflammatory chemicals called *prostaglandins.* Not all prostaglandins are "good" ones that ward off inflammation and pain—some actually cause inflammation. The diet you eat to a large degree governs whether you make "good" ones or "bad" ones, and therefore whether you increase inflammation and pain in arthritic joints or whether you relieve it. Please turn to the full discussion of these essential fats and the way that diet can control their effect in Section I, eicosinoids, pages 24–27. Recommendation: Take 2 EicoPro capsules, 1 to 3 times daily, or if you are unable to obtain this product, you can make a reasonable substitute by taking 500 mg evening primrose oil along with 1000 mg EPA fish oil and 100 IU vitamin E 1 to 3 times a day. (Warning to diabetics: EPA fish oil can cause blood sugar fluctuations in some diabetics. Carefully monitor your blood sugar if you use this supplemental oil and discontinue its use if your blood sugar becomes difficult to control.)

• *S-Adenosyl-L-Methionine (SAMe)* isn't an herb or hormone. In fact, it is a chemical compound found in all living cells. In most people, the body manufactures all the SAMe it needs from the amino acid methionine, found in soybeans, eggs, seeds, lentils, and meat. SAMe appears to regulate more than 35 different mechanisms and helps the body maintain cell membranes, remove toxic substances, and produce mood-enhancing neurotransmitters. Studies have shown that patients with osteoarthritis benefit in pain relief, increased ability to move around, and less stiffness as greatly with this nutrient derivative than with prescription anti-inflammatory medications such as ibuprofen (Motrin), naproxen (Naprosyn), or indomethacin (Indocin), but with fewer side effects. Recommendation: Take SAMe twice a day on an empty stomach. Since dosage depends on many factors, check with your physician for the correct amount. Studies have shown that it doesn't appear to cause adverse effects, even at high dosages.

Herbal remedies

• On every continent where it grows, *stinging nettle* has gained a reputation as an effective treatment for arthritis. As far back as biblical times, people have been enjoying the effects of nettle. Most people, even today, chose urtication—grasping the plant in a gloved hand and actually swatting their stiff, swollen joints—as a treatment method instead of eating the herb. It works; it really does. Dr. James Duke, author of *The Green Pharmacy,* claims to have seen swelling subside within minutes after the stings were administered.

• *Ginger* provides relief from arthritic pain and swelling. Although it causes pain on the tongue, *red pepper* inhibits pain perception elsewhere in the body, which also makes it good for headaches. The active constituent, capsaicin, can be found in creams available over-the-counter. Apply the cream directly to the skin and you should experience relief. If your skin becomes irritated, discontinue use.

• *Oregano* is a potent antioxidant that helps prevent cell damage caused by free radicals. Free radical reactions are involved in inflammation, degenerative arthritis, and the aging process in general. There is evidence that antioxidants relieve osteoarthritis and rheumatoid arthritis.

• *Willow bark* is the original herbal aspirin. Its active chemical, called salicin, was eventually made into little white tablets by the Bayer Company and promoted as pain-relieving aspirin. Willow bark has pain-relieving and anti-inflammatory effects similar to those of aspirin without the nasty side effects. Caution: If willow upsets your stomach, combine it with licorice, which will alleviate any gastrointestinal problems caused by the willow bark.

• *Alfalfa* may help arthritis because it contains the minerals necessary for bone formation.

Dosages may vary, depending on the duration and severity of your symptoms. Consult a qualified herbal practitioner. Let your physician know of your decision to treat your condition with herbs. Not all herbal remedies can be used in combination with conventional pharmaceuticals.

What makes it worse?

• *Food sensitivities*—especially to the foods from plants in the nightshade family that contain the chemical *solanine*—can produce severe arthritic joint pain. These plants include white potatoes, tomatoes, all peppers except black pepper, eggplant, and tobacco. And although the nightshades are common offenders, you could just as easily become sensitive to the particular chemicals found in any food.

The devil of this situation is that regular use of the over-the-counter and prescription anti-inflammatory medications—the very things you may be taking to alleviate your joint pain—can cause irritation to the lining of your gastrointestinal tract, which can make it easier for you to absorb certain chemicals from foods, and which can in turn increase your risk of becoming sensitized to foods you eat. Once sensitized to a particular food, you could suffer worsening of your arthritic symptoms each time you eat that food. Recommendation: If possible, consult an allergy specialist to discover which specific foods you react to on testing. Then, in a systematic way, go about eliminating each of these food suspects one at a time. Totally avoid that food for 3 to 4 weeks to see if your symptoms improve. If they don't, that food probably was not causing the problem. Move on to test another food. If you do feel better not eating that food for 3 to 4 weeks, then you must test the response by eating the food again. If you develop symptoms when you try it the second time, then you've found your food culprit—or at least one of them.

Asthma

What is it?

If you suffer from episodes of shortness of breath, wheezing sounds when you breathe, a feeling of tightness in the chest, and chronic coughing of thick clear or white phlegm, you may be one of the 4% of Americans who have asthma. During an attack of asthma, the bronchial tubes constrict or spasm, making it difficult for you to get in enough air. When the spasm of the airway is mild, you may just feel a little tightness or wheezing, a little cough—a tolerable nuisance. But sometimes, attacks can cause severe spasm, and then asthma can be life-threatening if not treated correctly and in time. Any asthmatic who has had this kind of severe attack should be under a physician's watchful care.

Just as there are many degrees of asthma severity, there are many causes for asthma. Some people develop asthma with allergy to pollens, pets, dust, foods, or medications. Some people wheeze when they exercise, or only when they have a respiratory infection. Although prescription medication may still be the cornerstone of asthmatic care, can vitamins and minerals help? Yes.

What helps it?

• *Caffeine* in coffee and its cousin, theobromine, found in tea, both act as effective bronchodilators (substances that relax and open up the bronchial tubes). In fact, the prescription bronchodilator theophylline, long used in asthmatic treatment, is really nothing more than an altered form of caffeine (but about twice as potent). Recommendation: Unless you avoid caffeine for other health reasons (heart problems), you can help to relieve mild wheezing and constriction of asthma with the amount of caffeine contained in 3 or 4 6-ounce cups of regular coffee throughout the day. Each cup contains about 150 mg caffeine. Warning: If you currently take a prescription theophylline bronchodilating medicine, you must take great care in using caffeine, since the two are related. Toxic amounts of theophylline can build up when you combine these substances. Toxic symptoms include shaking tremors, nausea, vomiting, irritability, sleeplessness, and hyperactivity.

• Asthmatic wheezing increases when the diet is low in *niacin*. Especially when the wheezing occurs because of allergy, niacin supplementation helps to relieve symptoms, probably by keeping the mast cells from releasing their histamine (see Section II, Allergies, page 176). Recommendation: Take 100 mg niacin daily.

• *Vitamin B*$_6$ (pyridoxine) levels in asthmatics may be low, especially in people who take theophylline bronchodilator medicines. Supplementation of the vitamin seems to help asthmatic wheezing, sometimes significantly. Recommendation: I would begin at a 50 mg dose once or twice daily. If after 3 to 4 weeks your asthmatic attacks become less severe and occur less often, remain at that dose. If your response has been less dramatic at this level, you can increase the dose to 100 mg twice daily, but do not increase beyond that point, and immediately discontinue use of the supplemental dose of the vitamin if you develop numbness or tingling of your feet and hands. At higher doses, vitamin B$_6$ can occasionally cause nerve irritation that can persist if you continue to supplement the vitamin at the high dose. The 200 mg dose—which some researchers have used even in children—should offer no problem to you, but better to err on the side of safety with this vitamin. Some people have this reaction and some do not, but there's no way ahead of time to predict who will and who won't.

• *Vitamin B*$_{12}$ has proven an excellent relief for asthmatic wheezing in numerous research tests in people of all age categories, including even toddlers. Exactly how the vitamin helps to relax the bronchial tubes is unclear, but it appears quite effective in improving your ability to tolerate exercise and allergens, substances that stimulate allergic symptoms. Recommendation: If your physician will assist you, the best route of administration is to take 1000 *micro*grams by injection weekly for 4 weeks, then monthly to every 3 to 4 months as needed to maintain control of symptoms. Failing that, look for the drug in sublingual form (dissolves under the tongue) and keep to the same schedule. All ages, in the research testing, took the same dose.

• *Vitamin C* deficiency may cause an increase in asthmatic symptoms (wheezing and tightness), especially in asthma that occurs with allergy and with exercise, possibly by reducing histamine release or by stimulating the body to produce "good" eicosinoid messengers. (See discussion in Section I on vitamin C, pages 50–54, and eicosinoids, pages 24–27, for more details.) Attacks become less frequent and less severe in people who respond, although I hasten to add that some people do not respond to this therapy. Recommendation: Take 500 mg to 1000 mg prior to exercising, if you wheeze after exercise. Take a daily dose of at least 1000 mg (1 gram) to improve ongoing asthma symptoms.

• *Vitamin C plus niacin in combination* seem to assist one another in reducing asthmatic wheezing. By using the two together, you can reduce the doses of each vitamin and still get relief of asthmatic symptoms. Recommendation: Take 90 to 110 mg of niacin (as nicotinic acid) along with 250 to 300 mg vitamin C daily.

• Tests on blood samples taken from people during asthmatic attacks often show a deficiency in *magnesium*. This is an extremely important supplement, because it opens the bronchioles and relaxes the muscles inside the air tubes, which stops an acute asthma attack quickly. As a preventive measure, asthmatics can benefit from large doses taken orally. Because magnesium has a laxative effect, it is best taken throughout the day with meals. Recommendations: Adults can take between 1000 and 1500 mg daily; children and infants can tolerate 100 to 400 mg. It is worthwhile to note that when taken with calcium, vitamin C, and the B vitamins intravenously, serious asthmatic symptoms subside within minutes. Although this is not something you can do at home, you may want to discuss injections with your doctor.

• *Coenzyme Q10* resembles vitamin E in its healing abilities, though it may be an even more powerful antioxidant. It relieves asthma symptoms because it has the ability to counter histamine. Recommendation: Take 100 mg daily.

• *Molybdenum* deficiency occurs quite often in people who have an allergic sensitivity to sulfites (found in wine and eggs). It is a mineral necessary to the detoxification of the sulfite, and lacking it, you will be more severely troubled by your sensitivity. If you develop asthmatic wheezing when you consume these foods, you may be able to improve your tolerance for these foods by adding molybdenum into your diet. Recommendation: Begin with 250 *micro*grams of molybdenum twice weekly, then increase to 500 *micro*grams twice weekly, and finally, if necessary, you may increase to 750 *micro*grams twice weekly to achieve the maximum response. Remain at the lowest dose at which you see improvement in your symptoms.

• Physicians have relied on *N-acetylcysteine,* a modified amino acid or protein building block, in a form breathed in as a mist to thin the thick, sticky secretions in their asthmatic patients. In this inhaled mist form, the drug works very well. It doesn't always give as good a result taken as a pill or capsule by mouth; however, it works quite well for some people to help thin the thick mucus. Although cysteine probably won't alleviate all your asthmatic symptoms by itself, if it works for you, you should be able to reduce the doses of bronchodilator medications necessary to control your other asthmatic symptoms. Recommendation: Begin by taking a dose of 200 mg twice daily, then increase to 3 times daily after a week. If you have not seen a good response at that level, take 400 mg twice daily. If you have not responded at that level, you can increase to 500 mg twice daily; however, I would not recommend your going beyond that point, because the likelihood of your getting a good response by doing so is small.

• *Essential fatty acids,* important in the body's regulation of inflammatory prostaglandins, can help reduce the swelling and spastic hyperreactivity of the bronchial tubes in allergic asthma especially. Please refer to the complete discussion of eicosinoids in Section I, pages 24–27, to learn about these powerful natural anti-inflammatory agents and how they work. Recommendation: Supplementing your diet with a tablespoon or two of corn oil, canola oil, or cold-pressed virgin olive oil made into a light vinaigrette dressing may prove beneficial. Two additional sources of omega-6 essential fatty acids can be found in evening primrose oil capsules and in a product called EicoPro (available from Eicotec, Inc., 21 Tioga Way, Marblehead, Massachusetts 01945), 2 capsules daily. To get maximum benefit, reduce your intake of refined sugars and starches as well. If you cannot obtain this combination product, you can make a reasonable substitute by combining evening primrose oil capsules (which provide essential linoleic acid or GLA) with fish oil capsules (which provide EPA), plus vitamin E (which protects these essential oils from oxidation and damage). Take 500 mg of evening primrose oil (a source of linoleic acid in capsule form), plus 1000 mg EPA fish oil, plus 100 IU vitamin E 1 to 3 times a day. (Warning to diabetics: EPA fish oil can cause blood sugar fluctuations in some diabetics. Carefully monitor your blood sugar if you use this supplemental oil and discontinue its use if your blood sugar becomes difficult to control.)

Herbal remedies

• *Ephedra* is considered one of the world's oldest medicines. Scientists isolated the active chemical constituents in 1887. But it wasn't until after World War I that doctors began prescribing these substances in the United States. Ephedra has a stimulant effect, so I don't recommend using it to treat asthma in children. And it does have side effects, such as insomnia, anxiety, restlessness, and aggravation of high blood pressure. However, it is very effective in treating asthma; just be sure to use the herb carefully.

• Australians have used *stinging nettle* to treat asthma for many years. Americans were slow to catch on, and it has only been a short while that we have recognized the herb for its antihistamine properties.

• *Licorice* soothes the throat and is often recommended for treating asthma. Long-term use has some side effects, such as headache, lethargy, sodium and water retention, loss of potassium, and high blood pressure. If you decide to use licorice on an ongoing basis, I recommend the deglycyrrhizinated extracts, which cause fewer problems. This form is available over the counter.

• *Ginkgo* works by interfering with platelet-activating factor, a protein that helps trigger bronchospasms. The leaves contain low concentrations of the active constituents, so low that to get an effective dose, you'd have to eat about 50 leaves. I recommend using an extract, available in health food stores and pharmacies everywhere.

• *Lobelia* is a bronchial smooth muscle relaxant and expectorant. Use this herb during an attack, but refrain from using it regularly.

• *Mullein oil* stops coughs, unclogs bronchial tubes, and helps clear up asthma attacks. It is said to have an almost immediate effect when taken in tea or fruit juice.

• Other useful herbs include *fennel, cayenne, juniper berries, goldenseal, and slippery elm bark tablets.*

Dosages may vary, depending on the duration and severity of your symptoms. Consult a qualified herbal practitioner. Let your physician know of your decision to use herbs; not all herbal remedies can be used in combination with conventional pharmaceuticals.

What makes it worse?

• *L-trytophan,* one of the essential amino acid building blocks of protein, may aggravate the spasm of the bronchial tubes and increase wheezing in people with asthma. Recommendation: Do not take supplemental tryptophan (currently unavailable on the market) and reduce the amount of dietary tryptophan to 300 mg per day for 2 weeks to see if your symptoms improve. A rule of thumb is that 60 grams of protein (from meat, eggs, milk) contains about 600 mg. This would mean that you would have to reduce your intake to a mere 30 grams of protein from these sources. This level is too low for virtually all adults (refer to the section on macronutrients, page 23). But by adding protein from nonanimal sources, such as tofu, you can eat enough high-quality protein to meet your body's needs for muscle repair and maintenance and still keep the tryptophan low. If after 2 to 4 weeks you have seen no improvement in your asthmatic symptoms, you will not likely respond by continuing for a longer period of time, and you may return to your usual sources of high-quality protein.

• *Alcohol* in its pure form acts as a mild bronchodilator and, in that sense, can actually *help* asthmatic constriction to a certain degree. However, we rarely drink it in its "pure" form; rather, it is usually an additive in beverages, such as beer, wine, or distilled spirits. If you suffer from allergies to foods, and if your asthmatic symptoms worsen because of these allergies, you could develop asthmatic wheezing from the other substances in alcoholic beverages—remnants of the hops, the malt, the grapes, the barley, sulfites in wines, or the corn from which the liquor was made. Recommendation: Although a modest amount of alcoholic beverage (a glass of wine, an ounce of distilled liquor, or a beer per day) might not bother you, or might even help to relax your airway, proceed with caution. Just as with other foods, you need to check your response with an elimination trial to be sure it doesn't make your tightness, wheezing, and cough worse.

• A diet high in *sodium* can increase the spastic constriction of your bronchial tubes that histamine causes. Recommendation: Not adding extra salt into your diet—by that I mean don't salt your food—will help. However, you can reduce salt retention even more dramatically by eating a basic diet that will discourage your body from holding salt. A diet high in concentrated sources of starch and sugars can cause you to retain salt and fluid, too. (The basic dietary principles I described in the discussion about macronutrients in Section I, page 23, would work quite well for this purpose.)

—— Autoimmune Disorders ——

What are they?

Your body's defense network, the immune system, is designed to protect you from infection by the viruses, bacteria, and fungi in the world around you, from your own body's cells that have gone haywire and could develop into cancers, and from all things that are not a part of you. Your immune system's defenders and killer cells can normally tell the difference between what is you—the *self*—which they will ignore or leave alone, from what is not you—the *non-self*—which they will attack and destroy. The defenders recognize the *self* by protein markers (sort of like "name tags") on the surface of every cell that is yours. Foreign cells or particles don't have these markers on their surfaces, and the immune fighters go after them. That's how it should work, at least, but sometimes the surface markers change, and the immune system becomes confused. Without the ability to recognize the self, the defenders will attack their own body's tissues as if they were foreign. When this happens, an autoimmune (meaning the body's turning on itself) disorder develops. There are a number of these kinds of disorders of the immune system: lupus erythematosus, multiple sclerosis, Raynaud's syndrome, rheumatoid arthritis, scleroderma, various myopathies, and various nerve- and muscle-degenerating disorders. I have included a brief description of each of these in the A to Z, but because the vitamin and mineral therapies for them are very similar, I have included only one listing here for them all.

What helps them?

• *Essential fatty acids* play a more significant role in alleviating the symptoms of autoimmune disorders than perhaps any other nutrient. I refer you to the discussion of the eicosinoid messengers (Section I, pages 24–27) for details about how essential fats reduce inflammation and pain. Nutritional help for your symptoms begins here. Recommendation: Begin with the proper basic dietary framework (see the discussion about macronutrients, Section I, page 23) to pave the way for best results. To that sound base, add 240 mg of gamma-linoleic acid to 960 mg of EPA fish oil—a ratio of 1:4 (GLA:EPA) 2 to 6 times daily. The EicoPro essential fatty acid product manufactured by

Eicotec, Inc. of Marblehead, Massachusetts, contains ultrapure sources of linoleic acid and fish oils already combined in the proper ratio. If you cannot get that product, you can purchase linoleic acid in a product called evening primrose oil at most health and nutrition stores, and EPA fish oil as well. Because it is not as pure a form, the milligram dosing will be different. You can make a reasonable substitute by combining evening primrose oil capsules with fish oil capsules plus vitamin E. Take 500 mg of evening primrose oil (a source of linoleic acid in capsule form), plus 1000 mg EPA fish oil, plus 200 IU vitamin E 1 to 3 times a day. (Warning to diabetics: EPA fish oil can cause blood sugar fluctuations in some diabetics. Carefully monitor your blood sugar if you use this supplemental oil and discontinue its use if your blood sugar becomes difficult to control.)

• Although the medical research is sketchier, there is some evidence to suggest that *vitamin C* may slow the progression of autoimmune disorders and so may help. On the other hand, this vitamin plays a key role in the production of collagen, the chief structural protein in the body, which may already be produced in excess in many of the autoimmune disorders (especially scleroderma). Could increasing vitamin C be counterproductive? In that light, possibly so, but I could find no hard science to confirm that theory. I would still recommend that you add some extra vitamin C in your diet for its many other benefits to your health. Recommendation: Unless some other condition arises for which a higher dose of vitamin C would be of value, keep your intake at no more than 500 mg to 1000 mg per day.

• *Vitamin E* has proven beneficial in patients suffering from autoimmune disorders. Notable improvement in symptoms usually occurs in 4 to 6 weeks in those who respond. Recommendation: Begin with 100 IU daily, increasing weekly to 200 IU, 400 IU, then 800 IU of vitamin E (as d-alpha-tocopherol succinate) daily. Some people require doses of 1200 IU to 1600 IU per day, but these higher doses can cause elevation of blood pressure in some people. Be certain, if relief of your symptoms requires a dose in this range, to check that your blood pressure is in the normal range (no higher than 140/90). There is no value in increasing your dose beyond 1600 IU if you have not responded by 4 to 6 weeks.

• Adding *selenium* in a small amount to your daily vitamin E dose will allow you to take a smaller dose of E if your blood pressure increases. Again, allow 4 to 6 weeks to judge your response. Recommendation: Take 140 *micro*grams of selenium (as sodium selenite or selenium aspartate) along with 100 IU vitamin E (as D-alpha-tocopherol succinate) daily.

Herbal remedies

• *Astragalus* boosts the immune system and generates anticancer cells. It is a potent antioxidant as well.

• To enhance overall immune response, consider *bayberry, fenugreek, hawthorn, horehound, licorice root, and red clover.* Caution: Licorice can elevate blood pressure and should not be used daily for more than 7 consecutive days.

• The liver is king when it comes to detoxification, and you should treat it royally. *Black radish, dandelion, and milk thistle* cleanse the liver and bloodstream.

• Germanium is a trace element that aids immune function and has anticancer properties. It can be found in *boxthorn seed, ginseng, suma, and wisteria.* Caution: Ginseng can elevate blood pressure.

• *Echinacea* boosts the immune system and enhances lymphatic function.

• *St. John's wort* is a natural blood purifier.

• Strengthen the immune system using *goldenseal.* This herb also cleanses the body and has antibacterial properties.

Dosages may vary, depending on the duration and severity of your symptoms. Consult a qualified herbal practitioner. Let your physician know of your decision to use herbs; not all herbal remedies can be used in combination with conventional pharmaceuticals.

What makes them worse?

• A diet high in *saturated fat* may hasten the onset of such disorders and worsen the symptoms. Recommendation: The basic guidelines you should follow are to eat 30% of your daily calories as lean protein, 40% of your calories as low-glycemic carbohydrate, 20% of your calories as polyunsaturated fats, and limit your intake of saturated fats to 10% of your total calories per day. Please refer to the discussion in Section I, on macronutrients, page 23, for more complete instructions on how to compose this kind of eating program.

——————— Binge Eating ———————

What is it?

Binge eating is one of the three major eating disorders, along with anorexia and bulimia. People suffering from binge-eating disorder feel driven to rapidly eat large volumes of high-calorie foods in a short period of time, sometimes 8,000 or 10,000 calories (3 to 5 days' worth of calories for an average adult) in an hour or two. You may suffer from binge-eating disorder if you feel at least some sense of being out of control, or of anxiety during the binge, and a sensation of emotional numbness as a result of the bingeing. The aftermath? Waves of guilt for having succumbed to the desire to binge, usually accompanied by a vow to never do so again, often followed before long by another binge, numbness, guilt, and another vow. The binge cycle after a time can destroy self-esteem and ruin health through tremendous weight gain. The problem is not one of willpower, but a complex interplay of psychological and emotional needs, physical changes, brain chemical–driven cravings, social conditioning, and addiction to the emotional numbness brought on by the binge. Although the disorder may require a period of psychological support (therapy with a knowledgeable counselor) to rehabilitate self-esteem and learn new coping skills, there are a number of important nutritional factors that can help curb the physical cravings the binge brings on. Let's take a look.

What helps it?

• Concentrating on *proper daily nutrition* can be your best food ally in combating the desire to binge. Eat on a preset schedule, dividing your intake throughout the day, if possible. And don't skip meals. Recommendation: Carefully read the macronutrient discussion in Section I, page 23. You should follow the specific instructions there to construct for yourself a basic diet providing plenty of high-quality lean protein to support your muscles (about 30% of your total day's calories); another 40% of calories each day should be from low-glycemic carbohydrate (about 40% of your day's calories) found in fibrous vegetables, green leafy vegetables, fruit, rice, and oats. Your diet should contain no refined sugar, corn syrup, honey, or other concentrated simple sugar sources or foods made from them, and you should also *limit* potatoes, wheat, corn, and foods made from their meals or flours (this means bread, rolls, pasta) because of their unfavorable effect on your blood sugar and your hunger. The last component of your diet comes from polyunsaturated fats, such as olive oil, canola oil, sunflower oil, and the oils from cold-water fish such as mackerel, herring, salmon, flounder, sardines, and tuna; these should make up about 20% of your day's calorie total, with the final 10% coming from the saturated (animal) fat found in lean meats, poultry, dairy products, and eggs. Divide your day's calories into 4 parts, and try to schedule one-fourth of the total about every 4 to 5 hours while you are awake. Try to never let yourself go for long periods without eating, and plan what you will eat (the right choices), when you can stop to eat, and where you intend to eat. Take your food with you in an insulated lunch bag if needed.

• *Zinc* is often deficient in people who binge. Taking zinc is especially important to battle this disorder because it increases the appetite and aids the sense of taste. Recommendation: Take 50 to 100 mg of zinc daily. Do not exceed this amount. To balance the zinc, take 3 mg of *copper* as well.

• *Tryptophan,* an animo acid protein building block, may help to curb desires to binge in some people. Your brain takes this amino acid and turns it into the brain chemical *serotonin,* which curbs the desire to eat carbohydrates (starches and sugars). Much research into this area has turned up evidence that a need for serotonin may be behind abnormal patterns of eating, such as binge-eating disorder. Recommendation: The FDA has ordered the removal of all supplemental tryptophan from the shelves following an outbreak of a severe muscular disorder called EMS, eosinphilia myalgia syndrome. This disorder was caused by a contaminant in the tryptophan supplements from a single manufacturer, but all tryptophan was recalled and has not yet been allowed back onto the shelves. In the event that the FDA finally decides to allow harmless supplemental tryptophan to be sold again, you may follow this regimen. Take tryptophan in a dose of 50 mg at bedtime. If it doesn't make you sleepy, I would encourage you to take half that dose twice or even 3 times a day. For safety's sake, however, I caution you not to use any old tryptophan you may have bought in the past.

What makes it worse?

• *Sugars* and *concentrated starches,* because they play havoc with the hormones of metabolism, can cause your blood sugar to swing wildly up and down. These substances make up foods that are typical "binge foods" for most people: candy, cookies, pastries, ice cream, and breads. Falling blood sugar levels stimulate your brain to release chemicals that drive the hunger center, sending out a "need to feed" signal, making you want to eat. (Emotional or physical stress causes the same phenomenon.) Recommendation: Work to eliminate the simple sugars (table sugar, honey, corn syrup) and foods made with these products and the concentrated starch sources (potato, corn, wheat) and foods made from these or their meals or flours from your daily diet.

Bleeding Gums
(see Capillary Fragility)

Blood Sugar Stabilization
(see Diabetes and Hypoglycemia)

Bone Health
(see Osteoporosis)

Breast Cancer

What is it?

Cancers develop from normal cells in the body that have been damaged and as a result have gone haywire. These renegade cells no longer obey the body's commands, no longer perform their usual functions, and grow in a haphazard and disorganized fashion to infiltrate and overtake the normal tissues around them. Every day, a few of the billions of cells that make up the body sustain this kind of damage and go haywire. When all is working as it should, your ever-vigilant immune system recognizes these troublemakers and destroys them before they can take root. When that defense system breaks down, however, a cancer forms.

In the breast, these cancers can occur early in life (before the menopause, or premenopausal) or later in life (after the menopause, or postmenopausal). The two kinds of breast cancer differ dramatically. The breast cancer that develops early in life has a strong genetic component, by which I mean it runs in the family. You inherit a tendency for the cells of the breast tissue to go haywire, whereas the late-life cancers don't have such a strong family tendency. The early-life cancers tend to be much more aggressive when they do develop; they grow more quickly and don't respond to treatment as readily as the late-life kind. For all their differences, however, the nutritional factors that affect them are remarkably similar. I would like to insert a word of caution at this point: Nutrition is a tool to improve risk of cancer and enhance your response to conventional cancer treatments. It is not, alone, a treatment for breast cancer. So, in addition to conventional treatment methods, what does nutrition have to offer? Let's take a look at the nutrients involved.

What helps it?

• *Vitamin C,* in its role as an antioxidant, helps reduce the formation of free radicals (see discussion in Section I, pages 19–23) that inflict the kind of damage that could turn a normal breast cell into a renegade. For this reason, if you have a family risk for breast cancer, you should supplement your diet with vitamin C. If you have already developed a breast cancer and are in (or have been in) treatment for it, you will want to supplement with vitamin C to an even greater degree to help heal and repair the damage caused by both surgical treatment and postoperative X-ray therapy and chemotherapy. Recommendation: Before you proceed, read the Section I listing for vitamin C. Although it comes in tablet or capsule form, I recommend you purchase your vitamin C in the crystalline (powdered) form, because you can more easily adjust your dose and it is not as hard on your stomach at higher doses. Begin with ¼ to ½ teaspoon of the crystalline powder (mixed in a citrus beverage) once daily for an intake of 1000 mg to 2000 mg per day. Remain at this dose for several days before increasing. Now take the same dose twice daily for several days. At this point, you will be taking 2000 mg to 4000 mg (or 2 to 4 grams) per day. A daily intake of 4 to 8 grams is sufficient for most people to prevent the formation of free radicals. Larger people (and most adult men) may need to be at the higher end of that range, so begin to slowly increase the amount you take at each dose until you reach a total of 8 grams. If you are currently recovering from breast cancer surgery and postoperative treatment, you will need a little more. Continue to increase your daily dose to about 12 grams (that's 1 teaspoon taken 3 times a day).

• *Vitamin D* appears to be a factor in improved survival from breast cancer, although the reasons for this effect remain unclear. The vitamin does seem to inhibit the growth of cancer cells in the laboratory, and this may be a part of why it helps. Recommendation: Take 400 IU to 600 IU per day. Warning: Vitamin D is a stored vitamin, which means that it can build up to toxic levels if you take too much. Refer to the Section I listing for vitamin D to reacquaint yourself with the possible side effects.

• *Vitamin E* appears to reduce your risk of developing precancerous breast lumps (those that in time can often become cancers). It also aids in hormone production and immune function. Women with breast cancer often have a zinc deficiency. Recommendation: Begin with 100 IU vitamin E (as d-alpha-tocopherol succinate) daily. Remain at that dose for 2 weeks. Check your blood pressure to be certain you are not one of the people for whom vitamin E causes a blood pressure rise. If your blood pressure remains in the normal range, increase your daily dose to 200 IU for 1 week, then 400 IU, then finally 800 IU per day. Between each increase in dose, check your blood pressure again to be sure all is well. Do not increase to a higher dose if your average blood pressure rises above 140/90.

• *Selenium* is a powerful free radical scavenger that assists vitamin E in its antioxidant work to reduce cancer risk. Taking the two nutrients together will allow you to reduce the amount of vitamin E required to do the job, which may be especially important if you cannot tolerate an increase in vitamin E because of blood pressure consequences. Recommendation: Take 140 *micro*grams of selenium along with 100 IU to 200 IU vitamin E once daily. You may increase this dose to twice daily if your blood pressure remains normal.

• *Essential fats.* The relationship between fat and breast cancer development is a confusing one, so let me try to clarify it. Some studies suggest that dietary fat increases risk for late-life breast cancers, and others find no significant association. The confusion in part arises because all fats are not created equal; some kinds of fat are "good" because of their importance for maintaining a healthy immune system, while others cause some trouble. (See the discussion of the fats that worsen risk of breast cancer under the heading "What makes it worse?") And even a "good" fat, heated to the high temperatures needed for frying, can become a "bad" fat, because the heating alters the structure of the fat molecule, making it unusable to the body.

Another factor that makes the research concerning fat intake and breast cancer risk difficult is that diets high in fat tend to also be high in many other breast cancer–promoting culprits, such as sugar and total number of calories.

The essential fatty acids that lead to the production of "good" eicosinoids (see discussion, Section I, pages 24–27) are crucial to reducing your risk of breast (and other) cancer and improving response to X-ray therapy and chemotherapy in people under treatment for cancer. Dietary sources of unheated linoleic acid (GLA) and fish oils (EPA) in the proper proportions will ensure that you will make more of the "good" kind of eicosinoid and keep your immune system strong.

Recommendation: Avoid deep-frying food in any kind of oil. Begin with a solid macronutrient framework (see the discussion of macronutrients, Section I, page 23), and to that sound base add 240 mg of gamma-linoleic acid to 960 mg of EPA fish oil—a ratio of 1:4 (GLA:EPA) 2 to 6 times daily. The EicoPro essential fatty acid product manufactured by Eicotec, Inc. of Marblehead, Massachusetts, contains ultrapure sources of linoleic acid and fish oils already combined in the proper ratio. If you cannot get that product, you can purchase linoleic acid in a product called evening primrose oil at most health and nutrition stores, and EPA fish oil as well. Because it is not as pure a form, the milligram dosing will be different. You can make a reasonable substitute by combining evening primrose oil capsules with fish oil capsules plus vitamin E. Take 500 mg of evening primrose oil (a source of linoleic acid in capsule form), plus 1000 mg EPA fish oil, plus 200 IU vitamin E 1 to 3 times a day. (Warning to diabetics: EPA fish oil can cause blood sugar fluctuations in some diabetics. Carefully monitor your blood sugar if you use this supplemental oil and discontinue its use if your blood sugar becomes difficult to control.) Another good dietary source of essential fats is cold-pressed virgin or extra-virgin olive oil or canola oil. I would recommend that you use this oil when cooking and that you lightly sauté foods, never deep-fry them.

• *Fiber* may contribute to lowering your risk of developing breast cancer by binding to the female hormone estrogen in the intestine and allowing it to be removed from the body, thus lowering your estrogen levels somewhat. Since estrogen stimulates growth of breast cancers, the modest reduction in estrogen that fiber provides may be important if you have a family risk for cancer. This reduction of estrogen is especially important, however, if you currently are a breast cancer survivor. Recommendation: The cornerstone of increasing your fiber intake should be to concentrate your efforts on eating more high-fiber fruits and vegetables, such as the green leafies, broccoli, cauliflower, asparagus, and green beans. And fewer of the starchier ones, such as potatoes, refined flours and meals, and the breads and pastries made from them. Instead, choose whole grains, rice, oats, and legumes. To further increase your fiber intake, you may want to add a commercial vegetable fiber bulking product (such as Konsyl, Metamucil, or Citrucel), beginning with a small dose of $1/2$ teaspoon in fruit juice or an artificially sweetened, fruit-flavored beverage each night. Slowly increase your dose to 1 teaspoon nightly, then morning and night, then 2 teaspoons morning and night, until you reach a combined fiber (food fiber plus commercial fiber) intake of at least 40 to 50 grams per day. I caution you to proceed slowly with your incremental increases. Allow yourself to become accustomed to each new level before moving on. Don't try to do it all in one week or you will suffer from bloating, stomach cramping, and gas from the rapid change in fiber level and wonder why you ever thought you wanted to increase your fiber intake.

• *Beta-carotene,* when taken with *vitamin A,* has been shown to have a positive effect on breast cancer. In animal studies, vitamin A has been shown to slow the spread of breast cancer to other parts of the body. In a study of women with breast cancer undergoing chemotherapy, women with higher blood levels of vitamin A responded twice as well to the therapy as did women with lower levels. There are two possible reasons for this result: Vitamin A may have helped protect the women for the drugs' toxicity, or it may have interacted with the drugs in a way that increased their effectiveness. Although studies using beta-carotene alone have shown that it is not effective in treating breast cancer, when paired with vitamin A, it seems to fight the good fight. Recommendation: You may already have increased your intake of green and yellow vegetable sources for the higher fiber content they contain, and as a consequence you will already be eating a diet higher in beta-carotene. If you cannot eat these foods, you may want to add beta-carotene in a dose of 10,000 and 25,000 IU per day to make up the dietary lack. Also supplement with 50,000 IU vitamin A daily.

• In areas of low *iodine* intake, breast cancers and precancerous breast lumps occur more frequently. Supplementing the diet with iodine may help decrease this risk. Recommendation: Use iodized table salt in cooking to prevent deficiency.

• *Two nutritional regimens from the work of Dr. Linus Pauling appear to improve survival of breast cancer:*

(1) Vitamin C 12 grams per day, niacinamide 1.5 to 3 grams per day, pyridoxine 250 mg per day, B-complex (suggested dose 100 mg per day), vitamin E 800 IU per day, beta-carotene 30,000 IU per day, selenium 2 at 500 *micro*grams per day, plus at least the RDA for all other vitamins and minerals. This regimen improved the survival time of breast cancer patients from an average of 5.7 months to 122 months.

(2) To a basic diet of reduced red meat, increased green vegetables, and no sugar, coffee, cocoa, or milk products, add a daily dose of: B-complex 50 mg, niacinamide 1.5 to 3 grams, vitamin A 25,000 to 50,000 IU, vitamin C *at least* 12 grams, vitamin E 800 IU, magnesium 500 mg, selenium 4 to 500 *micro*grams, zinc 30 to 50 mg, beta-carotene 30,000 to 60,000 IU per day. On follow-up checks done at 5 years from onset of this regimen, 4 of 6 patients were still alive.

Herbal remedies

• More than 1500 plants contain anticancer compounds. Obviously, these are too numerous to include here, but the following are helpful in preventing cancer and are easy to find, as well: *astragalus, echinacea, burdock root, dandelion root, milk thistle, red clover, ginkgo, licorice root, sage, cumin, garlic, onion, primrose oil, flaxseeds, rosemary, and cayenne.*

Dosages may vary, depending on the duration and severity of your symptoms. Consult a qualified herbal practitioner. Let your physician know of your decision to use herbs; not all herbal remedies can be used in combination with conventional pharmaceuticals.

What makes it worse?

• *Saturated fat* has for years been said to promote the development of breast cancers that occur in later life, but not the early-life cancers. Although study after study in the research laboratory has pointed to this dietary fat–cancer connection in animals, recent medical investigations in people appear to contradict this long-held view. The reason for the contradiction may lie in the fact that a diet of *high calories* promotes breast cancer, too. And in the real world, the two usually occur together—it's hard to eat a diet high in fat that isn't also pretty calorie rich. Also, we humans rarely eat just fat; no one would crave a big glob of butter or lard by itself. But mix that butter with powdered sugar and what do you get? Cake frosting.

That, we sweet-toothed Americans *will* definitely eat. So the human fat–breast cancer connection has been confounded over the years because dietary fat occurs with calories and with sugar—both suspect in promoting cancer themselves—much of the time. So where does that leave you in trying to reduce your risk? Recommendation: Don't overeat. Reduce your intake of fatty meats and egg yolks (not whites). Reduce total calories to a level that will let you reach and then maintain your ideal weight and body-fat percentage. Refer to the discussion in Section I on macronutrients for dietary guidelines and to the section on calculation of lean body weight. Strive for an approximate body-fat percentage of 15 to 20% if you are male and 22 to 28% if you are female. The two sources mentioned for calculation of lean body weight will also describe how to calculate your body-fat percentage.

• *Alcohol* increases your risk of several cancers, including breast cancer. Even moderate levels (3 or more oz. of alcohol per day) can increase the risk. Although less potent in alcohol content, beer drinking appears to increase your risk of developing breast cancer (or of having a breast cancer recur) than distilled spirits. Recommendation: If you have a family risk for breast cancer or have survived breast cancer yourself, reduce or eliminate your consumption of alcohol. A level equivalent to 1 glass of wine or 1 ounce of distilled liquor no more often than 3 times weekly is probably safe.

• *Sugar* promotes the development of breast cancers in both animals and people. Reducing intake of sugar is especially important when you live in America, where sugar contributes more calories to the diet than any other substance—more than meat, more than milk, more than vegetables. Recommendation: Sharply reduce or eliminate sugar from your diet. This means table sugar that you sprinkle on, sugar added to commercially prepared foods, corn syrup, molasses, and honey. Don't be misled into thinking that just because it's "natural" or "raw" sugar or that a bee makes it it's not every bit as damaging to your health risk. Use sugar with great caution—respect it for the potent chemical that it is.

• *Iron.* Cancer cells need nutrition to grow, and one of the critical nutrients they appear to need is iron. One hypothesis suggests that taking increased iron may increase the chances that cancer cells can survive your immune system's defenses and flourish. Recommendation: If you have a family risk for breast cancer, of if you are a breast cancer survivor, I would recommend that you not add any additional iron to your diet unless you are truly iron deficient and anemic.

• Eating a diet containing greater than 30 to 35% of calories as *polyunsaturated fats,* such as commercially prepared corn oil and safflower oil, may have a weakening effect on the immune system and may thus worsen your risk of developing breast cancer. Eating the same amount of calories as fat, but keeping approximately equal portions of polyunsaturated fats (corn oil, safflower oil, some vegetable oils) to monounsaturated fats (olive oil, fish oil, evening primrose oil) to saturated fat (butter, milk fat, animal fat) is less damaging. The problem arises because the polyunsaturated oils are chemically unstable, making them easy targets for damage by oxidation. (Refer to the discussion of oxidation in Section I, pages 18–19.) If you eat a diet in which the majority of your fat and oil consumption comes from these polyunsaturated sources, it increases your body's need for antioxidant protection, such as you would get from vitamins C and E. Without this protection, a high intake of polyunsaturated fats and oils can damage your tissues and your immune function, and thereby increase your risk for breast cancer.

Also, to keep these chemically unstable oils on the consumer shelf longer without "going bad," food manufacturers usually heat them to high temperatures. This heating rearranges the chemical structure of the oil molecules, creating new compounds and more stable oils, but ones that recent scientific research suggests may be cancer promoting themselves. This same kind of heating damage occurs at extreme cooking temperatures—such as would occur in deep-frying. Recommendation: Choose cold-pressed virgin or extra-virgin olive oil, canola oil, or sunflower oil for your cooking and baking needs. Try to include more cold-water fish (tuna, mackerel, herring, salmon) to provide a counterbalance to the polyunsaturated oils. See the recommendations about vitamins C and E. And don't deep-fry your food.

Breast Disease, Benign

What is it?

Many women suffer from painful, lumpy breasts throughout their reproductive years. The symptoms in some women worsen and improve in a pattern that follows the menstrual cycle, but in others, the problem seems to obey no rules and symptoms occur without regard to menstrual hormonal surges. Some women suffer symptoms most of the time. These women, especially, might argue with calling these disorders of the breast *benign,* which generally means "good" or "kind," or at least "not bad." What the designation *benign* actually means in this case is merely *not cancerous.* If you suffer with any of the benign breast diseases—fibrocystic breast disease, chronic mastodynia, or cyclic mastalgia—you would probably agree that they're certainly not good.

Fibrocystic breast disease occurs most commonly in women between the ages of 30 and 50, rarely occurring after menopause. These fluid-filled cysts and lumps tend to be quite painful, increasing and decreasing in size through the menstrual cycle each month. Younger women more commonly develop nontender solid, rubbery lumps called fibroadenomas. Just because these lumps cause little pain, they should not be ignored, even in young women.

On that score, let me insert a word of caution. Some benign lumps of the breast sometimes can develop into cancers, and for that reason, you should never ignore any kind of breast lump in the hope that it will go away. If you suffer from benign breast disease, I strongly advise you to maintain regular contact with your personal physician, who can keep a close watch on your breast lumps. Absolutely no breast lump—even in women who get them often—should go unexamined by a trained physician who knows when to recommend mammogram, ultrasound, or biopsy if the lumps fail to respond to nutritional or conventional therapy. With that, let's look at what nutrition has to offer for this problem.

What helps it?

• *Vitamin E* appears to improve the symptoms of most (but not all) women with benign breast disease, including reducing the size and number of painful cysts in fibrocystic breast disease. Recommendation: Because in some people vitamin E can cause a rise in blood pressure, begin at 100 IU per day for 1 week and check your blood pressure. If your reading remains below an *average* (taken on 5 different occasions and averaging the values of the first number and then of the second number) of 140/90, increase your vitamin E dose to 200 IU per day, then 400 IU, then 600 IU. Check your blood pressure again each time you move your dose up. Remain at a dose of 600 IU for 3 months. For most women, this dose will be sufficient to improve symptoms. If you should require a higher dose, you may increase to 1000 IU or at most 1200 IU per day. If you have not seen a response by this time, increasing to a higher one probably will not help.

• *Coenzyme Q_{10}*, a powerful antioxidant, is similar to vitamin E in action, but is even more potent. Recommendation: 100 mg daily.

• *Essential fatty acids* of the type found in evening primrose oil (linoleic acid or GLA, primarily) also appear to decrease breast tenderness in mastalgia and chronic mastodynia and to reduce the pain, number, and size of cysts in fibrocystic breast disease. This remedy works through providing your body with the forerunner of the "good" group of eicosinoids (see Section I, pages 24–27) that control pain and inflammation. By combining the essential fatty acids found in evening primrose oil (the GLA) with some of the kinds found in cold-water fish oil (EPA), you can take less of each and better control the process. Recommendation: Begin with a solid macronutrient framework (see Macronutrients, Section I, page 23), and to that sound base add evening primrose oil capsules, fish oil capsules, plus vitamin E. Take 500 mg of evening primrose oil, plus 1000 mg EPA fish oil, plus 200 IU vitamin E 1 to 3 times a day. The EicoPro essential fatty acid product manufactured by Eicotec, Inc., of Marblehead, Massachusetts, contains ultrapure sources of linoleic acid and fish oils already combined in the proper ratio. Of this product, take 2 capsules 1 to 3 times daily. Because it is a purer form, the milligram dosing on the label will be different from that recommended above. (Warning to diabetics: EPA fish oil can cause blood sugar fluctuations in some diabetics. Carefully monitor your blood sugar if you use this supplemental oil and discontinue its use if your blood sugar becomes difficult to control.)

• Some medical research has shown that dietary *iodine* deficiency can increase the development of benign breast lumps and cysts in both animals and people, and that supplementation will reverse this process. Recommendation: You may enlist the aid of your physician to prescribe the product SSKI, which provides 30 mg iodine per drop. You should take 1 to 3 drops per day. You should note some response in pain and swelling as early as 3 months; however, complete response may take as long as 1 to 3 years. You may also experience a period of transient worsening of tenderness during the course of treatment as the cysts and lumps begin to soften. *Warning: Do not use the antiseptic iodine products designed for cleaning cuts and scrapes as a liquid nutritional supplement!*

Herbal remedies
• Please refer to the box on nutraceuticals, pages 93–97.

What makes it worse?
• *Dietary saturated fat* and a diet *high in calories* also appear to be connected in some way to the development of painful breast lumps and cysts, perhaps through increasing the output of female hormones. Recommendation: Reduce total calories to a level that will let you reach and then maintain your ideal weight and body-fat percentage. Refer to the discussion in Section I on macronutrients for dietary guidelines and to the section on calculation of lean body weight. Strive for an approximate body fat percentage of 15% to 20% if you are male and 22% to 28% if you are female. The two sources mentioned for calculation of lean body weight will also describe how to calculate your body-fat percentage. Reduce your intake of dietary fats to 30% of your total day's calories with approximately equal parts coming from saturated (animal fat, egg yolks), monounsaturated (olive oil, canola oil, sunflower oil, fish oil), and polyunsaturated (corn oil, safflower oil, other vegetable oils) sources.

• Through the years, medical evidence has suggested both that *caffeine* did worsen benign breast disease and that it did not. When there is research that supports both sides, what conclusion can you come to if you suffer from the problem? That it can for some women and not for others, and therefore it *might* for you and is worth looking into. Caffeine (found in coffee, some soft drinks, and chocolate) and its relative theobromine (found in teas) act as stimulators to the activity of many glands in the body, including the milk glands in breast tissue. This increased activity, without the stimulation from the hormones released in pregnancy to cause the glands to produce milk, may instead result in the production of fluid-filled cysts and lumps. And discomfort. Recommendation: If you suffer from painful breast lumps, try to eliminate all sources of caffeine (and theobromine) from your diet and remain free of caffeine for at least 3 to 4 months to judge your response. Most research shows that simply reducing your intake is not enough; you'll probably have to go to zero caffeine. If, after that period of total abstinence, you cannot tell a difference in your breast problems, you are one of the women for whom caffeine makes little or no difference.

When you begin your caffeine-elimination trial, please heed this warning: Don't go off caffeine "cold turkey." Begin to *slowly* taper your intake or risk developing (as I did) a world-class headache that lasts for days and that nothing except caffeine will cure. If you're a big coffee drinker (which, I must confess, I am), the easiest and most painless method is to first reduce the amount of caffeine per cup by using a "blend" of half-caffeinated and half-decaffeinated coffee, of which there are several brands on the grocery shelf. After you have accustomed yourself to the 50/50 blend, then mix 1 part of that 50/50 store blend with 1 part of a fully decaffeinated coffee to get a 25% caffeinated/75% decaffeinated blend. Use that strength for a week or two, then cut it again. Use 1 part of the 50/50 store blend and add 2 parts of decaf, which now brings you down to 12.5% caffeine and 87.5% decaf. From there, the jump to total decaffeinated becomes a small hop, and you should suffer no ill effects. Remember, you must be forever vigilant in screening other foods and medicines: choose caffeine-free soft drinks, avoid chocolate (for which you can substitute carob), and read the labels on over-the-counter and prescription pain remedies, which may contain caffeine.

Bruising

(see Capillary Fragility)

Bulimia Nervosa

What is it?

Bulimia nervosa is a condition occurring mostly in young women in which they binge on large amounts of high-calorie (usually also high-sugar and high-fat) foods until they feel gorged and numb, then purge their bodies of the calories they've eaten by vomiting, enemas, abuse of laxatives, or excessive exercise. You will find more information about bingeing under the related disorder Binge Eating in this section. The two disorders are quite similar, except that bingers who do not purge gain tremendous amounts of weight, and bulimics damage their normal-weight bodies by purge techniques. The stomach acid brought up in vomiting erodes tooth enamel, burns the lining of the esophagus and throat, and causes disturbances of fluid balance and electrolytes such as sodium and potassium. Chronic use of laxatives or enemas can also damage the colon and cause the loss of fluid and electrolytes from daily diarrhea. Extreme exercising can lead to stress fractures of the bones of the feet and legs.

Most young women (or men) who suffer from bulimia should receive counseling from a qualified psychotherapist to help them recover their self-esteem and to overcome their fears of weight gain if they eat normally. But in addition to competent mental health care, nutrition can also help.

What helps it?

• Please refer to the listing for Binge Eating, as the dietary recommendations are nearly identical for these two disorders.

• Engaging in bulimia can deplete your blood of *potassium* and *sodium,* and I would recommend that you ask your personal physician to do a thorough physical examination, including laboratory testing, to be sure you have not done so. Recommendation: If your blood values are reasonably normal, eat proper amounts of foods rich in potassium, such as broccoli, spinach, tomatoes, oranges, and bananas. In addition, you may want to replace lost fluids using GatorAde Light, which contains both potassium and sodium.

What makes it worse?

• See Binge Eating.

Burn

What is it?

When you injure some or all of the layers of the skin by heat, caustic chemicals, or friction, you suffer a "burn." The same general kind of damage can result from a wide variety of activities: spending too long a time in the sun (thermal or heat burn), handling jalapeño peppers with ungloved hands (chemical burn), skidding across pavement in a fall (friction burn). But whether you burn yourself by one of these means or a spill of boiling water or a splatter of hot grease, even minor injury to the skin causes redness and pain. We call this a *superficial burn* or by its older name, a first-degree burn. Burns of slightly greater magnitude—that is, burning to deeper layers of the skin—cleave the layers of the skin, causing the formation of fluid-filled "water blisters." Blistering burns, once called second degree, we now refer to as *partial thickness burns.* If you should sustain either of these types of burns, your first order of business is to apply cold water. Never use any kind of oil, butter, or any oily first-aid spray, because these remedies only hold in the heat and worsen the injury.

If you should suffer a burn that does greater damage than to make small blisters, apply cold water quickly and seek immediate treatment by a physician. Injury to all the layers of the skin is called a *full thickness burn,* which may require treatment in the hospital (if a large area is burned) and may heal properly only with a surgical skin graft.

Although quite obviously nutrition has little to offer in the way of preventing a burn, many nutrients help to speed healing and improve scarring after the fact. Let's take a look at these.

What helps it?

• *Vitamin C* is required for making the collagen (chief protein of fibrous and scar tissue) needed to heal the burned skin. Under the stress of injury, the demand for vitamin C rises, and so does your requirement. Recommendation: 10,000 mg immediately after the burn occurs; 2000 mg 3 times daily until healed. One tablespoon of powdered vitamin C added to 1 quart of cold water and sprayed on the burn enhances healing as well.

• *Vitamin E* taken both internally and applied as the topical oil can help healing and prevent scarring after a burn. Recommendation: Increase your intake of vitamin E by 200 IU to 400 IU per day under the stress of a moderately severe burn or sunburn (as described above). After the skin has begun to heal—that is, no longer raw, moist, or open—begin to apply the vitamin E oil from the capsules directly to the new pink skin. To cover a larger area of skin, mix the contents of a capsule of vitamin E with a puddle of a good emollient lotion (such as Nivea, Alpha Keri, Lubriderm, or Vaseline Intensive Care) in your palm and apply twice daily to the new pink healing areas.

• During the healing phase of bigger burns—ones that may have required hospital treatment or surgery—because physical and emotional stress increases the demand for the *B vitamin complex* as well, you will need to increase your intake. Recommendation: Take an extra 100 mg to 150 mg of B-complex daily. You may also want to take an injection of 1000 *micro*grams of vitamin B$_{12}$ weekly for 1 month if your physician will assist you. You will absorb the vitamin more effectively in shot form than by mouth.

Herbal remedies

• *Echinacea* boosts your immune system, and an enhanced immune system is more resistant to infection. Apply a few drops directly to the burn.

• Worldwide, people have used *garlic* and its relatives (chives, leeks, and scallions) to treat burns. Mash the plant and apply directly to the burn as a paste. The herb's antiseptic qualities will go right to work.

• *Gotu kola,* when taken with foods high in vitamin C, is useful in treating burns. It may even stimulate collagen synthesis.

• *Lavender* oil relieves the pain from burns and helps reduce scarring. Although other oils, such as chamomile, geranium, peppermint, rosemary, and sage, have been used in burn treatments, aromatherapists value lavender oil most highly.

• Germany's Commission E, the board of scientists that advises the German government about herbal treatment, promotes *St. John's wort* as an anti-inflammatory external treatment for first-degree burns. Studies show it speeds up healing time and reduces scarring. Tinctures are readily available in the United States; salves are nearly impossible to find. Either one works well.

Dosages may vary, depending on duration and severity of symptoms. Follow package directions, or consult a qualified herbal practitioner.

What makes it worse?

• I know of no nutrient that specifically makes a burn worse.

Avoid reinjuring your burn. This means you should keep burned skin out of strong sun, hot water, and high-temperature environments, as well as away from potent chemicals and cleansers.

Bursitis

What is it?

Around your bigger joints, nature has provided a sack, called a *bursa,* that in the event of injury or overuse can swell with fluid to

act as an internal cushion or splint. Sometimes this protective cushion becomes inflamed from the injury or excessive use, and it hurts.
With the pain, you may find the area around the joint warm to touch
and, occasionally, even swollen and red. Often, the offending bursa
is one cushioning the shoulder, and you may tend to think of bursitis as being a shoulder problem. In truth, any bursa can develop such
an inflammation—the hip, the elbow, or the knee. The underlying
problem is one of inflammation, much like arthritis, and many of the
nutrients helpful in alleviating arthritic symptoms will help bursitis
as well. You may want to read over that listing for more information,
but let's look at some information specific to soft-tissue inflamma-
tions, like bursitis.

What helps it?

• *Vitamin B$_{12}$* appears to reduce the inflammation and pain of
bursitis, sometimes within the space of just a few hours. Even in
cases of calcific bursitis, a form of the disorder in which calcium deposits form inside the bursa, this vitamin offers some help. Recommendation: In this instance, your best bet is to take the vitamin by
the shot route, and for that you will need the help of a physician.
Take 1000 *micro*grams (that usually is 1 cc of the solution) daily for
7 days, then three times weekly for 2 to 3 weeks, and then twice
weekly for 2 to 3 weeks. If you cannot arrange to take the vitamin
by injection, then try the sublingual dose form. Take 1000 *micro*-
grams in these tablets designed to dissolve under the tongue. Along
with either dose form of the B$_{12}$, also take a *vitamin B-complex*
tablet or capsule providing about 100 mg per day. You should expect
to see relief in 5 to 7 days if you are responsive to this therapy.

• Your requirement for *vitamin C,* required for healing the tissues,
naturally increases following injury and overuse of joints, as well as
when the tissues become inflamed. Recommendation: If you already supplement with vitamin C, increase your daily intake in 500
mg increments twice daily. Under stress, you may easily be able to
tolerate double or triple your usual dose. If you do not already supplement with vitamin C, purchase the vitamin in crystalline or powdered form. Each teaspoon of the crystalline powder provides
4 grams (4000 mg) of ascorbic acid (vitamin C). Begin with ½ teaspoon in the morning mixed in a citrus beverage (a carbonated beverage works best). After a few days, increase to ½ teaspoon at
morning and night. Slowly increase your doses until you reach your

bowel tolerance level (see Vitamin C, Section I, page 50). Most adults will tolerate between 4 and 8 grams under normal conditions but will tolerate considerably more under stress or injury. Once the inflammation has subsided, you may return to your usual level of intake.

Vitamin C acts as a good preventive treatment for inflammation, as well. After a particularly strenuous workout, unaccustomed physical activity (raking the leaves, moving, weekend sports), or in the event of an injury, immediately increase your vitamin C dose as specified above to reduce the development of joint, bursa, and muscle soreness afterward.

• *Vitamin E,* through its antioxidant abilities as well as its ability to prevent the body's defense fighters from releasing as many of their toxic, inflammatory chemicals into an injured area, helps to shorten recovery time following injury and to lessen the inflammation that develops in the bursa. Recommendation: Take 400 IU to 800 IU of vitamin E (as d-alpha-tocopherol succinate) at the onset of bursitis. If you currently take a dose of this magnitude, increase your regular dose by 200 IU per day until the inflammation and pain subside.

• *Quercetin* and other *bioflavonoids* slow down or prevent the transformation of arachidonic acid (a fatty acid) into the "bad" eicosinoids that promote inflammation and pain. Reread the discussion on eicosinoids on pages 24–27 in Section I for a full explanation of these chemical messengers. Recommendation: Take 500 mg to 1000 mg twice daily.

• *The essential fatty acids,* linoleic acid (GLA) and fish oils (EPA), are the basic nutrients from which your body makes potent natural anti-inflammatory chemicals called *prostaglandins.* Not all prostaglandins are "good" ones that ward off inflammation and pain—some actually cause inflammation. The diet you eat to a large degree governs whether you make "good" ones or "bad" ones and therefore whether you increase inflammation and pain in an injured joint and its bursa or relieve it. Please turn to the full discussion of these essential fats and the way that diet can control their effect in Section I, on eicosinoids, pages 24–27. Recommendation: Take 2 EicoPro capsules 1 to 3 times daily, or if you are unable to obtain this product, you can make a reasonable substitute by taking 500 mg evening primrose oil along with 1000 mg EPA fish oil and 100 IU vitamin E 1 to 3 times a day. (Warning to diabetics: EPA fish oil can cause blood sugar fluctuations in some diabetics. Carefully monitor your blood sugar if you use this supplemental oil and discontinue its use if your blood sugar becomes difficult to control.)

Herbal remedies

• *Willow bark* is the original aspirin; meadowsweet and wintergreen produce similar results. They contain salicylates, which are natural precursors of aspirin. You can take these in the form of tea or tincture. Caution: If you are allergic to aspirin, you probably don't want to try these herbs.

• *Licorice* is as effective for bursitis as hydrocortisone, but without the nasty side effects. It acts as an anti-inflammatory. Caution: Long-term use can result in headache, lethargy, sodium and water retention, loss of potassium, and high blood pressure.

• To repair tissue and stimulate healing, try *horsetail* extract.

Dosages may vary, depending on duration and severity of symptoms. Consult a qualified herbal practitioner. Let your physician know of your decision to use herbs; not all herbal remedies can be used in conjunction with conventional pharmaceuticals.

What makes it worse?

• I know of no specific nutrients that worsen bursitis.

──────────── **Calf Cramps** ────────────

(see Atherosclerosis and Muscle Cramps)

──────────── **Canker Sores** ────────────

(see Aphthous Stomatitis)

──────────── **Capillary Fragility** ────────────

What is it?

If you tend to bruise easily—sometimes without even knowing what you did to cause the bruise—you may have fragile capillaries.* Or perhaps you notice a little bleeding from your gums when you brush your teeth or use dental floss or a Water Pik. Maybe you've

───────────────────

*Easy bruising and bleeding can also be early warning signs of more serious health problems. Before you undertake nutritional therapy to alleviate these symptoms, please consult your personal physician about them.

always been troubled by occasional nosebleeds that come on without warning. You may not think much about these symptoms, but their cause may certainly be nutritional. The bleeding may occur because the tiny blood vessels (the capillaries) in the gum tissue, the skin, or the lining of the nose have become so weak that now minor trauma—as little as your brushing your teeth or a minor blow—can break them. The weakness is usually the result of poorly made collagen that tears more easily, a weakened structure that comes about from certain dietary deficiencies.

What helps it?

• Deficiency of *vitamin C* plays a greater role than any other nutrient in causing weak capillaries that bleed easily. One of the earliest (and least dangerous) signs of the deficiency of vitamin C— scurvy—is bleeding of the gums. You may find it interesting to read the discussion in Section I about the discovery of scurvy. In the A-to-Z Nutrient listings in Section I, you will also find a more detailed discussion of how vitamin C works in the production of strong collagen. Recommendation: If possible, purchase vitamin C (ascorbic acid) in crystalline (powdered) form. Each teaspoon should contain 4 grams of vitamin C. Begin with ⅛ teaspoon (500 mg) once a day. After a few days, increase to ¼ teaspoon (1000 mg or 1 gram) once a day. Then take that dose (¼ teaspoon) twice a day. After you have reached this dose level, which gives you 2000 mg (or 2 grams) of vitamin C per day, begin to increase the amount taken at each dose (½ teaspoon next) or the frequency of dosing (3 times a day, 4 times a day) until you reach your bowel tolerance level (see Vitamin C, Section I, page 54) or reach a daily dose of 4 to 8 grams. By this time you should no longer be seeing bleeding gums or frequent nosebleeds, and you should find that you bruise less easily.

• The action of vitamin C on capillary fragility is improved if you add *bioflavonoids* to it. The bioflavonoid *hesperidin* works well in this regard. Recommendation: Take 200 mg hesperidin plus 200 to 250 mg vitamin C with each meal and at bedtime (4 doses spaced throughout the day) for 2 weeks. Then reduce your dose to 100 mg of each 4 times a day (still at meals and bedtime) until your symptoms disappear. Then maintain your intake at 200 mg of each taken only once per day.

• In bruising rashes (called purpura) brought on by infection, reactions to medications, or other allergic reactions, which all act to make the capillaries fragile, *vitamin E* seems to speed clearance of the rash. Let me stress that I do not intend to imply that vitamin E treats the causes of these rashes, only that it will help to clear the rash that develops because of them. Recommendation: Take 400 IU to 600 IU vitamin E (as d-alpha-tocopherol) daily for 3 weeks.

• A deficiency in *zinc* may contribute to the fragility of blood vessels in the thinned skin of older people. Recommendation: 100 mg chelated zinc daily for 3 to 6 months. Warning: Supplementation of zinc in its ionic form can create deficiencies of other minerals, such as copper, by competing with them for absorption from the intestine. Chelation of the minerals (see pages 30–31, Section I, on chelation) prevents this competition, allowing you to fully absorb each of the minerals.

Herbal remedies

• *Arnica* has pain-relieving, antiseptic, and anti-inflammatory properties. Use it topically to treat bruises. Commercial products that contain up to 15% arnica oil should do the job if you follow directions on the label.

• Among the oldest skin problem remedies is *comfrey*. This herb contains allantoin, a chemical that promotes skin repair. Commission E in Germany discovered evidence that this herb is also anti-inflammatory. If applied quickly, comfrey can prevent some discoloration. Apply a bandage soaked in comfrey tea. Do not ingest this herb.

• *St. John's wort* is useful for treating bruises and other wounds. Steep 1 to 2 teaspoons of dried herb in vegetable oil for a few days, then apply directly to the bruise. Tinctures and salves also work well.

Dosages may vary, depending on the duration and severity of your symptoms. Follow package directions, or consult a qualified herbal practitioner.

What makes it worse?

• I know of no nutrients that of themselves worsen capillary fragility.

Aspirin decreases the ability of blood to clot and may worsen bruising and prolong bleeding with injury.

——————— **Cardiac Arrhythmias** ———————

What are they?

The most enduring and dependable muscle in your body is your heart. It contracts and relaxes at an average rate of about 60 to 80 times every minute of every hour of every day of your life. Imagine any other muscle—one in your arm or your calf, for example—flexing and relaxing once a second, day and night, without stopping. Now imagine the terrible muscle soreness and cramps from use that even an hour of such extreme overwork would cause the next morning in your arm or calf muscles. And yet your heart does it, usually without complaint, if you're thoughtful enough to provide it with good nutrition and plenty of oxygen. The beating of the heart depends on the transmission of regularly spaced nerve impulses from a structure called the pacemaker. It sends a sort of electrical signal to organize contracting the muscle fibers, so that they work as a unit in a coordinated fashion. When something causes a short-circuiting of these nerve impulses, the electrical signal doesn't transmit properly, and the garbled signal causes disruption of the normal regular heart rhythm. The disruption results in skipping of beats, fluttering or twitching of the heart muscle, extra beats, or racing of the heart rate—what your doctor would call a heart rhythm problem, or cardiac arrhythmia. There are a number of nutrients that the heart requires to do its 24-hour-a-day job and some that worsen the rhythm problems. Let's take a look at these.

What helps them?

• *Vitamin D* is important in making calcium (which is necessary to generate the electrical signal) available to the pacemaker of the heart, although the exact nature of its role is unclear. Deficiency of the vitamin appears to make rhythm problems more difficult to treat. Refer to the discussion of this vitamin in the A-to-Z listings in Section I and read it thoroughly. Recommendation: Aim for 400 IU to 800 IU vitamin D per day to prevent deficiency. Remember that the manufacturers of milk products usually add vitamin D to their dairy foods, so your supplemental need will depend on how much you eat of low-fat dairy sources. Strive for a total daily intake of 400 IU to 800 IU.

• *Vitamin E* makes the heart muscle fibers resist developing abnormal rhythms from the short-circuited electrical nerve impulses. This effect is especially important if you have poor heart circulation and angina (see Atherosclerosis). Recommendation: Begin with a dose of 100 IU per day and remain there for 1 week. Because in some people vitamin E can increase blood pressure, be sure to have your blood pressure taken before you move on to a higher dose. If your average blood pressure has not risen above 140/90, increase your daily intake to 200 IU and then to 400 IU of vitamin E (in the form of alpha-tocopherol succinate) daily. Larger adults may increase to 800 IU per day as a maximum dose.

• *Magnesium* can reduce or stop abnormal heart rhythms in some cases. This effect is especially beneficial in arrhythmias that occur because of taking too much digitalis* or after heart muscle damage from a heart attack, but may also help abnormal rhythms due to other causes. Recommendation: Take magnesium in a dose of 200 to 400 mg daily. The mineral works best when taken along with its related mineral, calcium, and I would therefore recommend an intake of about 500 mg calcium for each 250 mg magnesium.

• *Potassium,* another mineral important to normal electrical function of the heart, can cause rhythm changes when your blood levels of potassium fall too low or become too high. It's another of those body chemicals that needs to stay in the "just right" range. The vast bulk of the potassium in your body is inside the individual cells, which act as a giant reservoir to keep the level in your blood pretty constant under normal conditions. Those conditions change, for example, if you take certain medications, like diuretics (fluid pills), which cause your kidneys to lose potassium, and you can become deficient in potassium. Or the conditions change if you have kidney damage and cannot eliminate an excess of potassium, putting you at risk for elevated blood levels. Under normal circumstances, however, your kidneys and the storage reservoir inside your cells work together to keep you in the right range. Recommendation: Under normal conditions, eating foods rich in potassium, such as broccoli, bananas, tomatoes, and oranges, should be sufficient. If you take diuretic pills, however, you may need to increase your potassium

---

*Digitalis (digoxin, or Lanoxin) is a drug used to make the heart muscle contract more effectively when it has become weakened after heart attack damage. The drug has what is called a narrow therapeutic range, meaning that the amount of the drug necessary to do the job is just a short jump away from the amount of drug that is deadly. One of the effects of too much digitalis is the development of abnormal heart rhythms.

intake. Use a product called NO SALT, which is an over-the-counter salt substitute, available in most grocery stores, containing potassium chloride and potassium bitartrate. One-fourth of a teaspoon will provide enough potassium, sprinkled on your food or added in when cooking. Or you can take potassium gluconate tablets, available at most health and nutrition stores, at a dose of 99 mg each.

• *Coenzyme Q_{10}*, a bioflavonoid, may help to reduce the frequency of PVCs—the early beats, extra beats, or skipping of beats of the heart's ventricles (the muscle tissue making up the main pumping chambers of the heart)—in some people. Recommendation: Take coenzyme Q_{10} in a dose of 50 to 100 mg per day. You should see improvement (fewer PVCs) after 1 to 2 weeks if your arrhythmia is going to respond to this treatment.

• *Essential fatty acids* also seem to help reduce the risk of arrhythmias, probably through the "good" prostaglandins made from them. Among the many other effects that make these chemical messengers so good for you is their ability to relax the muscle layer in the walls of the arteries supplying blood to the heart muscle itself: Relaxed arteries bring more blood, which carries in more oxygen, which keeps the heart healthy and happy. Supplementing your diet with essential fats is especially important. Recommendation: Begin with a solid macronutrient framework (see Macronutrients, Section I, page 23), and to that sound base add gamma-linoleic acid (GLA) to EPA fish oil in a ratio of 1:4 (GLA:EPA) 1 to 3 times daily. The EicoPro essential fatty acid product manufactured by Eicotec, Inc., of Marblehead, Massachusetts, contains ultrapure sources of linoleic acid and fish oils already combined in the proper ratio. If you cannot get that product, you can purchase linoleic acid in a product called evening primrose oil at most health and nutrition stores, and EPA fish oil as well. Because it is not as pure a form, the milligram dosing will be different. You can make a reasonable substitute by combining evening primrose oil capsules with fish oil capsules plus vitamin E. Take 500 mg of evening primrose oil (a source of linoleic acid in capsule form), plus 1000 mg EPA fish oil, plus 200 IU vitamin E 1 to 3 times a day. (Warning to diabetics: EPA fish oil can cause blood sugar fluctuations in some diabetics. Carefully monitor your blood sugar if you use this supplemental oil and discontinue its use if your blood sugar becomes difficult to control.)

Herbal remedies

• *Angelica* contains at least 14 anti-arrhythmic compounds.

• Quinidine is standard anti-arrhythmic medication and is also a compound found in *cinchona*. This herb contains about 12 other helpful compounds as well.

• Studies show that *hawthorn* strengthens the heart muscle, improving blood circulation throughout the heart and reducing the heart's need for oxygen. Unlike other herbs, it is important to use the correct extracts of hawthorn. The recommended extracts contain 1.8% vitexin-4-rhamnoside or 10% oligomeric procyanidins (OPCs) in dosages of 120 to 240 mg 3 times daily. If the extracts are standardized to 18% OPCs, the recommended dosage is 240 to 480 mg once daily. You must consult a naturopath to get these extracts. Caution: There have been reports that hawthorn may increase arrhythmias in some cases. It is of vital importance that you be monitored by a doctor should you choose to use this herb.

• According to Dr. Melvyn Werbach, of the University of California, Los Angeles, School of Medicine, *barberry* helps prevent and treat ventricular arrhythmias. One study showed the herb reduced arrhythmias by more than 50% in more than half the people who used it. I recommend a standard herbal extract.

• Like *hawthorn*, *ginkgo* improves blood flow to the heart and lessens the demand for oxygen. It certainly can't hurt in treating arrhythmias. Caution: In high amounts, this herb may cause diarrhea, irritability, and restlessness.

• *Horehound*, best known for its treatment for coughs and colds, also has a normalizing effect of heart rhythm.

• Chinese studies show that *motherwort* slows a rapid heartbeat, tranquilizes the nervous system, and generally improves cardiac activity.

• *Reishi* is a heart tonic that has effects similar to hawthorn and ginkgo.

• Though best known as a sleep enhancer, *valerian* also contains anti-arrhythmic compounds, and has been used to treat related disorders since Roman times. It also lowers blood pressure and increases blood flow to the heart.

Dosages vary, depending on duration and severity of symptoms. Some herbal remedies are not to be combined with conventional pharmaceuticals. Consult a qualified herbal practitioner, and tell your physician before starting any herbal regimen.

What makes them worse?

• *Alcohol* slowly damages the heart muscle, making it weaker and more susceptible to rhythm disturbances, although it may take 10 years of chronic abuse of alcohol before signs of heart muscle damage show up. Fluttering of the heart may be one of the early signs of this kind of damage. Recommendation: Stop drinking alcohol. If you are a social or occasional drinker, quitting should present no problems. However, if you've been drinking multiple drinks on a daily basis for many years, stopping abruptly can sometimes be dangerous. I would recommend your getting some help to quit from your physician, from a community or regional alcoholic treatment program, or at least with the help of your local chapter of Alcoholics Anonymous.

• *Caffeine* seems to make abnormal heart rhythms worse for some people, but not for others. No clear-cut reason emerges from the medical research to explain these contradictory responses. My advice to you is to listen to your body to determine whether your heart rhythm problems get worse when you drink caffeine-containing beverages (coffee, tea, and many soft drinks) or eat chocolate. Recommendation: If you find that these foods do give you problems, then I would recommend you avoid them. If, on the other hand, caffeine seems to cause you no ill effect, then the medical evidence at this point really doesn't support a need for you to give up your morning coffee.

• *Saturated fat* intake can make your heart's electrical system more susceptible to the production of short-circuited signals. Recommendation: Decrease your consumption of saturated fats to 10% of your total caloric intake. Substitute monounsaturated oils, such as cold-pressed, virgin, or extra-virgin olive oil or canola oil in cooking and salad dressings for animal fat, lard, bacon drippings, or butter. Avoid deep-frying foods, even in polyunsaturated fats or oils. Use leaner cuts of meat or poultry: Trim away all visible fat, remove the skin of chicken, and cut down on fatty meat products such as sausage, bacon, or hot dogs. Increase the amount of fish and seafood you eat—but don't batter it and deep-fry it or you'll defeat the purpose. Use low- or nonfat dairy products as much as possible.

• *Food allergies and sensitivities* may also cause fluttering or skipping symptoms in the heart. If you are a person who suffers from allergies, and if you also have heart rhythm problems, the two may be connected, and you may wish to ask your allergist or personal physician to investigate the possibility. Recommendation: Begin to systematically avoid foods you think may cause the problem one at a time. If your symptoms disappear, you're home free. If they do not, however, continue your step-by-step search. Typical offenders are chocolate, strawberries, wheat, various food dyes, and sugar, but any food is possible.

——————— Cardiovascular Disease ———————

What is it?

Cardiovascular disease is the number-one cause of death in the United States, claiming more than 1 million lives annually. An estimated 50 million Americans are afflicted with heart and blood vessel disease, though many show no symptoms and so are unaware of the condition.

There are many types of cardiovascular disease, including angina, heart attack, hypertension, heart failure, arrhythmias, and valvular disease. Let's take a quick look at each of these:

• Angina refers to a heavy, tight pain in the chest that occurs after some type of exertion. It happens when the blood vessels narrow and fail to supply the heart with a sufficient amount of oxygen.

• Heart attacks occur when the coronary arteries that carry oxygen and nutrients to the heart muscles become obstructed. Signs of heart attack include pain in the chest that can extend to the shoulder, arm, neck, and jaw. Other signs include sweating, nausea, vomiting, shortness of breath, dizziness, fainting, anxiety, ringing in the ears, loss of speech, and difficulty swallowing. Not everyone experiences the same degree of pain. In fact, many people mistake the signs for indigestion. Others have no symptoms at all, a situation referred to as a "silent heart attack."

• Hypertension is also known as high blood pressure and is very common. It is usually caused by a decrease in the elasticity or a reduction in the interior diameter of the arteries. This form of cardiovascular disease is basically painless. By the time a person experiences the symptoms—rapid pulse, shortness of breath, dizziness, headaches, and sweating—the condition is more difficult to treat. If untreated, it drastically increases the risk of heart attack, heart failure, and kidney failure.

• Heart failure occurs when there is an inadequate flow of blood from the heart. Symptoms include poor color, fatigue, shortness of breath, and edema.

• Arrhythmias are disturbances in the normal rhythm of the heartbeat. Some are dangerous while others are harmless, though annoying.

• Valvular disease is a term used for disorders that impair the functioning of one or more of the heart's valves. Cardiovascular disease often reaches an advanced stage before detection of symptoms. Experts estimate that 25% of people who have heart attacks had no warning signs or symptoms. Yet every minute, someone in America dies of a heart attack.

The good news is that cardiovascular disease is not an inevitable result of aging, and there are many preventive measures you can take. Controllable factors that can contribute to heart disease include smoking, high blood pressure, cholesterol problems, stress, obesity, a sedentary lifestyle, and diabetes.

What helps it?

• *Coenzyme Q10* increases oxygenation of heart tissue and has been shown to prevent recurrences in individuals who have had a heart attack. Recommendation: Take 50 to 100 mg 3 times daily.

• *Calcium* and *magnesium* are necessary for proper functioning of the cardiac muscle. Recommendation: Supplement calcium at 1500 to 2000 mg daily, in divided doses. Take 750 to 1000 mg daily of magnesium, in divided doses. Use the chelate form of each.

• To lower blood pressure and thin the blood, consume *garlic*. Recommendation: Take 2 capsules 3 times daily.

• *L-carnitine* reduces fat and triglyceride levels in the blood while it increases oxygen uptake. Recommendation: Take 500 mg twice daily on an empty stomach.

• *Dimethylglycine* acts as a building block for a number of important substances, including hormones, neurotransmitters, and DNA. It also enhances the utilization of oxygen. Recommendation: Take 50 mg 4 times daily.

• *Potassium* is important if you are taking cortisone or blood pressure medication because it keeps your electrolyte level in balance. Recommendation: Take 99 mg daily.

• A deficiency of *selenium* has been linked with heart disease. Recommendation: Take 200 *micro*grams daily.

• *Vitamin E* strengthens the heart muscle, improves circulation, and destroys free radicals. Recommendation: Start with 100 to 200 IU daily and slowly increase by 100 IU each week until your daily dosage reaches 800 to 1000 IU. Warning: Use this supplement only under the supervision of a physician, and do not exceed 400 IU daily if you take an anticoagulant drug.

• *Vitamin B_1* is important for strength of the heart muscle. A deficiency has been linked to heart disease. Recommendation: Take 50 mg daily.

• To lower cholesterol and improve circulation, supplement your intake of *vitamin B_3*. Recommendation: Take 50 mg daily. Warning: Do not take niacin if you have a liver disorder, gout, or high blood pressure.

• A deficiency of vitamin B_6 has been linked to heart disease. Recommendation: Take 50 mg daily.

• *Vitamin C* is very important in treating cardiovascular disease because it has been shown to reduce serum cholesterol. Some experts even think that vitamin C plays a role in moving cholesterol from the arteries to the liver, where it is converted into bile acids and then eliminated along with fiber. Vitamin C helps repair damaged arterial walls, which prevents cholesterol deposits from forming. Recommendation: Supplement 1000 mg 3 times daily using a vitamin C/bioflavonoid combination.

• *Chromium* depletion has been implicated in cardiovascular disorders because of its role in insulin production and glucose regulation. Recommendation: Take 400 to 600 *micro*grams daily.

• *N-acetylcysteine* (NAC) seems to be useful in treating and preventing this disorder. It lowers levels of lipoprotein (a), which is important because high levels of lipoprotein (a) have been associated with an increased risk of cardiovascular diseases. Recommendation: Supplement with 1 to 3 grams daily of NAC.

Herbal remedies

• *Suma* can be made into a tea. Drink 3 cups daily, and take with it ginkgo extract as directed on the label.

• Other herbs that may be beneficial include *barberry, black cohosh, butcher's broom, cayenne, dandelion, ginseng, hawthorn berries, and valerian root.* Caution: Do not use barberry or black cohosh if you are pregnant. Do not use ginseng if you have high blood pressure.

Dosages may vary, depending on the duration and severity of your symptoms. Consult a qualified herbal practitioner, and talk to your doctor before beginning herbal remedies. Some remedies cannot be used in combination with conventional pharmaceuticals.

What makes it worse?
• Abnormally high blood *copper* levels are often found in people who have experienced a heart attack. The reason is not totally clear, but it may be that increased levels of copper play a role in the development and progression of this condition, or perhaps the body circulates more copper in an attempt to deal with the condition. Recommendation: Ask your physician for a routine blood test if you want to check your blood copper level. Eliminate all *sodium* sources from your diet. Any products whose label includes "soda," "sodium," or the symbol "Na" should be avoided.

• Eat a well-balanced *diet* that contains plenty of fiber. Get your protein from low-fat sources such as broiled fish and skinless turkey or chicken.

• Although the FDA claims that taking 1 baby aspirin daily can reduce the risk of heart attack without side effects, a Harvard Medical School newsletter asserts that there is no sufficient evidence to support this. If you do use aspirin, remember that it can cause internal bleeding and stomach ulceration.

─────────── **Carpal Tunnel Syndrome** ───────────

What is it?
The medical name for the bones of your wrist are the carpals or carpal bones. At the bend of your wrist, a thick fibrous band of tissue forms the roof of a "tunnel" across the carpals to make a protected path, or "tunnel," through which the nerves, veins, arteries, and tendons travel on their way from your arm into your hand. This is the carpal tunnel. Occasionally, the area becomes inflamed from injury or repetitive use, during pregnancy, and in inflammatory arthritic conditions, such as rheumatoid arthritis. Swelling from the

inflammation puts pressure on the nerves running in the tunnel, "pinching" them and causing the syndrome: pain, numbness, stiffness, weakness, and loss of use of the hand and, oddly enough, the arm as far as the elbow and even the shoulder. The ultimate treatment for this syndrome may require surgery to relieve the pinch on the nerve, but before that point, the vitamin shelf may offer some help.

What helps it?

Medical studies on people suffering from carpal tunnel pain have often shown them to be deficient in *vitamin B_6* (pyridoxine). When that is the case, taking the vitamin gives some relief of symptoms. Recommendation: Take 100 mg daily (along with B-complex as described below). Although some relief may begin in a few weeks, you should continue the treatment for 12 weeks. Warning: I would not advise your increasing your dose beyond this level. At doses as little as 200 mg per day over several years, some people develop nerve damage, and the potential for benefit is simply not worth that risk. In order to use vitamin B_6, your body must have a sufficient supply of *riboflavin* (vitamin B_2) and the other members of the B-complex group. Recommendation: Take 100 mg B-complex 3 times each day.

Herbal remedies

• *Willow bark* is the original aspirin that relieves pain and reduces swelling. Caution: I don't recommend this herb if you are allergic to aspirin.

• Although *chamomile* is best known for its ability to calm your nerves, is also has powerful anti-inflammatory action. An herbal tea works well in this case.

• *Cumin* has 3 pain-relieving compounds, as well as numerous anti-inflammatory substances. Add this spice to your food liberally.

• *Sage* is another spice with anti-inflammatory compounds.

Dosages may vary, depending on the duration and severity of your symptoms. Consult a qualified health practitioner before beginning any herbal regimen.

What makes it worse?

• I know of no nutrient that worsens carpal tunnel syndrome or hastens its development.

• Carpal tunnel syndrome can develop as a side effect of taking the

medication/mineral *lithium,* prescribed by physicians for the treatment of bipolar (manic-depressive) disorder. This side effect usually
occurs when control of symptoms requires high doses of the mineral.
Recommendation: Unless your physician specifically recommends
you continue lithium, if you suffer from carpal tunnel syndrome, a
trial period off medication to assess whether taking the drug worsens
your symptoms is probably prudent.

Cataract

What is it?

The lenses inside your eyes are crystal-clear structures that sit directly behind your pupil and help to bring what you look at into
focus. When you are young, your lenses are supple and their shape
is easily changed by the tugging of tiny muscles attached to them to
let you see clearly up close and far away. As the years pass, however,
the process of aging not only stiffens the lens, making it hard to see
close objects clearly, but causes opaque spots to form, like flaws in
a diamond, inside the clear lens. These flaws, or cataracts, are not
clear; they cause a fogginess to what you see. If left unattended to
the point that the entire lens becomes opaque, you could not see at
all from that eye. One of the truly miraculous advances in medicine
is that eye surgeons can remove the aged cloudy lens and replace it
with an artificial lens, restoring vision. Once the cataract has advanced to a stage where vision is greatly reduced, surgery is the only
option to clear vision. But earlier in life, several nutrients play a part
in preventing the formation of cataracts or in arresting their growth
before they reach a size to severely hamper your vision. Let's take a
look at these nutrients.

What helps it?

• Medical research has reported that people who eat diets low in
vitamin C have a greater risk for developing cataracts. The reason
for this connection very likely hinges on vitamin C's role as an antioxidant. Refer again to oxidation, free radicals, and antioxidants,
found on pages 18–23 in Section I, for more details. Even after you
have begun early development of cataracts, vitamin C helps slow or
stall the process and improve vision. Recommendation: If you do
not currently take vitamin C, begin with this regimen. If possible,
purchase vitamin C (ascorbic acid) in crystalline (powdered) form.
Each teaspoon should contain 4 grams of vitamin C. Begin with ⅛

teaspoon (500 mg) once a day. After a few days, increase to ¼ teaspoon (1000 mg or 1 gram) once a day. Then take that dose (¼ teaspoon) twice a day. After you have reached this dose level, which gives you 2000 mg (or 2 grams) of vitamin C per day, begin to increase the amount taken at each dose (½ teaspoon next) or frequency of dosing (3 times a day, 4 times a day) until you reach your bowel tolerance level (see Vitamin C, Section I, page 50) or reach a daily dose of 4 to 8 grams. If you currently take vitamin C in a tablet, pick up the regimen at the dose you currently take and increase from there. A combination of *vitamin A along with vitamin C* also seems to arrest the progression of cataracts and decrease the need for cataract surgery. The earlier in the process you begin, the better the response. Recommendation: Take 10,000 IU to 20,000 IU vitamin A per day along with at least 1 gram of vitamin C. Refer to the discussion of vitamin A and familiarize yourself with the symptoms of taking too much of this vitamin. Because your body stores the vitamin, toxic levels can build up. You must be very careful in taking vitamin A supplements to not overdo it.

• *Vitamin E,* another of the strong antioxidant, free radical scavenging vitamins, also plays a crucial role in protecting your lenses from the development of cataracts. If you have direct family members who have developed cataracts, you can reduce your risk of doing so by as much as 50% just by taking vitamin E daily. Recommendation: Begin with a dose of 100 IU per day and remain there for 1 week. Because in some people vitamin E can increase blood pressure, be sure to have your blood pressure taken before you move on to a higher dose. If your average blood pressure has not risen above 140/90, increase your daily intake to 200 IU and then to 400 IU of vitamin E (in the form of alpha-tocopherol succinate) daily. Larger adults may increase to 800 IU per day as a maximum dose for this condition as long as blood pressure remains normal for them.

• *Selenium,* the mineral that the body needs to produce its own potent free radical scavenger *glutathione peroxidase,* also helps reduce the aging of the lens of the eye. By taking a small dose of selenium, you can reduce the amount of vitamin E you take. This interaction is especially important in people who suffer from high blood pressure and may not be able to take a higher amount of vitamin E. Recommendation: Take 400 *micro*grams of selenium along with 100 IU to 200 IU of vitamin E daily.

• *Beta-carotene,* a forerunner and relative of vitamin A, also helps to protect the eye from oxidation and aging. Because beta-carotene is much less toxic than vitamin A, you may tolerate taking it with fewer side effects. Recommendation: First increase your intake of food sources rich in beta-carotene, such as orange, yellow, and dark green vegetables. Then add a daily supplement of 15,000 IU to 30,000 IU per day.

• People with early cataract development often prove to be deficient in *riboflavin (vitamin B_2)*. No clear evidence suggests that the deficiency causes the cataract, but one study found riboflavin deficiency in 80% of the people with cataracts, but in only 12% of those without cataracts. In a small study at the University of Georgia (1976), all the people treated with riboflavin reported improvement of symptoms in as little as 24 to 48 hours. Within 9 months of daily treatment, the cataract opacities had disappeared. But before you rush out to purchase riboflavin, let me add that in this case you can get too much of a good thing. Supplementation of greater than 10 mg per day increases the production of free radicals and could hasten cataract formation unless you counter the free radical attack by taking vitamins C, E, and selenium. Recommendation: Take 50 mg riboflavin along with the doses of vitamins C and E and selenium suggested in this section.

• Deficiency of *zinc,* necessary for normal glucose use by the cells of the lens, seems to promote the formation of cataracts in laboratory animals (including fish) and in people. Supplementation with zinc becomes especially important for the elderly, who frequently suffer from this mineral deficiency and more often develop cataracts. Recommendation: Take 50 mg to 100 mg of chelated zinc (zinc aspartate or zinc picolinate) daily for 6 to 8 weeks. Then reduce your daily dose to 25 to 50 mg per day. Warning: Supplementation of zinc in its ionic form can create deficiencies of other minerals, such as copper, by competing with them for absorption from the intestine. Chelation of the minerals (see pages 30–31, Section I, on chelation) prevents this competition to get into the body, allowing you to fully absorb each mineral.

Herbal remedies

• *Bilberry* improves night vision. This fruit and its relatives (blueberry, cranberry, huckleberry, blackberry, raspberry, grape, plum, and wild cherry) contain anthocyanosides, compounds that contribute to visual acuity. An Italian study shows that bilberry plus vitamin E halted the progression of lens clouding in 97% of people with early-stage cataracts. This herb can be found in standardized extract. You can also make a tea using 2 to 4 tablespoons of crushed berries, or just eat a cup of berries.

• *Rosemary* contains more than 12 antioxidants, 4 of which are known cataract fighters. Use it liberally in cooking.

• *Purslane* contains all the nutrients that help prevent cataracts: vitamins C and E, carotenoids, and other antioxidants. This herb is not easy to find, but you can grow it yourself, indoors or out.

• *Ginger* is an antioxidant as well as a very popular spice. Use it liberally in your cooking.

Dosages may vary, depending on the duration and severity of your symptoms. Consult a qualified herbal practitioner before beginning any herbal remedy.

What makes it worse?

• An article in *Science* magazine reported that the greatest cause of cataracts is the body's inability to cope with food *sugars*. The worst offender is lactose, followed by refined white sugar. Simple sugars include: table sugar and corn syrup (sucrose), honey (glucose), milk sugar (lactose), fruit sugar (fructose), and xylose, the sugar-like substance often used to sweeten "sugar-free" diabetic candies, chewing gum, and cookies. Recommendation: Sharply reduce or even eliminate your intake of sucrose and xylose products. Let the dietary sugars you do eat come mainly from fresh fruit and dairy sources, keeping the total amount of even these sugars at 30% to 50% of your daily carbohydrate intake. Refer to the discussion of macronutrients on page 23 of Section I for more dietary information.

• *Dairy products,* as mentioned above, and the simple sugar found in milk—lactose—can promote cataract formation, especially in some people who have inherited a difficulty in metabolizing lactose and its "cousin," galactose. If you have a family risk for such a lactose sugar metabolism disorder (and if you do, you will likely already know it), dairy products of all types will be a problem. Let me clarify that this kind of inherited problem with metabolizing lactose is not the same thing as "lactose intolerance" or "milk intolerance," which causes bloating, gas, stomach cramping, and diarrhea in some people when they eat dairy products. This latter kind of milk intolerance occurs in people who lack an enzyme in their intestine needed to break down the milk sugar and absorb it properly. And although these people may wish to avoid dairy products in order to avoid these unpleasant symptoms, they are not among the group at increased risk for cataracts because of high lactose intake.

———————— Cavities/Tooth Decay ————————

What is it?

Tooth decay and its related disorders are not natural processes but are caused by bacteria in the mouth that combine with mucus and food debris to create plaque. These bacteria feed on ingested sugars and produce an acid that sucks calcium and phosphate from the teeth. Tooth decay relies on three factors: the presence of bacteria, the availability of sugars, and the vulnerability of tooth enamel. Does nutrition play a role in prevention? You bet; let's see how.

What helps it?

• It should come as no shock that *calcium* is necessary for strong, healthy teeth. Recommendation: Take 1500 mg daily, in tandem with 750 mg of *magnesium*.

• *Vitamin A* is important for healing and for tooth formation. Recommendation: Take 10,000 IU daily. Warning: Do not exceed 8000 IU daily if you are pregnant.

• *Vitamin C* is useful in preventing and treating tooth decay because it protects against infection and inflammation. Recommendation: Supplement with 3000 mg daily, in divided doses. Warning: Do NOT use a chewable form, as it can erode tooth enamel. To help calcium absorption and to heal gum tissue, take *vitamin D*. Recommendation: Take 400 mg daily.

• *Vitamin E* is a powerful antioxidant that promotes healing. Recommendation: Take 600 IU daily.

• Zinc is a necessary nutrient in the process of bone formation. Recommendation: Take 30 mg daily in the form of zinc gluconate.

• *Raw fruits and vegetables* keep the saliva from becoming too acidic, which is another factor that puts you at risk for tooth decay.

Herbal remedies

• *Tea* contains quite a generous amount of fluoride. Because there are other anticavity compounds besides fluoride in tea, you don't need much to benefit from it.

• *Bay* has the potential to prevent tooth decay because it kills bacteria. Look for it in toothpaste that is carried at your natural foods store.

• Studies indicate that *bloodroot* reduces the amount of plaque and prevents it from adhering to teeth.

Dosages may vary, depending on the duration and severity of your symptoms. Follow package directions, or consult a qualified herbal practitioner.

What makes it worse?

• *Carbonated beverages* contain high levels of phosphates, which promote the loss of calcium from the tooth enamel. Recommendation: Sharply curtail or eliminate your consumption of carbonated drinks.

Celiac Sprue

What is it?

Probably better thought of as "gluten intolerance," celiac sprue is a disorder in which the lining of the intestine reacts to the protein (called gliadin) found in wheat, oats, barley, and rye. The irritated intestine ceases to function properly and becomes unable to absorb fat (and ultimately protein, starch, and water as well). The unabsorbed fat passes through, causing bulky, pale, frothy, greasy bowel movements that smell quite foul and float. Unfortunately, if you cannot absorb fat, you also cannot absorb a number of other crucial nutrients, such as the fat-soluble vitamins A, D, E, and K. Deficiencies of these vitamins, the B vitamin group, and important minerals, such as iron, zinc, and selenium, cause a whole host of medical problems for the person suffering with celiac sprue: anemia, depression, dry skin, swelling, cracking at the edges of the mouth, bruising, and weak bones, to name only a few. I invite you to review the discussion of each of these vitamins and minerals in the A-to-Z Nutrient listings to see how many and varied the symptoms occasioned by deficiencies that occur with celiac sprue can be. The treatment is quite straightforward: Totally eliminate gluten from your diet. With elimination, your symptoms will clear. If you eat gluten-containing foods, your symptoms will quickly return. I have included specific dietary recommendations on what foods you must avoid under "What makes it worse?" on page 247, but first let's see what nutrients you may need.

What helps it?

• *Folic acid* deficiency occurs frequently in people suffering with celiac sprue, although not to as severe a degree as in a similar bowel disorder called tropical sprue. Deficiency of folic acid contributes to anemia, and until the sprue symptoms respond to elimination of gluten, you should supplement folic acid. Recommendation: Take at least 5 mg folic acid daily. Warning: Read the discussion about this vitamin in Section I before supplementing. You may also need to take B_{12} in shot form at a dose of 1000 *micro*grams weekly for 4 weeks, then 500 to 1000 *micro*grams monthly for 3 to 6 months while supplementing folic acid.

• *Vitamin B_{12}* taken orally may not do much good, because the irritated intestinal lining can't absorb it very well. As noted above, you should take B_{12} by injection into the muscle.

• Your irritated intestinal lining may also not be able to absorb *vitamin B_6* (pyridoxine) to a normal degree. The emotional depression that many people with sprue develop will sometimes respond to supplementation of this vitamin. Recommendation: Take 50 to 80 mg of pyridoxine daily for 6 months. Warning: Take care increasing your dose beyond this point. There have been reports in the medical literature of nerve inflammation and damage occurring on doses of as little as 200 mg per day over a several-year period.

• In sprue, people become deficient in *vitamins A, D, E, and K,* because they are all fat-soluble vitamins. When the bowel cannot absorb fat, it also cannot absorb these vitamins very well. Until the symptoms of sprue subside with strict gluten elimination, you will need to supplement these vitamins in larger than normal amounts daily. Be sure to carefully read the discussion of each nutrient and its potential toxicity symptoms, which can develop quickly at these dosages as the intestine recovers normal function. Recommendation: Take 20,000 IU vitamin A per day, 10,000 to 20,000 IU vitamin D per day, and 1000 to 1200 IU vitamin E per day (reach this dose by slowly building up from 100 IU per day, as suggested in the Section I listing for vitamin E). You probably don't need to take vitamin K unless you are bruising extremely easily or if you tend to bleed for a prolonged period of time following minor cuts. As soon as your bowel symptoms begin to subside, cut these vitamin doses by half. Once your symptoms have cleared completely, you will probably not need to supplement vitamins A or D beyond what you can get from food sources. You may continue to supplement vitamin E at 400 IU daily.

• *Iron* deficiency occurs in sprue, again because of poor absorption by the irritated bowel lining. While you are waiting for the symptoms to subside on a gluten-free diet, you will need to supplement with iron. Once the bowel recovers its normal function, iron absorption will return to normal. Recommendation: Take iron glycinate in a dose of 20 mg daily until your sprue symptoms have cleared.

• *Selenium,* which is needed in greater amounts in states of stress and disease, becomes depleted in people suffering from sprue. The lower levels persist for quite some time even after the bowel has begun to recover on a gluten-free diet. Recommendation: Take 300 *micro*grams selenium per day until the symptoms subside. You may then drop your dose to 150 to 200 *micro*grams and remain there.

• In sprue, the use and loss of *zinc* increase, and you can become deficient in this mineral even though the bowel can still absorb it normally. Recommendation: Take 50 mg to 100 mg of chelated zinc (zinc aspartate or zinc picolinate) daily until the bowel has recovered and you are free of symptoms. Then reduce your daily dose to 20 mg per day. Warning: Supplementation of zinc in its ionic form can create deficiencies of other minerals, such as copper (which can already have become deficient through poor absorption) by competing with them for absorption from the intestine. Chelation of the minerals (see pages 30–31, Section I, on chelation) prevents this competition to get into the body, allowing you to fully absorb each of them.

Herbal remedies

• *Alfalfa* supplies vitamin K, which is often deficient in people with this disorder. I recommend getting your alfalfa in tablet form.

Dosages may vary; follow package directions.

What makes it worse?

• *Gluten,* the protein found in wheat, buckwheat, barley, oats, and rye, is the offending antagonist and the irritant that you must eliminate entirely from your diet. Recommendation: Strive for total avoidance of all products made from these grains or their flours/meals, including: breads, pastries, crackers, muffins, cereal, breading on fried foods, pasta, beer, malt, and many medication tablets that use gluten as a filler. Your grain sources become rice and corn. Fortunately, nowadays, many health and nutrition stores or specialty groceries carry rice flour, which you can use in baking in place of wheat flour.

• *Lactose,* the sugar found in dairy products, requires a special enzyme (called lactase) to be absorbed in the intestine. Although people with sprue have this enzyme, their irritated bowel lining can't make it properly. As long as the sprue is active, you may be intolerant to dairy products, and eating cheeses, milk products, or butter may cause diarrhea, cramping, and bloating. After bowel recovery using a strict gluten-free diet, you will most likely be able to tolerate dairy products once again. Recommendation: Until bowel symptoms subside, avoid dairy products. After you are symptom free, reintroduce them slowly into your diet, beginning with small servings of yogurt or cultured buttermilk, then if you tolerate those, moving on to milk, cheese, and butter.

Cervical Dysplasia

What is it?

The cervix is the knob-like end of the uterus (or womb) where it opens into the vagina. It is covered, as all exposed but still-internal body parts are, in a layer of skin-like cells that are tougher and designed to protect the deeper tissues from injury by chemicals, abrasion, and attack by viruses and bacteria. Your physician collects a sampling of these cells when you have your annual pelvic examination with a Pap smear to be sure they are healthy and normal. Occasionally, these cells in the skin-like (or epithelial) covering are injured themselves, and they begin to change. We call this change that we discover on an "abnormal" Pap smear *cervical dysplasia.* Because sometimes dysplasia leads to cancer of the cervix, you should never ignore it or downplay its importance. Many nutrients may help to reduce your risk for developing cervical dysplasia and some may even help to reverse it; however, let me stress that if you currently have an abnormal Pap smear, you must work closely with your physician, repeating Pap smears or colposcopy (a sort of magnified high-tech cell sampling technique) at 2- to 4-month intervals, or as he or she suggests, to be sure of your progress.

What helps it?

• *Folic acid* deficiency may not only increase your risk for developing cervical dysplasia, but supplementation can reverse the damage. Taking the birth control pill can cause deficiency of folic acid (see page 250), and thereby increase your risk for abnormal cervical changes. If you have had cervical dysplasia in the past and want to reduce your risk of recurrence, folic acid supplementation may be helpful. If you are at an increased risk for developing dysplasia because of frequent cervical infections (such as herpes simplex II or human papilloma virus or HPV), if you take oral contraceptive agents, or if your mother took the drug DES (diethylstilbestrol) during pregnancy, you, too, may wish to supplement with folic acid to reduce your risk of dysplasia. Recommendation: If you currently have dysplasia, take 10 mg folic acid per day for at least 6 months, following your progress with your physician at least every 8 to 12 weeks. If you want to reduce risk, take 5 mg folic acid per day. Warning: Read the discussion in the A-to-Z Nutrient listings in Section I about the need to check B_{12} levels or take extra B_{12} when you supplement folic acid.

• Many women who develop cervical dysplasia are found to have low levels of *vitamin C,* although whether the deficiency in vitamin C contributes to the development or is a consequence of it is unclear. It makes perfect medical sense that vitamin C, in its role as a potent antioxidant, prevents tissue damage from toxins and infections. On this basis, it very likely does play a role in preventing the development of dysplasia. Recommendation: Take at least 500 mg of vitamin C per day. That amount should be considered a bare minimum, and I would advise most adult women to take 2000 mg (2 grams) to 3000 mg (3 grams) per day. Read the discussion of this vitamin in the A-to-Z Nutrient listings, and about antioxidants and free radical scavengers in Section I (pages 19–23) for more information on the importance of vitamin C.

• Women who develop cervical dysplasia also tend to be deficient in *vitamin E,* another potent antioxidant and scavenger of free radicals. Recommendation: Begin with a dose of 100 IU per day and remain there for 1 week. Because in some people vitamin E can increase blood pressure, be sure to have your blood pressure taken before you move on to a higher dose. If your average blood pressure has not risen above 140/90, increase your daily intake to 200 IU, then to 400 IU, and finally to 600 IU of vitamin E (in the form of alpha-tocopherol succinate) daily.

• *Selenium,* important for the body to make its own natural free radical scavenger, glutathione, may also be deficient in women with cervical dysplasia. If you also take selenium, you can reduce the dose of vitamin E you take, which could be important if you cannot increase the dose of vitamin E because of blood pressure considerations. Recommendations: Take 100 to 150 *micro*grams of selenium per day along with 100 IU to 200 IU vitamin E.

• Studies show that many women who develop cervical dysplasia eat a diet lacking in *beta-carotene,* the retinol (vitamin A–like substance) found in dark green and yellow vegetables. Supplementing the diet with either beta-carotene or actual vitamin A may reduce your risk of dysplasia. Because your body stores vitamin A, supplementing it in large amounts can be fraught with dangers from toxicity. Recommendation: Take 15,000 to 20,000 IU of beta-carotene per day, or take no more than 5,000 to 10,000 IU of vitamin A per day.

What makes it worse?

• *Oral contraceptive agents* (birth control pills) deplete the body of folic acid, and that deficiency can increase your risk of developing cervical dysplasia. Recommendation: If you take "the pill," be certain to also take 1 to 5 mg folic acid per day. See specific instructions for folic acid on page 248.

• *Smoking* is another factor that increases your risk of dysplasia. Nicotene actually lodges in the tissue of the cervix. Then, when exposed to the virus, DNA can become abnormal.

Cheilosis

What is it?

Painful cracking that develops in the angles of the mouth can occur for a variety of reasons. Sometimes the cracks develop from deficiency or overuse of certain vitamins; sometimes they occur because of infection with yeast fungus (usually *Candida,* the same yeast that causes diaper rash and vaginal itching), or occasionally from bacterial infections (such as impetigo). The cracking brought on by bacterial or fungal infections will require specific treatment with antibiotic or antifungal medications or ointments, but certain nutrients can help speed healing these painful cracks and in some instances be the cure for them. Let's take a look.

What helps it?

• *Vitamin B_6* (pyridoxine) deficiency can cause cracking of the mouth angles. Recommendation: Take 50 to 80 mg vitamin B_6

(pyridoxine) each day. If you currently take a dose that approaches this amount, deficiency of this vitamin probably is not at the root of the problem. Warning: Doses of this vitamin above 200 mg per day over a period of years have resulted in nerve damage. If you develop tingling, pins-and-needles sensations, or numbness at any dose level, discontinue supplementation immediately.

• Another B vitamin, B_2, is often deficient in those with cheilosis. In fact, classic symptoms of such a deficiency involves the lips as well as other body parts. Recommendation: Supplement with 100 mg daily.

• *Essential fatty acids* have an ability to regulate inflammation, wound healing, the immune defense response, and pain. Even in cracking associated with infection, taking essential fatty acids can help speed healing. Refer to the discussion in Section I on eicosinoids for more information about how these chemical messengers work. Recommendation: Begin with a solid macronutrient framework (see macronutrients, Section I, page 23) and to that sound base add approximately 250 mg of gamma linoleic acid (GLA) and fish oil (EPA) in a ratio of 1:4 (GLA:EPA) 1 to 2 times daily. The Eico-Pro essential fatty acid product manufactured by Eicotec, Inc., of Marblehead, Massachusetts, contains ultrapure sources of linoleic acid and fish oils already combined in the proper ratio. If you cannot get that product, you can purchase linoleic acid in a product called evening primrose oil at most health and nutrition stores, and EPA fish oil as well. Because it is not as pure a form, the milligram dosing will be different. You can make a reasonable substitute by combining evening primrose oil capsules with fish oil capsules plus vitamin E. Take 500 mg of evening primrose oil (a source of linoleic acid in capsule form), plus 1000 mg EPA fish oil, plus 200 IU vitamin E once or twice a day. (Warning to diabetics: EPA fish oil can cause blood sugar fluctuations in some diabetics. Carefully monitor your blood sugar if you use this supplemental oil and discontinue its use if your blood sugar becomes difficult to control.)

• Although cheilosis is often associated with deficiencies of the B vitamins, one report indicated that an *iron* deficiency was present in a much higher percentage of sufferers. Iron supplementation is tricky, though; you don't want to get an excess of iron. Recommendation: If you suspect you have an iron deficiency, it is best to seek the advice of your physician. The suggested daily dosage is 18 mg for adults, but only if a deficiency exists.

What makes it worse?

• *Vitamin A* taken in too great a dose can build up in your body. One of the symptoms of toxicity for vitamin A is cheilosis. The amount of vitamin required to cause this side effect varies from person to person, and therefore, I can't really give you an absolute recommendation for maximum safe intake. I can tell you that from my own experience, I developed cheilosis on a daily intake of 10,000 IU, and it disappeared on an intake of 5000 to 6000 IU per day. Many of my patients tolerate 10,000 IU without difficulty. And it would be unusual for an adult to develop it on a dose of 5000 IU per day. Recommendation: If you supplement with vitamin A at any level and develop painful cracking around the mouth, decrease your intake to zero to determine if the cracking will subside. If it does (and it usually doesn't take but a few days to do so), then resume your dose at one-half its previous level or 5000 IU, whichever is lower.

—————— **Cholesterol Problems** ——————

What is it?

Although it has a bad reputation, cholesterol is important to a number of body functions. We need cholesterol to build membranes, manufacture bile acids, and produce hormones. So it isn't that cholesterol is *bad* for you; but too much of a good thing is never beneficial.

Cholesterol is produced in our body by the liver. It is then carried through the body to the cells, which take what they need. The excess is then transported back to the liver. If this excess isn't picked up promptly, it can stick to artery walls and eventually lead to cardiovascular disease.

High cholesterol levels are one of the primary causes of heart disease because cholesterol produces fatty deposits in arteries. Elevated cholesterol levels are also implicated in gall stones, impotence, mental impairment, and high blood pressure.

Diet and nutrition have a major influence on cholesterol levels.

What helps it?

• *Fiber* mops up excess protein and removes it from the blood. Recommendation: Eat food high in fiber, such as apples, beans, brown rice, fruits, and oats. Whole grain cereals are also good for this job. Remember that fiber also absorbs the minerals from the food it is in, so take extra minerals separate from the fiber.

• *Vitamin B_3* helps lower cholesterol. Recommendation: Eat leafy greens, wheat germ, tuna, and beans. Supplement with 300 mg daily. Warning: Do not exceed this amount. Do not use a sustained-release formula, and do not take niacin if you have a liver disorder, gout, or high blood pressure.

• Lower your total cholesterol levels with *chromium picolinate.* Recommendation: Take 400 to 600 *micro*grams daily.

• *Coenzyme Q₁₀* improves circulation. Recommendation: Take 60 mg daily.

• *Garlic* lowers cholesterol levels and blood pressure. Recommendation: Take 2 300 mg capsules 3 times daily.

• *Vitamin C* lowers cholesterol levels. Recommendation: Take a supplement of vitamin C with bioflavonoids at a dosage of 3000 to 8000 mg daily in divided doses.

• Improve circulation with *Vitamin E.* Recommendation: Start with 200 IU daily and slowly increase to 1000 IU daily. Use the emulsion form for rapid assimilation.

• *Essential fatty acids* reduce the LDL (the "bad" cholesterol) level and thin the blood. Recommendation: Take up to six 1000 mg capsules of the omega-3 fatty acids EPA and DHA (you can find supplements with a combination of these two fatty acids).Warning: Since fish oils can interfere with blood clotting, do not take if you are taking a blood thinner.

Herbal remedies

• *Cayenne, goldenseal, and hawthorn berries* help lower cholesterol levels. Caution: Do not take goldenseal internally on a daily basis for more than 7 consecutive days. Do not use it during pregnancy, and use it with care if you have a ragweed allergy.

Dosages may vary, depending on the duration and severity of your symptoms. Consult a qualified herbal practitioner, and talk to your doctor before beginning herbal remedies. Some remedies cannot be used in combination with conventional pharmaceuticals.

What makes it worse?

• *Saturated fat* includes all fats of animal origin as well as co-conut and palm kernel oils. Eliminate margarine, lard, and butter.

• *Meat and dairy products* are primary sources of dietary cholesterol. Recommendation: Center your diet around vegetables and fruits, which are cholesterol-free.

• *Coffee* can elevate cholesterol levels when consumed in large amounts. Recommendation: If you can't eliminate coffee, keep your daily intake to a maximum of 2 cups.

───────────── **Chronic Ear Infection** ─────────────

What is it?

Ear infections come in two varieties: infection of the middle ear and infection of the outer ear or ear canal, often called swimmer's ear. I will address middle ear infections here and discuss ear canal infections under Swimmer's Ear.

Middle ear infections, common in young children, occur behind the eardrum in the small cavity that houses the hearing bones. The eustachian tube provides a drainage port from the other side of that space down into the side of the throat. When this drainage port stops up from thick fluid, swelling from infection in the throat, or allergies, fluid builds up in the space and presses outward on the eardrum, causing pain and muffled hearing. The stagnant fluid in the middle ear makes a great place for bacteria to grow, and when they find their way up the eustachian tube and into the fluid, they usually set up an infection. The body sends in infection-fighting immune cells to defend against the bacteria, and the battle that then rages between the body and the bacteria makes pus. When the pressure becomes too great, the thin eardrum can rupture to let the pus drain. Many children suffer one bout of middle ear infection after the next from about age 3 months to 3 years and seem to spend most of their early lives on antibiotic medications. What can the nutritional shelf offer these children? Let's take a look.

What helps it?

• *Vitamin C* improves resistance to infection in children and adults through its role as an antioxidant. Recommendation: Give your infant (under age 1) a multivitamin drop containing 50 mg vitamin C per day. Your toddler, age 1 to 3, can take chewable vitamin C in a dose of 100 to 250 mg per day. Children 3 to 9 can take 250 to 500 mg per day in chewable tablets of vitamin C.

• *Iron* deficiency has been proven to increase the risk for respiratory and ear infections. Supplementation can reduce this risk. Recommendation: Multivitamin drops containing 1 to 2 mg of iron glycinate should provide enough additional iron for most infants. Give your toddlers and children up to age 9 a chewable multivitamin supplement with added iron.

Herbal remedies

• If you catch it early enough, *echinacea* will generally end the ear infection. Take the extract orally.

• Alleviate pain by placing a few drops of warm *garlic* oil in the ear, followed by a drop or two of *lobelia* or *mullein oil.* You can find mixtures of these in your natural foods store.

• *Ephedra* contains two decongestants that help drain fluid from the middle ear. Make a tea using 1 teaspoon of dried herb, or orally take 1 teaspoon of tincture. It is essential that you do not take more than these amounts; people have died of overdose. Give children less than half the amount recommended for adults.

• *Goldenseal* is a natural antibiotic. You can make tea using 1 teaspoon of the herb.

Dosages may vary, depending on the duration and severity of symptoms. Consult a qualified herbal practitioner, and inform your physician of your decision to use herbal remedies. Some herbal regimens are not meant to be used in combination with conventional pharmaceuticals.

What makes it worse?

• *Sugar* inhibits normal immune function. As little as 18 grams of sugar (about the amount contained in one-half a regular 12-ounce soft drink) can cause measurable reductions in the output of antibodies (immune chemicals directed against bacteria). Children in America consume more of their calories as sugar than as any other single food group—more than meat, more than vegetables, more than dairy products. They may eat as much as 40% of their calories as sugar! That statistic alone explains the rapid rise in ear and respiratory infections among our children today. Recommendation: If your child is still an infant, restrict sugar from the outset. They will not miss what they don't eat. If you have already got a sugar junkie on your hands, sharply reduce your child's sugar intake at least where you have control—in your home. Don't keep sugary treats, sugar-frosted cereals, or sugar-frosted pastries around the house. Try to prepare foods without using much sugar in the cooking. Fresh fruit, popcorn, nuts, or sugar-free puddings, ice pops, or ice cream work just fine as snacks or desserts.

• Children who suffer from chronic ear infections should be tested for *food allergies.* The relationship between allergies and chronic otitis media has been firmly established.

• *Lead toxicity* can increase susceptibility to all infections in children. The commonest source of low-level lead poisoning occurs in older homes painted with lead-based paints. Recommendation: If you live in an older home, and your child suffers from frequent infections, you may want to have him or her checked for high levels of lead.

• *Cigarette smoking* in the house where the child lives or in the car in which he or she rides markedly increases the frequency of colds and ear infections in babies and young children. Recommendation: Even if you or other family members smoke, you should do so outside the house and never in the car with your children, if you want to reduce the frequency of their ear infections.

——— Chronic Fatigue Syndrome ———

What is it?
Chronic fatigue syndrome (CFS), which rose to prominence in the 1980s, at which time everyone who was tired thought maybe they had it, was once thought to occur because of recurrence of an old dormant viral illness. It has been determined that many cases of chronic fatigue occur without any known preceding infection, and now researchers are looking for other possible causes. If a virus is involved, it may be Epstein-Barr (the mononucleosis virus) or human herpes virus type 6 (a relative of herpes simplex virus) or probably other as-yet-unidentified viruses. Other causes may include immune system problems or a defect in the mechanisms that regulate blood pressure. Some experts have even thought CFS is the result of anemia, chronic mercury poisoning from amalgam dental fillings, hypoglycemia, hypothyroidism, sleep problems, and fungal infections. Many people with CFS have been diagnosed with fibromyalgia, a muscle disorder. More than likely, the cause is a combination of factors. The syndrome strikes far more women than men, for reasons that are not clear, and causes a host of recurring and persistent symptoms over the space of 6 months to several years. These symptoms include: mild fever; sore throat; painful swollen lymph glands in the neck or under the arm; general body weakness; soreness of the muscles; fatigue lasting more than a day after little exertion; headaches; migrating joint pain (this joint now, another later, yet another some other day) without redness or swelling of the joints; emotional disturbances such as forgetfulness, depression, ir-

ritability, confusion, difficulty concentrating; light-sensitive eyes; and sleep disturbance (insomnia or excessive sleeping). The development of such symptoms should prompt a careful physical and laboratory evaluation by your personal physician. Before declaring the syndrome to be chronic fatigue, all other possible causes must be looked for. If after evaluation your physician deems you to have chronic fatigue, let's see what nutrition can offer.

What helps it?

• *Essential fatty acids,* through the production of "good" eicosinoids (see eicosinoids in Section I, pages 24–27), help to improve immune function and decrease inflammation and pain. Recommendation. Begin with a solid macronutrient framework (see macronutrients, Section I, page 23), and to that sound base add 250 mg of gamma-linoleic acid to 1000 mg of EPA fish oil in a ratio of 1:4 (GLA:EPA) 1 to 3 times daily. The EicoPro essential fatty acid product manufactured by Eicotec, Inc., of Marblehead, Massachusetts, contains ultrapure sources of linoleic acid and fish oils already combined in the proper ratio. If you cannot get that product, you can purchase linoleic acid in a product called evening primrose oil at most health and nutrition stores, and EPA fish oil as well. Because it is not as pure a form, the milligram dosing will be different. You can make a reasonable substitute by combining evening primrose oil capsules with fish oil capsules plus vitamin E. Take 500 mg of evening primrose oil (a source of linoleic acid in capsule form), plus 1000 mg EPA fish oil, plus 200 IU vitamin E 1 to 3 times a day. (Warning to diabetics: EPA fish oil can cause blood sugar fluctuations in some diabetics. Carefully monitor your blood sugar if you use this supplemental oil and discontinue its use if your blood sugar becomes difficult to control.)

• Some people suffering from chronic fatigue syndrome report that they feel less fatigue when they take *vitamin B_{12}.* I have found this to be true in my own medical practice; however, I have not seen any hard science to back up the claim. It is true that your need for B vitamins increases anytime your immune system is under attack, and so the connection is not without some scientific merit. Since B_{12} is so innocuous, a trial supplementation can't hurt. Recommendation: Take 500 to 1000 *micro*grams of vitamin B_{12} weekly for 1 month, then twice a month for 2 months, then monthly for 4 to 6 months. You will absorb it best in shot form from your doctor, but you can also take the vitamin in the sublingual (dissolves under the tongue) or swallowed tablet or capsule form.

• Deficiency of *magnesium* causes weakness, fatigue, sleepiness, personality changes, poor appetite, and soreness of muscles. Certainly, when such a host of symptoms plagues you already, compounding the problem with a deficiency causing much the same kinds of symptoms can only make matters worse. Recommendation: Ask your physician to check your magnesium level. If it is frankly deficient, he or she will probably prescribe a magnesium supplement product. If the level is on the borderline of low but still "normal," it may still contribute to worsening of your symptoms. You may supplement it over the counter with 200 mg magnesium aspartate once or twice daily.

• *Coenzyme Q_{10}* has proven to help relieve symptoms in people suffering from chronic fatigue. Recommendation: Take 30 mg of coenzyme Q_{10} as often as 2 to 4 times daily.

• A recent study at Johns Hopkins University Hospital identified a link between CFS and a problem with the body's ability to regulate blood pressure. In this study, 22 out of 23 subjects with CFS were found to have a syndrome in which the body responds inappropriately to periods of prolonged standing. A significant percentage of those in the study experienced an improvement when they were treated for the blood pressure problem.

Herbal remedies

• *Asian ginseng and Siberian ginseng* are natural energizers, used by Russian cosmonauts to reduce fatigue and improve alertness, coordination, and memory. Studies indicate that ginseng also boosts the immune system. Make a tea using 1 teaspoon of the dried herb.

• *St. John's wort* has antiviral properties. Many people diagnosed with CFS have been suffering from long bouts of viral infection.

• *Burdock root, dandelion, and red clover* promote healing and enhance immune function. Make a tea using a combination of these, or alternate among them. Drink 4 to 6 cups daily.

Dosages may vary, depending on duration and severity of symptoms. Consult a qualified herbal practitioner. Alert your physician to your decision to use herbs, as not all herbal remedies can be used in conjunction with conventional pharmaceuticals.

What makes it worse?

• I know of no nutrient that of itself makes the condition worse.

Circulation Problems

What are they?

With aging, many people develop problems such as dizziness, coldness of the hands and feet, flakiness and thinning of the skin on the lower legs, and loss of hair on the lower legs. Although these symptoms may have other causes, poor circulation is among them. People develop poor circulation because of hardening of the arteries. The blood vessels become narrowed by the buildup of deposits of cholesterol, calcium, and fibrous tissue that form hard plaques in the artery walls. Blood flow through these narrowed channels becomes more sluggish, which is another way of saying that the circulation is poor. I have discussed the process of atherosclerosis (hardening of the arteries) fully, and I would ask that you refer to it now.

What helps them?

• See Atherosclerosis.

Herbal remedies

• These herbs support the heart and circulatory system: *black cohosh, cayenne, ginkgo, goldenseal, hawthorn, horseradish, horsetail, licorice, rose hips, and wormwood.* Caution: Do not use black cohosh or wormwood if you are pregnant or suffer from any type of chronic illness. Do not use licorice for more than 7 consecutive days, and avoid it completely if you have high blood pressure. Wormwood can be habit forming if used on a long-term basis.

Dosages may vary, depending on the duration and severity of your symptoms. Consult a qualified herbal practitioner. Let your physician know of your decision to use herbs; not all herbal remedies are meant to be used in combination with conventional pharmaceuticals.

What makes them worse?

• See Atherosclerosis.

Claudication

(see Atherosclerosis)

——————————— **Cold Sores** ———————————

What are they?

Most cold sores or "fever blisters" on the lips are caused by infection with the herpes simplex virus (type I) or HSV type I. You "catch" the virus from another person who is currently infected with it, usually by eating or drinking after him or her, or by kissing or other close contact. Once the virus enters through your skin (a process made easier if your lips are already cut, cracked, scraped, or chapped), it sets up a local infection on the lips or inside the mouth. When your body's immune defense system gets wind of the infection, it sends fighters to the area to try to stop the attack. But usually by this time the virus has already done its dirty work, causing one or more clusters of painful, red, weepy blisters to form on the lips. As if that infection weren't bad enough, the virus can then travel up the tiny nerve fibers that provide sensation to that area of the lip and take up a permanent residence at the origin of the nerve fiber in a ganglion in the brain. There the virus "rests," usually not causing any trouble, until something activates or stimulates it. Such stimulators could be fever, a cold, lip trauma, chapping, or prolonged sun exposure—hence, another name they're known by: sun blisters. Once activated, the virus begins to multiply and send new viruses back down the nerve fiber to the same area of lip that blistered before. In the day or so before the blisters break out, you usually can feel a difference in that spot on your lip. You recognize it with an "Uh-oh, I'm getting one of those cold sores again." There are prescription medications that kill the viruses outside the brain and help to speed healing and prevent outbreaks of herpes virus cold sores—primarily the drug acyclovir or Zovirax—but even these drugs do not eradicate the viruses at "rest."

What helps them?

• *Vitamin C,* which through its role as an antioxidant helps reduce the frequency of many viral illnesses, also seems helpful in preventing recurrences of herpes cold sores as well as aborting early outbreaks. Recommendation: Read the discussion on Vitamin C in Section I for specific instructions on how to increase your dose. Begin with a dose of 500 mg per day and slowly increase to a dose of at least 2 grams per day. At the first tinglings or sensations that you recognize as an outbreak on the way, increase your dose to at least 4 grams or 5 grams per day, or to your bowel tolerance level.

• The combination of *zinc plus vitamin C* has shown some benefit in helping to prevent recurrent outbreaks. The zinc is required for normal functioning of your immune defenses. Recommendation: Take zinc picolinate or zinc glycinate in a dose of 100 mg along with 500 mg vitamin C twice a day for at least 6 weeks to assess your response. If the treatment fails to suppress your outbreaks, discontinue the regimen. Many people, however, will respond to the combination well, and their recurrences stop. Occasionally, a person will experience a dramatic "last" outbreak before the virus becomes dormant and outbreaks stop, so don't give up the treatment if you break out once, only if the outbreaks recur repeatedly. Warning: Supplementation of zinc in its ionic form can create deficiencies of other minerals, such as copper, by competing with them for absorption from the intestine. Chelation of the minerals (see pages 30–31, Section I, on chelation) prevents this competition to get into the body, allowing you to fully absorb each of the minerals.

• *Vitamin E,* applied topically with a cotton-tipped applicator, seems to give rapid relief of pain of the blisters and speed up the healing process. Recommendation: Squeeze the contents of a single 200 IU capsule of vitamin E (as d-alpha-tocopherol succinate) onto a cotton-tipped applicator and apply carefully to the blistered areas 3 to 4 times daily. Continue until the blister heals.

• The amino acid (protein building block) *l-lysine* has been used by many cold sore sufferers for years as a treatment to prevent recurrences. Medical evidence does back up the claim that this amino acid helps to reduce both the number of outbreaks as well as lessen their severity in some people. The critical factor in getting a good response seems to be the proper balance of the amount of l-lysine compared to another amino acid, arginine, in the diet. People who use l-lysine as a preventive treatment should avoid nuts, chocolate, seeds, cereal grains, gelatin, carob, and raisins (all high in arginine) and eat more of meat, milk, fish, chicken, beans, eggs, and brewer's yeast, which are foods that have the "proper" balance. Recommendation: Take 500 mg daily. If you need to treat a current outbreak of blisters, take 1 to 6 grams of l-lysine daily between meals (but along with some carbohydrate such as milk or yogurt) until the blisters heal, then drop to the daily dose of 500 mg to prevent recurrences.

• *Lactobacillus acidophilus,* the friendly bacterium used to culture yogurt or buttermilk, also helps some people's cold sores, although hard medical evidence is not exceedingly strong in this case.

At least one study showed relief of pain in 38 of 40 people within 48 hours, and since the treatment is quite harmless and inexpensive, it would be worth a try. Recommendation: Take 1 to 2 lactobacillus tablets 4 times daily. An alternative would be to increase your intake of cultured yogurt, cultured buttermilk, or sweet acidophilus milk daily.

Herbal remedies
• Apply *goldenseal* to the affected area.
• *Tea tree oil* is a potent antiseptic that can be applied to the affected area several times daily. Use it full strength if possible; if not, dilute it with distilled water. Do not get this herb into your eye.
• *Licorice* inhibits the growth and cell-damaging effects of herpes simplex. If you use this herb, increase your potassium intake. Caution: Do not use for more than 7 consecutive days. Avoid it altogether if you have high blood pressure.

Dosages may vary, depending on the duration and severity of your symptoms. Consult a qualified herbal practitioner.

What makes them worse?
• *Prolonged sun and wind exposure,* although not a nutrient, indeed increases the likelihood of an outbreak. Protect your lips with zinc oxide ointment when you engage in outdoor sports such as sunning, skiing, swimming, fishing, camping, hiking, or boating.

—————— Colon, Spastic ——————
(Colitis, Irritable Bowel Syndrome)

What is it?
Your colon, or large intestine, the final 3 or 4 feet of your bowel, functions mainly to absorb water from the bowel contents back into the body. The muscular wall of the colon moves the contents along by a coordinated squeezing of one small segment after another along the length in a rippling wave. When the muscles work properly, things move right along. Sometimes, however, the muscle activity becomes uncoordinated and poorly timed, and several segments squeeze down at once, trapping the contents between them; a "spasm" results. People who suffer with a spastic colon will have alternating bouts of constipation and diarrhea, accompanied by painful cramping and gas.

The colon is especially prone to spasm when its contents are not uniform in consistency. By that I mean some stool is compact and dry and some is watery, with pockets of gas residing in between the two. It's almost as though the muscle wall becomes confused, never knowing exactly how tightly to squeeze the contents beneath it. Let's see what nutrition has to offer you in alleviating the symptoms of a spastic colon.

What helps it?

• Eating a diet high in *soluble fiber* to keep the stool uniformly soft will do more than any medication to normalize your spastic colon. A soluble fiber is one that will dissolve in water; it works in the colon by drawing water to itself and holding it there in the colon contents to make the stool uniformly soft. Fruit pectin, oat bran, and psyllium powder (vegetable fiber) all fill this bill. Wheat bran, which is insoluble and will not dissolve in water, does not.

The trick to making fiber work for you is to be consistent with your intake. Recommendation: If you do not currently eat a diet with much fiber, I implore you to begin slowly. First concentrate on eating more foods rich in fiber: broccoli, cauliflower, asparagus, green leafy vegetables, brown or wild rice, oat bran, fresh fruit. Then to that basic diet, begin to add a commercial vegetable fiber "bulking agent," such as Konsyl, Metamucil, or Citrucel. Begin with a tiny dose—$1/4$ teaspoon at bedtime in juice or water. Each week, increase your dose, first to $1/2$ teaspoon, then 1 teaspoon. Then take the 1 teaspoon morning and night, then 2 teaspoons morning and night, then 1 tablespoon. Aim for a daily total fiber intake of 40 to 50 grams per day, but stop at the level at which your bowel movements are soft and bulky, but not liquid, and are occurring daily.

• *Folic acid* deficiency can cause chronic constipation, which only compounds the problem of an irritable or spastic colon. Recommendation: Begin with 10 mg folic acid daily. If after 2 to 3 weeks you have seen no response, increase your dose to 20 mg, 30 mg, or even 60 mg per day. Because it is a good idea to take all members of the B vitamin complex together, add a 100 mg tablet of B-complex along with your folic acid. Warning: Read the A-to-Z Nutrient discussion of folic acid, paying particular attention to its interaction with vitamin B_{12}. You must ask your physician to check a B_{12} level in your blood if you supplement with folic acid, because it can mask a deficiency in B_{12} with disastrous results.

• Deficiency of *pantothenic acid,* another of the B vitamins, also causes chronic constipation in some people, and supplementation relieves it. Again, constipation worsens spastic symptoms. Recommendation: Take 250 mg pantothenic acid daily for at least 3 to 4 weeks to assess response. Once your symptoms have improved, you may reduce your daily dose to 100 to 150 mg. And, again, take the other members of the B vitamin group along with it in a single 100 mg B-complex tablet.

Herbal remedies

• *Psyllium* absorbs fluids, making it useful for treating diarrhea. As it travels through the digestive tract, it exerts a soothing effect, which helps relieve cramping. Drink plenty of water if you use psyllium, and pay attention to your body's reaction. Some people are allergic to this herb.

• *Valerian* relieves spasms in smooth muscles such as the intestine. It can be taken in tablet form or as a tea. Other herbs reputed to relieve muscle spasms associated with irritable bowel syndrome, spastic colon, and colitis include: *chamomile, peppermint, and wild yam.*

• *Alfalfa* supplies the body with vitamin K, which is needed to build intestinal flora for proper digestion. It also provides you with chlorophyll for healing and cleansing the bloodstream. Take this in liquid or tablet form.

• *Aloe vera* heals and soothes the digestive tract. I'd recommend a juice in this case, which can easily be obtained at your natural foods store. Take ½ cup of juice 3 times daily, on an empty stomach.

Dosages may vary, depending on the duration and severity of your symptoms. Consult a qualified herbal practitioner. Let your physician know of your decision to use herbs. Not all herbal regimens are meant to be used in conjunction with conventional pharmaceuticals.

What makes it worse?

• *Constipating medications,* such as aspirin, codeine and its derivatives, and all narcotic pain medications, worsen the drying of the bowel movement and therefore increase the spasticity of your colon. Recommendation: Take these medications only when absolutely necessary.

• Take care with foods such as *cheese* that also tend to slow down the passage of food through the bowel, worsen constipation, and may stimulate spasm. Recommendation: Although cheeses offer a good source of complete protein, limit your intake to 1 to 2 ounces of cheese per day, and be certain to keep your fiber intake up as just recommended.

• Avoid *mucus-forming foods* such as animal fats, butter, carbonated beverages, caffeine, candy, chocolate, dairy products, fried foods, junk foods, margarine, nuts, orange and grapefruit juices, pastries, all processed foods, seeds, spicy foods, sugar, and wheat products. The secretion of mucus prevents the uptake of nutrients.

─────────────── **Colorectal Cancer** ───────────────

What is it?

Like all forms of cancer, cancer involving the large intestine (colon) and the rectum arises when some of the cells of those tissues go haywire, cease to function normally, no longer obey the body's normal controls, and grow in a rapid and haphazard fashion. The cells usually involved in this kind of cancer are from the mucus-producing glands in the lining of the bowel.

Colon and rectal cancers run in families and are especially common when there is a family tendency for colon polyps; these usually harmless growths on the inside wall of the colon can occasionally become cancerous. If you have such a family tendency or have developed polyps yourself, you will want to be especially vigilant in having your bowel checked regularly by your personal physician and in adhering to preventive nutrition that may help to reduce your risk for cancer.

But even without a tendency toward forming polyps, cancers of the colon and rectum occur quite commonly in the United States (more than 85,000 Americans are diagnosed with colon cancer each year, and that number is on the rise), and although they account for 15% of all cancer deaths, they are actually quite curable when discovered early. In colorectal cancer, perhaps more than in any other form of cancer, prevention through early detection is the name of the game. At least once a year, you should check your bowel movement for hidden bleeding with a chemical test card—called a hemocult or guaiac test—available at your local pharmacy. After age 40, your annual examination should include a rectal examination and, if you have an increased family risk, a sigmoidoscopic examination (done with a flexible lighted "scope" that allows the physician to actually "see" up into the colon). You should report any blood in the stool or other changes in your bowel habits that persist to your personal physician.

What does the nutritional shelf have to offer to reduce your risk for colorectal cancer? Let's see.

What helps it?

• *Vitamin C,* through its potent antioxidant effects, has proven value in reducing the risk of developing colon cancer. Recommendation: Take a dose of 3 to 10 grams per day or more, using ascorbic acid in crystalline form. Refer to the discussion of this vitamin in the A-to-Z Nutrient listings for specific recommendations on how to work your way up to an adequate dose of vitamin C. Most adults will easily tolerate a dose of 3 to 4 grams daily if taken in crystalline powdered form; larger people will be able to take even more before reaching bowel tolerance.

• *Vitamin E,* through its abilities to act as an antioxidant and scavenger of free radicals, reduces the levels of cancer-causing substances in the colon. Recommendation: Begin with a dose of 100 IU per day and remain there for 1 week. Because in some people vitamin E can increase blood pressure, be sure to have your blood pressure taken before you move on to a higher dose. If your average blood pressure has not risen above 140/90, increase your daily intake to 200 IU, then to 400 IU, and finally to 600 IU of vitamin E (in the form of alpha-tocopherol succinate) daily, checking blood pressure after each increase in dose.

• Some research suggests *combining vitamins C and E* works best at reducing the risk of cancerous change of colon polyps. Recommendation: Take 400 mg of each vitamin daily. Increase the vitamin E in small increments as suggested above to be sure your blood pressure does not increase on a larger dose.

• *Vitamins A, C, and E* have also been studied in combination in people who have had colon polyps removed and are more likely to develop more polyps, and are therefore at a higher risk for colon cancer. Among the people who followed the combined regimen for 18 months, fewer than 8% developed new polyps, as opposed to 41% of the people who did not use this vitamin regimen. Recommendation: The regimen used was a combination of 30,000 IU vitamin A, 1 gram vitamin C, and 70 mg vitamin E per day. Warning:

Vitamin A, taken in this dose, can cause toxic side effects. Please carefully read the discussion of vitamin A in the A-to-Z Nutrient listings and take this dose only under the supervision of your physician. If he or she is not willing to help you watch for untoward effects of too much vitamin A, reduce the dose of this vitamin to under 15,000 IU per day or substitute beta-carotene (the less toxic vitamin A relative) in a dose of 30,000 IU per day.

• *Beta-carotene* alone has shown promise as a means of reducing your risk for colorectal cancer. Recommendation: Increase your intake of dark green and yellow vegetables that are rich in beta-carotene. In addition, you may add supplemental beta-carotene in a dose of 15,000 IU to 30,000 IU per day.

• *Folic acid* deficiency may increase the risk of cancers of the rectum. Recommendation: If you have a family risk for colorectal cancer, take 1 mg to 5 mg folic acid per day; because the B vitamin family works best when all members are present, take 100 mg of B-complex along with it. Warning: Folic acid supplementation can mask deficiency of B_{12}. If you supplement with folic acid above $\frac{1}{2}$ mg per day, you should ask your personal physician to check the level of B_{12} in your blood or periodically administer an injection of B_{12}.

• A diet rich in both soluble and insoluble *fiber* keeps the consistency of the bowel movement soft and the frequency of bowel activity regular. The longer potentially cancer-causing substances remain in your colon, the higher the chance of their causing damage to the cells of the lining. Regular elimination of bowel contents shortens the time spent in contact with your tissues. Avoiding constipation helps improve the health of your bowel and its resistance to disease. Recommendation: Work your way up to an intake of 50 grams of fiber per day. See the discussion of how to do this without bloating and cramping under Colon, Spastic.

• *Calcium* may bind with certain types of fat in the colon and allow them to be harmlessly removed from the body in the waste. Studies also show that calcium may prevent precancerous cells from becoming cancerous. Recommendation: Take 1500 mg per day for at least 2 to 3 months, then 1000 mg indefinitely. Refer to the discussion of this mineral and its relationship to magnesium. You should take the two together in a ratio of 2 parts calcium to 1 part magnesium. Many health and nutrition stores stock combined products in roughly this ratio.

Herbal remedies
• See Breast Cancer entry, page 210.

What makes it worse?
• People who eat a diet high in refined *sugar (sucrose)* put themselves at a higher risk for developing cancers of the colon and rectum. A high sugar intake alters the environment for the "friendly" bacteria that live in the colon and slows down the passage of bowel contents through the colon. A diet high in sugar also weakens the immune system, which you depend on to be ever-vigilant to destroy any of your body's cells gone haywire. Recommendation: If you have a family tendency for polyps or colon cancer, you should sharply reduce or totally eliminate from your diet all refined sugars (table sugar, corn syrup, and high-fructose corn syrup) and all products made with these sugars.

• A *high animal fat or red meat* diet probably increases the risk for developing colorectal cancer. The possibility that simply a diet higher in calories (which is a natural consequence of a diet high in fat) may also be an important factor in promoting cancer development has not yet been discounted, nor have concerns about the cancer-promoting chemicals (nitrosamines and others) that develop from charred meat and fat. Recommendation: With the evidence currently available, I would advise you to reduce your intake of animal fats (lard, butter, egg yolk, fatty meat) to no greater than 8% to 10% of your total day's calorie intake. Reduce your consumption of red meats, relying on poultry, fish, dairy, and vegetable sources for your protein needs.

• A diet high in *sodium* may increase risk for colorectal cancer. Recommendation: Add no extra salt to your foods and limit your intake of salty foods such as salt-cured meats, pickles, salted nuts and seeds, chips, and sauerkraut.

• *Alcohol* increases your risk for developing colorectal cancer an average of 4 times if you are a man and nearly 2 times if you are a woman. The more you drink, the higher the risk. Recommendation: If you are at higher risk because of family tendencies or previous cancers or polyps of the colon and rectum, you should avoid alcohol entirely.

• *Iron* may be a mineral required for growth of cancer cells. If you have a risk for colorectal cancer because of a family tendency for polyp disease or have had removal of such a polyp or a cancer, you should be cautious about adding extra iron to your diet. Recommendation: Do not take iron supplements unless your physician documents anemia from iron deficiency. Do not take vitamins fortified with extra iron. And limit your intake of red meats and spinach to reduce iron consumption.

————————— **Common Cold** —————————

What is it?

Any of the several hundred identified cold viruses can cause the stinging-drippy-nosed, red-weepy-eyed, stuffed-up, achy, feverish, scratchy-throated misery that we've all come to recognize as "a cold." The huge number of viral culprits that can bring on these symptoms makes it difficult to find a medication that will treat them all or a vaccine to protect us from them all. And so conventional medicine struggles on, able to transplant hearts, but still unable to conquer the common cold.

Although a virus causing the cold symptoms may pave the way for bacterial invaders to set up a nasty sinus, ear, or throat infection that antibiotics will cure, the cold itself—in its pure form—will not respond to prescription antibiotic medications. So far, we physicians have no good medicines to kill the cold viruses, although vigorous new viral research may soon make that statement outdated.

You must therefore depend on your own immune defense system to corral and destroy the cold virus when it tries to invade your respiratory tract. And nutrition can be your greatest ally in building a healthy immune system to make you more resistant to catching a cold, as well as in combating the viral attack once one begins. Let's see how.

What helps it?

• *Vitamin C* holds the honor of the most famous of the nutritional cold remedies, thanks to the work of Dr. Linus Pauling. It is probably through the vitamin's antioxidant properties and its immune-boosting effect that it decreases the number and severity of colds if taken in adequate doses. When you are trying to fight off a cold virus (or any virus), the struggle creates a "drain" of vitamin C, increasing your need for it dramatically. The drain is especially large if you develop a fever with your cold. Because of this increased demand, when the early signs of a cold appear, you can probably tolerate double your regular intake of vitamin C without problem. Refer to the discussion of vitamin C in the A-to-Z Nutrient listings for basic recommendations of daily intake. Recommendation: When your child begins to develop a cold, immediately give him or her a 100 to 250 mg dose of chewable vitamin C. Repeat that dose 2 or even 3 times a day until the symptoms subside. If you develop the early signs of a cold, immediately take 1 to 2 grams of crystalline ascorbic acid powder ($1/4$ to $1/2$ teaspoon) mixed in a carbonated citrus beverage or citrus juice. Repeat that dose every 4 to 6 hours. If you already take the daily 4 to 8 grams recommended for an adult, double your daily total in divided doses throughout the day. In crystalline form, the vitamin absorbs very quickly and you will feel an almost immediate—if temporary—improvement.

• The struggle to fend off a cold or other viral attack also increases your demand for vitamins of the *B-complex.* Recommendation: At the start of a cold, you may want to switch your child over to a "stress formula" children's chewable that has higher amounts of the B vitamins. You, as an adult, should take an extra 50 to 100 mg of B-complex daily until your cold symptoms subside.

• Your need for *essential fatty acids,* critical to the production of the "good" eicosinoids needed in normal functioning of your immune defense system, also increases under viral attack. You may wish to read the discussion about eicosinoids, the "good" chemical messengers in section I, pages 24–27, to better understand their role in protecting you from viral illnesses. The essential fats are linoleic acid (GLA) and fish oil (EPA). The two work in concert, when taken in the proper amounts, to enhance the production of the "good" messengers. Recommendation: Begin with a solid dietary framework (see macronutrients, Section I, page 23), and to that sound basic diet add gamma-linoleic acid and EPA fish oil in a ratio of 1:4 (GLA: EPA) 2 to 6 times daily. The EicoPro essential fatty acid product manufactured by Eicotec, Inc., of Marblehead, Massachusetts, contains ultrapure sources of linoleic acid and fish oils already combined in the proper ratio. If you cannot get that product, you can purchase linoleic acid in a product called evening primrose oil at most health and nutrition stores, and EPA fish oil as well. Because it is not as pure a form, the dosing will be different from the combined product, but you can make a reasonable substitute by combining evening primrose oil capsules with fish oil capsules plus vitamin E. Take 500 mg of evening primrose oil, plus 1000 mg EPA fish oil, plus 200 IU vitamin E 1 to 3 times a day. (Warning to diabetics: EPA fish oil can cause blood sugar fluctuations in some diabetics. Carefully monitor your blood sugar if you use this supplemental oil and discontinue its use if your blood sugar becomes difficult to control.) If you already take a single daily dose of essential fats for other conditions, take an additional 1 to 2 doses daily at the start of cold symptoms. Do not take the combination more than 3 times daily.

Herbal remedies

• German research shows that *echinacea* strengthens the immune system against cold viruses. Experts disagree on how often this herb should be taken. One group believes it should be taken on a daily basis; the other believes this enhances a person's immunity to the herb and so a better plan is to take it only when you feel a cold coming on or when people you live with have a cold. Check out numerous labels and see what they have to say. There are probably benefits to both schools of thought.

• *Garlic* contains many useful compounds, the most important one being allicin. This substance is one of the most powerful antibiotics. It is most effective to eat garlic raw, or use it in cooking. You can buy capsules that have little odor, but experts claim they are less effective.

• *Ginger* contains about a dozen antiviral compounds. This herb relieves cold symptoms by reducing pain and fever, suppressing coughs, and enhancing rest and sleep. Pour boiling water onto a couple tablespoons of fresh, shredded ginger and enjoy this hot tea.

• The Chinese people have long depended on *forsythia and honeysuckle* to fight colds and other viruses. Mix the two herbs with lemon tea, which also has antiviral action, and you have a relaxing concoction. Drink throughout the day, but be sure to sip a cup before bedtime.

• Commission E in Germany supports the use of *anise* as an expectorant for getting rid of phlegm. Drink a cup of tea in the morning and at night.

• *Ephedra* is a powerful decongestant that inspired the commonly known over-the-counter drug Sudafed. Caution: This is a powerful herb, and one that has led to the death of people trying to get high off of it. Use it responsibly, and consult a physician to find a safe dosage to avoid the many potential side effects.

• Take advantage of the antiseptic and immune-stimulating action of *goldenseal*. It activates white blood cells that destroy bacteria, fungi, viruses, and tumor cells. Caution: I don't recommend ingesting this herb if you are pregnant.

• *Marshmallow* relieves cold-related coughs and sore throats. It soothes inflamed mucous membranes due to its anti-inflammatory and antiseptic compounds.

• Brew a tea made from *mullein* leaves. It's guaranteed to soothe the throat and relieve the cough.

• *Slippery elm* relieves sore throats and suppresses coughs. You can buy this herb in tablet form, or make a tea from the dried herb.

• Commission E advises using 2 to 3 teaspoons of dry *watercress* to make a tea that will relieve your runny nose and cough.

• *Willow* is nature's aspirin. Its pain-relieving and anti-inflammatory fever-reducing action works wonders on the common cold. White willow doesn't contain as much salicin (the active constituent). Other species work better: violet willow, crack willow, and purple osier. But if you need to, take about $1/2$ teaspoon of dried herb and make it into a tea. Caution: Do not take this herb if you are allergic to aspirin, and never give it to children with colds. It could lead to the potentially fatal condition known as Reye's syndrome.

Dosages may vary, depending on duration and severity of symptoms. Follow package directions, or consult a qualified herbal practitioner.

What makes it worse?
• Foods high in *arachidonic acid,* such as red meat and egg yolk, promote the production of the group of "bad" eicosinoid messengers, which can worsen inflammation and depress immune function slightly. When you are under viral attack, your immune system doesn't need anything to make its job more difficult, and a diet with too much arachidonic acid can do that. Recommendation: At the onset of a cold, do eat your good protein, but make it egg *white,* fish, and poultry until the cold passes. By those rules, the old tried-and-true cure for colds—chicken soup—fills the bill nicely!

———— Congestive Heart Failure ————

What is it?
The heart is a muscle that works continuously, around the clock, every day of the year. Its job is to pump the blood around the body to provide oxygen and nourishment to all your tissues. Sometimes,

after many years of service, or after a heart attack damages it, the heart muscle may weaken a bit. It can't squeeze with its usual vigor, and as a result of the weak pumping, fluid may back up into your lungs, causing you to be short of breath, or it may pool in your legs and feet, causing them to swell and hurt. The pooled fluid, called "congestion" of the lungs, gives the disorder its name.

Congestive heart failure is a potentially life-threatening medical condition, and I urge you to use nutritional therapy as an aid to the conventional therapy that your personal physician prescribes and to inform him or her of all medications and nutrients you take.

What helps it?

• *Magnesium* levels in the heart muscle may be low in congestive heart failure, and the deficiency can increase the risk for abnormal heart rhythms (see Cardiac Arrhythmias) and constriction of the blood vessels in the arms and legs, elevating the blood pressure. Trying to pump against this higher pressure puts an even greater strain on the already weakened heart muscle. Deficiency in magnesium also contributes to sodium buildup and to deficiency in potassium, which is critical for normal electrical function of the heart. Recommendation: Ask your physician to check your magnesium level. If it is low, he or she will likely recommend a prescription form of magnesium for you.

• *L-carnitine* is often called an amino acid but is actually a vitamin-like nutrient that helps power the heart. A deficiency has been linked to congestive heart failure. Recommendation: Take 2 grams daily.

• *Potassium* deficiency, which can occur easily in congestive heart failure, can become quite serious if you take diuretic medications (fluid pills) to help reduce the swelling. You may also be taking the prescription medication digitalis (Digoxin, Lanoxin) to improve the strength of the heart muscle, and low potassium can cause problems there, as well. If your potassium falls too low, your heart becomes prone to potentially dangerous electrical changes made more likely by the digitalis. Be on the lookout for symptoms of low potassium: You may feel shortness of breath and more worn-out than usual with little exertion if your potassium is falling too low. Recommendation: Ask your physician to check the potassium level in your blood. If it is deficient, you will need to take more potassium. You can add some potassium into your diet by eating more foods rich in it, such as broccoli, tomatoes, orange juice, and bananas. Or you can add potassium to the foods you cook by using the product NO SALT, which is potassium in two forms. Use $1/4$ to $1/2$ teaspoon per day.

• *Coenzyme Q_{10}* has proven beneficial in strengthening weak heart muscles, improving the pumping action of the heart and decreasing the "congestion" in the lungs, and reducing the amount of angina (heart muscle pain) in people with congestive heart failure. Recommendation: Take 30 mg of coenzyme Q_{10} 1 to 3 times daily for at least 2 months to assess benefit. Warning: Do not discontinue this medication abruptly! You can suffer a rebound of symptoms from doing so. If you elect to stop taking this medication, do so in small increments: Decrease your dose by half, then by half again, then go to every other day, and then every third day, and finally off. While doing so, ask your personal physician to monitor your blood pressure and follow you closely through this period.

• People on prescription therapies for congestive heart failure seem to be relieved of some of their shortness of breath, heart fluttering, lung congestion, and swelling when they also take the amino acid *taurine.* Although taurine has not yet been classified a "true" vitamin—that is, essential to human health—it is considered to be a "vitamin-like" nutrient. Dietary taurine comes chiefly from muscle meats and shellfish. Recommendation: Take 2 grams taurine 3 times daily for at least 1 month to assess your response.

• *Essential fatty acids,* the forerunners of the "good" prostaglandins (see eicosanoids on pages 24–27 and macronutrients on page 23 for more information), help to take some strain off the heart muscle by dilating the blood vessels and reducing blood pressure. These good messengers also improve the strength and function of the muscle itself. The improvement realized by careful diet control and the use of essential fatty acids can be remarkable: In one instance, this kind of regimen took a professional football player who had so destroyed his heart (by abusing anabolic steroids for muscle bulking) that his physicians put him on the list to receive a heart transplant or die to a man once again able to lift well over 300 pounds. Recommendation: Begin with a solid macronutrient framework (see macronutrients, Section I, page 23), and to that sound base add gamma-linoleic acid and EPA fish oil—in a ratio of 1:4 (GLA:EPA) 1 to 3 times daily. The EicoPro essential fatty acid product manufactured by Eicotec, Inc., of Marblehead, Massachusetts, contains ultrapure sources of linoleic acid and fish oils already combined in the proper ratio. If you cannot get that product, you can purchase linoleic acid in a product called evening primrose oil at most health and nutrition stores, and EPA fish oil as well. Because it is not as pure a form, the milligram dosing will be different. You can make a reasonable substitute by combining evening primrose oil capsules with fish oil capsules plus vitamin E. Take 500 mg of evening primrose oil (a source of linoleic acid in capsule form), plus 1000 mg EPA fish oil, plus 200 IU vitamin E 1 to 3 times a day. (Warning to diabetics: EPA fish oil can cause blood sugar fluctuations in some diabetics. Carefully monitor your blood sugar if you use this supplemental oil and discontinue its use if your blood sugar becomes difficult to control.)

Herbal remedies

• *Pigweed* is high in calcium, a mineral that significantly reduces the risk of heart attack. It is also high in fiber. Add it to salad, soup, and mixed vegetable dishes.

• Salicin is the herbal precursor of aspirin and can be found in *willow*. People use the bark of white willow, but crack willow and purple osier contain higher concentrations of salicin. White willow will work, though, so use it if that's what is available to you. Brew a tea with 1 teaspoon of bark to 1 cup boiling water. Steep for 15 minutes and strain. Try drinking 1 cup daily. Caution: Don't take this herb if you are allergic to aspirin.

• *Angelica* contains 15 compounds that are calcium channel blockers. These blockers are known to prevent heart attacks. By no means should you trade in your prescribed channel blocker in favor of angelica, but you could add it to your regimen.

• *Hawthorn* is a well-known heart tonic. It is especially useful in treating congestive heart failure. However, it also prevents heart attack. It opens the coronary arteries, increases the heart's ability to deal with a loss of oxygen, and keeps the heart beating regularly. This is a very powerful herb. Naturopaths do not recommend taking the raw herb for treatment of heart disease; if you decide to take it, do so only after consulting your physician.

• The omega-3 fatty acids that prevent blood clots are available in abundance in the herb *purslane*. This herb also contains many antioxidants, calcium, and magnesium. Eat it like spinach, either raw in a salad or lightly steamed.

• Egyptian researchers have discovered two benefits of *chicory:* It slows a fast heartbeat, and it has a heart-stimulating effect. Chicory can be found as a coffee substitute here in America.

Dosages may vary, depending on the duration and severity of your symptoms. Consult a qualified herbal practitioner, and alert your physician to your decision to use herbs. Herbal remedies cannot always be used in combination with conventional pharmaceuticals.

What makes it worse?
• *Sodium,* especially in the heart muscle itself, can reach high levels in congestive heart failure. The buildup of sodium contributes to the swelling and the lung congestion. Recommendation: Eat a diet that promotes loss of sodium and fluid (see macronutrients, page 23) and don't add extra salt to your foods.

Constipation

What is it?
In medical terms, constipation means the passage of abnormally infrequent or extremely hard and dry bowel movements. In point of fact, however, the frequency and consistency of bowel movements varies so widely from one person to another, it's sometimes difficult to say what "normal" is. The best measure of normalcy, however, is your own established frequency—that is, what's normal for *you.* Sometimes nutritional deficiencies can contribute to constipation, and supplementation can correct the problem. I have discussed these nutrients fully under Colon, Spastic.

What helps it?
• See recommendations: Colon, Spastic.

Herbal remedies
• See recommendations: Colon, Spastic.

What makes it worse?
• See recommendations: Colon, Spastic.

Crohn's Disease

What is it?
Also called granulomatous colitis, this inflammatory disorder of the intestine causes cramping, diarrhea, and weight loss in people

who suffer from it. What causes the inflammation to set in remains a mystery; the body simply "turns" on its own intestinal tissues. Current research suggests that the trigger that sets the immune system off may be a viral or bacterial infection and a case of mistaken identity. Nature designed your immune defense system to recognize its own body's tissues by specific markers on their surfaces (peculiar only to you), and to protect its own from infection or invasion by attacking and destroying anything "foreign"—that is, anything not a part of "you." Sometimes bacteria or viruses have markers very similar to your own. If you happen to become infected with one of these invaders, immune confusion can result, with the defense your immune system sets unintentionally misdirected at your own tissues. This may be what happens in Crohn's disease and the very similar inflammatory bowel disorder ulcerative colitis. Symptoms caused by these two disorders are virtually the same, as are the nutritional therapies that will help you if you suffer from either of them. Let's take a look at what nutrition can offer.

What helps it?

• Eating a diet *low in carbohydrate* but adequate in lean protein sources and dietary fiber improves symptoms for patients with both Crohn's disease and ulcerative colitis. Recommendation: Refer to the dietary guidelines under macronutrients, Section I, page 23. Construct a diet that provides you with ½ gram of lean protein for every pound of your lean tissues (I've given you methods to estimate your lean weight in the macronutrient discussion). Lean meat, fish, poultry, and egg white should constitute 35% of your day's caloric intake; another 35% should come from high-fiber vegetables (greens, squashes, broccoli, cauliflower, asparagus), whole brown rice, and dairy products. The final 30% should come from essential fats, mostly the polyunsaturated and monounsaturated oils, such as olive, sunflower, and canola.

• *Folic acid* deficiency occurs commonly in these bowel disorders, both from low intake and from poor absorption by the inflamed intestinal tissues. Medications used to treat these disorders (such as sulfasalazine) can further deplete folic acid. Adding the vitamin back into the diet helps to reduce the diarrhea that comes when the condition flares up. Recommendation: Take 1 to 5 mg of folic acid daily, along with the other members of the B vitamin family as discussed on page 278.

• Intake and absorption of the other *B-complex* vitamins (especially riboflavin, thiamine, and pyridoxine— B_2, B_3, and B_6) are important to normal bowel health and function. Recommendation: Take 100 mg of B-complex once or twice daily. Increase the dose to 3 times daily during flares.

• *Vitamin B_{12}* sometimes absorbs poorly by mouth, and that is especially true when your intestine is inflamed and not functioning normally. You can bypass the need to absorb the vitamin in the intestine by taking it in shot form. Your physician can administer the shots every 2 to 4 weeks, or occasionally, he or she will instruct a family member on correct shot technique and you can take the vitamin by injection at home. Recommendation: Take 500 to 1000 *micro*grams weekly for 4 weeks, then every 2 to 4 weeks thereafter.

• Your body uses more *vitamin C,* which is a potent antioxidant (see antioxidants in Section I, page 20) when it is under attack and inflamed. Your intake of the vitamin should, therefore, increase to keep up with the demand. Recommendation: Purchase vitamin C (ascorbic acid) in the crystalline (powdered) form. One teaspoon of the powder usually provides 4 grams of vitamin. Begin with $1/4$ teaspoon dissolved in a carbonated citrus beverage, taken at bedtime for 1 week. Next, increase your dose frequency to morning and night (still $1/4$ teaspoon at each time), and then begin to increase each dose to $1/2$ teaspoon, $3/4$ teaspoon, then 1 teaspoon at weekly intervals until you reach your bowel tolerance level. Refer to Vitamin C in the Nutrient listings for more information about determining your bowel tolerance.

• *Vitamin D* deficiency of at least a mild degree occurs commonly in people who suffer from these bowel disorders, again, likely from poor absorption by the inflamed bowel. Refer to this vitamin both in the discussion of the classic deficiency disorders, under Rickets, and in the A-to-Z Nutrient listings to learn about how you can increase your body's production of vitamin D through exposure to sunshine. Although you may need to take some supplemental vitamin D, soaking up a little sunshine will go a long way to keeping levels of vitamin D in the normal range. It can do so, however, only if the sunlight hits your skin; it will do you no good if you bundle up like an Eskimo, wrapped from head to toe. Recommendation: In good weather, spend 30 minutes every day sitting, walking, or exercising in the sun. During the winter months, if you live in an area that is too cold to allow more than face exposure when outside, you may want to look into purchasing a full-spectrum sunlight bulb, called a Vita-Lite, for the rooms you spend the most time in. These inexpensive bulbs, available for both regular and fluorescent fixtures, provide natural sunlight during the course of a full working day equal to your spending about half an hour in the sun on a pretty day at noon. For more information, contact the Duro-Test Company in North Bergen, New Jersey.

• Poor absorption by the inflamed intestine, lack of sufficient vitamin D, and increased loss in the bowel waste cause *calcium* deficiency in people with Crohn's disease and ulcerative colitis. Steroid medications used to control the inflammation during flare-ups worsens the calcium loss. Recommendation: Take a total of 1500 mg of calcium as 500 mg doses of calcium gluconate 3 times a day.

• *Iron* intake may be adequate, but deficiencies still occur because of chronic loss of small amounts of blood during symptom flare-ups. The amount lost can be so small as to be undetectable by your eye, but still enough on a regular basis to deplete your iron stores. Your physician will probably be checking iron levels regularly and will prescribe supplementation if they are low. Recommendation: Unless you *are* deficient in iron, I would not advise supplementation. Eating iron-rich foods, such as liver, kidney, fish, clams, oysters, asparagus, figs, dates, and nuts, will supply enough to keep your iron stores up. Because vitamin C improves iron absorption, you also need to be certain to get plenty of it along with these foods. You should already be taking extra vitamin C (see recommendations on page 278).

• *Magnesium* deficiency occurs with great regularity in people with inflammatory bowel conditions—again, from poor absorption, low intake, and increased loss when diarrhea occurs. The low levels of this mineral probably account for many of the unpleasant symptoms you may experience: weakness, loss of appetite, low blood pressure, confusion, muscle twitches and spasms, and even seizures. Recommendation: Take 750 to 1000 mg of magnesium daily. Refer to the discussion of interactions between magnesium and its close mineral ally calcium. You should take them together in a ratio of twice as much calcium as magnesium. The calcium recommendation above will fill that bill.

• *Selenium* is required for your body to produce glutathione, its own potent antioxidant and free radical scavenger (see antioxidants and free radicals on pages 19–23). You may become deficient, especially if you tend to eat a diet high in sugar (which you absolutely should not—see "What makes it worse?" below). Recommendation: Take 100 to 150 *micro*grams of selenium daily.

• *Zinc* deficiency, sometimes of severe degree, can occur in bowel inflammation through poor absorption, increased loss because of diarrhea, and decreased intake from lack of appetite. Because zinc is of critical importance to the immune system, as well as a host of other chemical reactions in the body, including a normal sense of taste, you probably need to supplement this mineral. Recommendation: Take 150 mg chelated zinc 3 to 4 times daily. Warning: Supplementation of zinc in its ionic form can create deficiencies of other minerals, such as copper, by competing with them for absorption from the intestine. Chelation of the minerals (see pages 30–31, Section I, on chelation) prevents this competition to get into the body, allowing you to fully absorb each of them.

Herbal remedies
• *Aloe vera* softens stools and heals the digestive tract. Drink ½ cup of aloe vera juice 3 times daily.
• Other useful herbs include: *burdock root, echinacea, fenugreek, goldenseal, licorice, marshmallow root, red clover, rose hips, milk thistle, and slippery elm.* Caution: Do not use licorice on a daily basis for more than 7 consecutive days. Do not take goldenseal on a daily basis for more than 1 week at a time, and avoid it completely during pregnancy.

Dosages may vary, depending on duration and severity of symptoms; consult a qualified herbal practitioner. Let your physician know of your decision to use herbs. Herbal remedies cannot always be used in conjunction with conventional pharmaceuticals.

What makes it worse?
• Compared to people without inflammatory bowel problems, people with Crohn's disease tend to eat significantly more *sugar* and *refined starches* (flour, meal, and food items made with them, such as bread, pastries, pasta, cakes, and pies). Elimination of these kinds of refined products from the diet results in rapid and sustained relief of symptoms. Recommendation: Refer to the basic dietary guidelines under macronutrients, Section I, page 23. Staying within that basic framework, construct a diet specific to your needs by elimi-

nating foods that you feel may worsen your symptoms but containing about 30% of your day's total calories as lean meat, fish, chicken, dairy products, or egg; 40% high-fiber carbohydrates; 20% monosaturated essential fats (olive oil, canola oil, sunflower oil); and 10% animal fats. Try to eliminate all sugar, corn syrup, molasses, and high-fructose corn syrup; white flour products; and refined meals. Limit potato, wheat, and corn products.

• People with Crohn's disease are often histamine-intolerant. Foods that are high in histamine include dairy foods (including cheese), hard sausage, fish, pickled cabbage, and yeast products. Milk and other dairy products also contain carrageenan, which has been shown to induce ulcerative colitis in lab animals. You may want to eliminate these foods from your diet and assess any improvement of symptoms.

• People who suffer from inflammatory bowel disorders have an increased immune response against some foods. *Food sensitivities* can contribute to abdominal cramping, diarrhea, bloating, and further bowel irritation. You may wish to read under Allergies for additional information about how such sensitivities develop. You may also need to enlist the aid of an allergy specialist to help you sort out what foods may cause your problems. Common offenders are milk, wheat, soy, egg protein, nuts, raw fruit, corn, tomatoes, carbonated beverages, shellfish, and pickles. Recommendation: With the help of an allergist, attempt to identify food allergies and sensitivities. On your own, you may undertake an elimination trial (see discussion in Food Allergy), beginning with the common foods listed above, one at a time.

Cystitis

(see Urinary Tract Infections)

Depression

What is it?

At some time in our lives, most of us suffer some degree of depression because of the physical and emotional stresses that are a part of adult life. We suffer losses of loved ones and friends, disappointments in our relationships and careers, and endure threats to our physical health or that of our parents, spouses, or children. And sometimes we stagger under the emotional weight of these typical stresses of adult living and become depressed. This situational or re-active kind of depression, clearly a result of a psychologically bur-densome event, may require nothing but time, patience, and supportive love to resolve itself as long as the symptoms do not be-come too severe or last too long. But when the typical symptoms—sadness of mood, guilt feelings, feelings of worthlessness or hopelessness, difficulty concentrating or making decisions, loss of interest in work or social life, loss of energy, headaches and other physical complaints, sleep disruptions, change of appetite, and de-creased sexual drive—interfere with your ability to carry on with your daily activities, you may need the assistance of a qualified and compassionate counselor to help you find your way out of the de-pression. Other causes for depression have physical roots—for ex-ample, the hormonal upheaval that women often experience during menopause may bring on quite a severe depression. Oftentimes, however, this kind of depression responds quite readily with re-placement of female reproductive hormone (estrogen). Some people experience depression during the winter months, when the available sunlight decreases. To alleviate this kind of depression, called SAD or seasonal affective disorder, you need only to spend more time in full-spectrum sunlight, provided by the sun or by a full-spectrum sunlight lightbulb. But some depressions have no discernible cause; they simply come on and often persist for many years. Struggling to overcome this kind of disorder of mood, called an endogenous de-pression, often demands enormous time and patience and the help of a qualified and compassionate counselor with whom you feel at ease. I encourage you, if you feel you have become depressed, with or without obvious cause, to explore your feelings with a therapist who can, like a guide on any journey, help you find your way more quickly and safely than if you try to go it alone. The need for ther-apy or prescription medications notwithstanding, nutrition may also play an important role in contributing to the development of depres-sion, as well as worsening or alleviating its symptoms. Let's see how.

What helps it?

• Deficiency of *biotin* can cause depression in only a few months. Although this deficiency usually does not occur in people eating a balanced diet, it may occur in people who subscribe to the "athlete's breakfast" of raw eggs, which contain a substance that destroys biotin. Recommendation: Take biotin in a dose of 300 *mi-*

*cro*grams per day for a period of 4 to 6 weeks to assess your response.

• A diet high in *complex carbohydrates* prevents serotonin depletion. Eat plenty of raw fruits and vegetables, and include soy products, brown rice, and legumes in your diet.

• Depression occurs commonly in people deficient in *folic acid,* perhaps because a deficiency of this member of the B vitamin group causes low levels of the brain chemical serotonin, important in maintaining a happy or contented mood. Recommendation: Take 2 to 5 mg of folic acid daily. Take a 50 to 100 mg dose of vitamin B-complex along with your folic acid. The B vitamins are a tight-knit group and work best together. Warning: Taking this level of folic acid daily could obscure a deficiency of vitamin B_{12}. If you supplement with folic acid, you should ask your personal physician to check the level of vitamin B_{12} in your blood periodically and supplement extra vitamin B_{12} in shot form if your levels are low.

• Your body requires *vitamin B_6 (pyridoxine)* to produce the mood-elevating brain chemical serotonin as well as other brain chemicals important in maintaining a stable, contented mood. Deficiency of this B vitamin could lead to deficiency of these brain chemicals and a worsening of depression, and the converse is that supplementing this vitamin may be important in overcoming depression. Recommendation: Take 100 to 150 mg of vitamin B_6 along with 50 to 100 mg of vitamin B-complex daily for 4 to 6 weeks. After that time, you may reduce your dose of B_6 to 50 mg per day. Warning: Do not increase your dose of this vitamin beyond the amount recommended. Doses of 200 mg per day over a several-year period have resulted in permanent nerve damage.

• Deficiency of *thiamine* and *riboflavin* may also contribute to depressive symptoms; however, hard science doesn't make as compelling a case for these members of the B vitamin group. Recommendation: Take 50 to 100 mg of B-complex daily to provide sufficient supplementation with all the B vitamins.

• Deficiency of *vitamin B_{12}* occurs more often in people suffering depression than it does in "normal" (i.e., not depressed) people. Recommendation: Take sublingual (dissolves under your tongue) vitamin B_{12} in a dose of 500 *micro*grams weekly for 4 to 6 weeks, then monthly if you respond with a lightening of your mood. Take a 50 mg tablet of B-complex daily along with your vitamin B_{12}.

• One of the earliest detectable symptoms of deficiency of

vitamin C is depression. Chronic depression, fatigue, and loss of the sense of well-being can occur even with mild deficiency of vitamin C. When mild to moderate deficiency causes depression, people of all ages respond to supplementation with this vitamin. Recommendation: Adults should take a minimum of 1 gram (1000 mg) of vitamin C (and up to 5 grams) per day to help combat depressive symptoms. Take 500 mg of time-release vitamin C twice a day. (Children ages 5 to 12 should take a total of 250 to 500 mg divided into 2 doses each day.) See the discussion of this important vitamin in the A-to-Z Nutrient listings for more information about its many benefits.

• *Iron* deficiency causes depression along with anemia, and anemia responds to iron replacement more rapidly than the sadness of mood. Recommendation: Taking supplemental iron when you are not deficient can cause problems of its own, and I would, therefore, recommend that you ask your personal physician to check you for iron deficiency and only supplement if your levels are clearly low. In that event, you may take a chelated iron replacement, such as iron glycinate, in a dose of 20 mg per day. If you cannot find a chelated iron product, you may take 90 mg ferrous sulfate 3 times per day, along with 500 mg of time-release vitamin C, which will enhance your absorption of the iron.

• *S-Adensyl-L-Methionine (SAMe)* isn't an herb or hormone. In fact, it is a chemical compound found in all living cells. In most people, the body manufactures all the SAMe it needs from the amino acid methionine found in soybeans, eggs, seeds, lentils, and meat. SAMe appears to regulate more than 35 different mechanisms and helps the body maintain cell membranes, remove toxic substances, and produce mood-enhancing neurotransmitters. It has proven effective in treating various stages of depression. Although studies haven't indicated that SAMe is significantly more effective than prescription antidepressants, it is less toxic. Recommendation: Take it twice a day on an empty stomach. Since dosage depends on many factors, check with your physician for the correct amount.

• *L-tyrosine* is a mood-elevating amino acid that can cause depression when deficient. Almonds, avocados, bananas, dairy products, and sesame seeds contain L-tyrosine. Recommendation: Increase your consumption of these foods and take 50 mg per pound of body weight daily. Take on an empty stomach at bedtime.

• A diet deficient in the *essential fatty acids,* because they are the raw materials from which your body makes a group of chemical messengers, called prostaglandins, important in maintaining a happy and contented mood, can contribute to depression. Please refer to the Yin and Yang of Human Health, and the eicosinoids, pages 24–27; for more information about these powerful substances. Recommendation: To facilitate the best response from essential fatty acids, begin with the proper macronutrient framework (refer to macronutrients on page 23 for more information). Then to that nutritionally sound base add gamma-linoleic acid (GLA) and EPA in ratio of 1:4 fish oil (GLA:EPA) 1 to 3 times daily. The EicoPro essential fatty acid product manufactured by Eicotec, Inc., of Marblehead, Massachusetts, contains ultrapure sources of linoleic acid and fish oils already combined in this ratio. If you cannot get that product, you can purchase linoleic acid in a product called evening primrose oil at most health and nutrition stores, and EPA fish oil as well. Because it is not as pure a form, the milligram dosing will be different. You can make a reasonable substitute by combining evening primrose oil capsules with fish oil capsules plus vitamin E. Take 500 mg of evening primrose oil (a source of linoleic acid in capsule form), plus 1000 mg EPA fish oil, plus 200 IU vitamin E 1 to 3 times a day. (Warning to diabetics: EPA fish oil can cause blood sugar fluctuations in some diabetics. Carefully monitor your blood sugar if you use this supplemental oil and discontinue its use if your blood sugar becomes difficult to control.)

Herbal remedies

• Despite the fact that *licorice* has more antidepressant compounds than any other herb, it does not have the popularity of St. John's wort in the treatment of depression. At least 8 compounds are MAO (monoamine oxidase) inhibitors. Licorice can easily be added to your diet; just add it to any of the herbal teas suggested in this book. Caution: Do not use on a long-term basis (more than 7 consecutive days).

• *St. John's wort* has a long history in the treatment of depression. It has fewer side effects than any pharmaceutical drug, and some experts say it has no side effects at all. This herb improves the quality of sleep. I recommend a tea made by steeping 1 to 2 teaspoons of dried herb in 1 cup of boiling water for 10 minutes. St. John's wort is most effective if you drink 1 to 2 cups of tea daily for 4 to 6 weeks, according to Varro Tyler, Ph.D. Caution: Do not take this herb if you are pregnant. Stay out of the sun, as your skin is more sensitive to sunlight.

• *Ginger* has also been used for centuries to treat anxiety and depression. It even tastes good. Use it liberally in your cooking, or make a tea from it.

• *Rosemary* oil contains cineole, which stimulates the central nervous system. A therapeutic massage using rosemary oil certainly can't hurt.

• *Ginkgo* has been shown to relieve depression, particularly in elderly populations. Studies also reveal its ability to reduce memory loss and enhance circulation. If you want to try ginkgo, use the standard preparation, a 50:1 extract, which uses 50 parts leaves to arrive at 1 part extract. You can take 60 to 240 mg daily, but that's it. Any higher, and you run the risk of diarrhea, irritability, and restlessness.

• *Siberian ginseng* has the action of an MAO inhibitor. It improves the depressed condition. I recommend capsules or extract.

As always, consult a qualified health professional before beginning any herbal program. Dosages vary depending on duration and severity of symptoms.

What makes it worse?

• Abnormal levels of *magnesium,* whether too high or too low, can increase depression, and for that reason, you may need to enlist your personal physician's help to determine by blood testing whether your magnesium level is normal. Recommendation: If your level is too high, stop taking any supplements containing magnesium as well as any over-the-counter products, such as Milk of Magnesia and magnesium-containing antacid liquids and tablets. If your levels are low, take 250 mg magnesium aspartate once or twice daily until your levels return to normal.

• People who drink large amounts of *caffeine* (3 to 4 cups of regular coffee per day or more) usually score higher on tests designed to measure depressive symptoms. The higher the score, the more depressed the person taking these kind of tests. This connection may not be one of cause and effect, however, but simply that depressed people tend to spend more time sitting and thinking and drinking coffee because they're depressed. In other words, caffeine abuse may be a symptom of depression and not a cause. Other studies have shown, however, that depressed mood improves with caffeine reduction in as little as a week's time. Recommendation: If you are depressed or tend toward depression, I would recommend that you decrease your consumption of caffeine slowly (following the regimen I have outlined under Breast Disease, Benign) and, once decaffeinated, spend a few weeks to a month assessing your response. If you find that your mood lightens considerably off caffeine, then you should continue to abstain from it, or at least to curtail your intake to a single cup of coffee per day.

• Many people in the throes of depressed mood turn to sweets as a solace; however, medical studies have shown that the intake of *sugar* increases depression, fatigue, and moodiness. Recommendation: Eliminate or sharply reduce your intake of all refined sugars, including table sugar, corn syrup, high-fructose corn syrup, molasses, and all products made with these substances for a minimum of 4 to 6 weeks to assess your response.

• Eating a *high-fat diet,* especially fats coming from meat, may increase the risk for suicide during depression. Recommendation: Refer to macronutrients, Section I, page 23, where you will find information about constructing a diet that provides about 30% of your day's calories in lean protein (choose primarily from poultry, fish, egg white, and dairy products); about 40% of your day's calories from fruit, low-starch vegetables, rice, and oats; and the final 30% from polyunsaturated and monounsaturated fats and oils (about 20%) and fats from animal origin (about 10%).

• *Wheat products* have been linked to depressive disorders. Cut back or eliminate your intake of wheat.

• *Food sensitivities or allergies* can play a role in worsening depressive feelings, and when they do, eliminating the culprit foods helps to lift your mood. Recommendation: Because almost any food could be a problem food, you may want to enlist the aid of an allergy specialist, who can perform skin and blood testing to narrow your list of suspects. Armed with that information, you will need to test each food suspect in its turn, by conducting an "elimination trial." You will find the details of how to undertake such an experimental regimen under Food Allergies. Also limit your intake of the amino acid *phenylalanine.* It contains phenol, a highly allergenic chemical. Avoid aspartame (found in Equal and NutraSweet) for the same reason.

──────────── **Dermatitis** ────────────

What is it?

Dermatitis means "inflammation of the skin," a rash. Alone, dermatitis doesn't tell you anything about why the skin is inflamed, merely that it *is* inflamed. For example, contact with poison ivy breaks some people's skin out in red, itching blisters—called a contact dermatitis. Cold dry winter air causes redness and scaling of the skin—a winter dermatitis. Some people inherit a tendency for a condition that causes redness and flaking of the skin on the bridge of the nose, the scalp, the eyebrows, and the ears, which we call a seborrheic dermatitis. Others inherit a tendency to have the skin of the scalp, elbows, and knees erupt in patches of thick silvery white scales, and that's a psoriatic dermatitis, or psoriasis. And highly allergic people may break out in red itchy rashes when they eat, drink, or breathe in substances they have allergy to—an allergic or atopic dermatitis. Sometimes, allergic problems can break the skin out in hives (an urticarial dermatitis).

They're all dermatitis of some sort, but very different from one another in cause and in cure. In this discussion, I will address the *allergic or atopic* kinds of dermatitis. You can find information about other kinds of dermatitis under the listings Psoriasis, Seborrheic Dermatitis, and Urticaria (hives).

An allergic rash (sometimes also called allergic eczema) tends to occur most commonly in younger children (up to about age 10) and then disappear until adulthood (age 20 or so), when it may return. This form of dermatitis usually makes an itchy, weeping, or leathery rash that occurs especially on the face, neck, upper body, wrists and hands, and in the creases behind the knee and at the bend of the elbow. Most people troubled by allergic dermatitis also suffer from typical seasonal respiratory allergies to pollen, dust, weeds and grasses, and may also be sensitive to some foods. What does the nutritional shelf have to combat this kind of problem? Let's look.

What helps it?

• *Vitamin C* improves allergic skin symptoms most likely through its antioxidant effects (see discussion of Vitamin C, Antioxidants) as well as through encouraging the production of the "good" eicosinoids (see discussion of eicosinoids, pages 24–27). Recommendation: Children ages 2 to 3 may take chewable vitamin C (ascorbic acid) 100 to 250 mg per day; ages 4 to 6 may take chewable tablets up to 500 mg per day; and ages 7 to 10, up to 1 gram per day. Adults should take 4 to 8 grams per day to their bowel tolerance level. Follow instructions for how to begin and to increase your dose in the discussion of Vitamin C in the A-to-Z Nutrient listings.

• The B vitamins are needed for healthy skin and proper circulation as well as for reproduction of cells. Recommendation: Take 50 to 100 mg of *vitamin B complex* 3 times daily with meals. Supplement with extra *vitamin B* at a dosage of 50 mg 3 times daily. People suffering from skin disorders are frequently deficient in this vitamin.

Essential Fatty Acids

• *Oleic acid,* a fat found in olive oil, has been shown to inhibit histamine release, which worsens the itching of the dermatitis. Recommendation: Use this oil where possible in cooking.

• *Linoleic acid (GLA) and fish oils (EPA)* also inhibit the inflammation that causes swelling and irritation from allergies, contributing to the itching, redness, and scaling of your skin. Refer to eicosinoids (Section I, pages 24–27) for more information about these fats. Recommendation: The combined GLA and EPA product called EicoPro provides ultrapure sources of these oils ready for consumption. You can obtain this product from Eicotec, Inc., Marblehead, Massachusetts. Take 2 capsules 1 to 3 times daily. You can construct a reasonably crude substitute for this combined product with a daily intake of 500 mg of evening primrose oil (a source of linoleic acid in capsule form), plus 1000 mg EPA fish oil, plus 200 IU vitamin E. Take this combination 1 to 3 times a day. (Warning to diabetics: EPA fish oil can cause blood sugar fluctuations in some diabetics. Carefully monitor your blood sugar if you use this supplemental oil and discontinue its use if your blood sugar becomes difficult to control.)

• *Selenium,* necessary to make the body's own natural antioxidant glutathione, has shown variable results in treating allergic dermatitis. Some people improve and others do not, for reasons that are not entirely clear to me. I do not recommend that you give selenium to children with allergic dermatitis. Recommendation: You (as an adult) can take a dose of 200 *micro*grams daily. Take this dose for 6 to 8 weeks to assess your response. You may continue to take 100 to 200 *micro*grams daily thereafter if you get a good response.

• *Zinc* has shown benefit in some people who suffer allergic dermatitis and not in others, for reasons that are not clear. In cases in which it does work, complete clearing of rashes often occurs. Recommendation: Take 50 mg chelated zinc 3 times daily. You should be able to see some response in 4 to 6 weeks, although complete clearing may take several months. Warning: Supplementation of zinc in its ionic form can create deficiencies of other minerals, such as copper, by competing with them for absorption from the intestine. Chelation of the minerals (see pages 30–31, Section I) prevents this competition to get into the body, allowing you to fully absorb each of them.

• *Vitamin A* supplementation may improve the dry scaling of skin in children with allergic dermatitis, but the vitamin is quite toxic at high doses and most children can't tolerate taking it without side effects. The vitamin A relative, beta-carotene, may be a similar, but safer, alternative. Recommendation: Give an allergic 3- to 5-year-old child 5,000 IU beta-carotene per day. Increase to 10,000 IU for children 6 to 10 years old. Adults can take 30,000 IU per day.

Herbal remedies
• To relieve itching and promote healing, mix *goldenseal root powder* with *vitamin E oil,* then add a little honey. Apply the paste to the affected area.
• Take these herbs in capsule or tea form: *dandelion, goldenseal, myrrh, and red clover.* For best results, alternate among them.

What makes it worse?
• *Copper* levels in the skin and hair of people with chronic allergic dermatitis may be elevated. Whether this elevation plays a role in worsening the skin condition is unclear; however, there may certainly be a connection considering the fact that supplementation of zinc (see above) seems to help some people. Zinc and copper interact with one another such that if you absorb too much of one, you may become deficient in another. Perhaps the elevated copper occurs because of enhanced absorption and perhaps more copper absorption results in too little zinc. I have seen no hard science to back that theory up, but it's worth examination. Recommendation: Avoid taking supplemental vitamin and mineral preparations with added copper.
• *Raw eggs* contain avidin, a protein that binds biotin and keeps it from being absorbed. Biotin is necessary for healing skin and scalp disorders.

• Many people are sensitive to *gluten* and don't realize it. Research shows that people suffering from any skin disorder find their symptoms improved on a gluten- and dairy-free diet.

• *Continued exposure* to whatever triggered the allergic rash will, of course, keep the rash active. Recommendation: Remove or eliminate offending foods, pollens, pets, and dust. Identifying the offending items by allergy testing is the first order of business.

Diabetes Mellitus

What is it?

The disorder called diabetes mellitus is actually two very different diseases that share a common feature: high blood sugar. The kind of diabetes that usually develops in childhood (juvenile-onset diabetes or Type I diabetes) occurs because something—a viral infection or a chemical toxin—has destroyed the cells in the body that produce *insulin.* Without enough insulin, the hormone that controls blood sugar, the body cannot store the calories coming in, and they run right through the body as "sugar" in the urine. A person with this kind of diabetes will develop weight loss, ravenous appetite and thirst, and constant urination. This kind of diabetes requires that the person take injections of insulin and be under the care of a knowledgeable physician. A person suffering from Type I diabetes can certainly improve with proper nutrition and regular exercise, but without the ability to make insulin, he or she cannot treat the disease by diet alone.

The other kind of diabetes that comes on in adulthood (adult-onset or Type II diabetes) develops not from lack of insulin but from overabundance of it. In all of us, when we eat, our blood sugar rises and this signals the gland that makes insulin (the pancreas) to do so. The insulin acts on sensors in the tissues to allow them to take up the sugar from the blood to use or to store away, and the blood sugar falls to normal. In some people, the pancreas overresponds to the call for insulin, providing too much of it. The high levels of insulin, over time, damage the sensors in the tissues, making them insensitive or unresponsive to that amount of insulin. Then the pancreas must make more, and more, and more to make the sensors respond to bring the blood sugar back to normal. As long as the pancreas can make more insulin, it will, and the body can control blood sugar; however, at some point, the sensors become so damaged that the full capacity of insulin available from the pancreas is no longer enough to bring blood sugar back down to normal. Once that point comes, the blood sugar begins to rise, and adult-onset diabetes mellitus has developed.

The overabundance of insulin can cause other mischief in adult-onset diabetics: the production of cholesterol, triglycerides (other blood fats), heart disease, hardening of the arteries, high blood pressure, salt and fluid retention, and the storage of excess body fat. This disorder, if caught and treated in time, will respond virtually completely to nutritional rehabilitation and the symptoms will come under control. But diabetes is an unforgiving disorder—*keeping* it controlled requires constancy and vigilant adherence to your nutritional regimen. You can learn to control it, but the metabolic tendency to produce too much insulin in response to diet always remains. Given access to the wrong kinds of foods, your diabetic state will return, and with it the whole host of medical maladies that were present before.

One final word: If you are an adult-onset diabetic, already taking insulin shots or medication by mouth to control your sugar, you must undertake this kind of nutritional regimen only under the care of your personal physician, who can help you adjust the doses of these medications safely as your blood sugar control improves. The control will happen quickly if you adhere strictly to the regimen, and in order to check your sugar and blood pressure (which will also drop quite precipitously) frequently, you may want to invest in (and learn to use) a home blood glucose testing machine and a blood pressure cuff. That way, you can monitor your readings, record them, and report them to your physician, who can help you reduce your medications safely. You could develop insulin shock or severe low blood sugar or blood pressure if you continue to take the same doses of medication on this kind of nutritional regimen. I also strongly recommend you find, read, and reread a copy of the book *Diabetes Type II* (Prentice Hall, 1990) by a diabetic physician named Richard Bernstein, which is by far the best book currently available on controlling this disease. But now, let's look at what nutrition can do to help you.

What helps it?
• *The right diet* can work miracles in adult-onset diabetes. But the diet usually recommended to treat this disorder can make mat-

ters worse. Conventional medical wisdom has for years deemed the best diabetic diet to be made of 55 to 60% complex carbohydrate, 30% polyunsaturated fat, and 10 to 15% protein. A quick analysis of that diet, beginning with protein intake, shows the fallacy in thinking. Look at this with me for a moment.

Let's take as an example an adult man weighing 195 pounds with a lean body mass of 140 pounds. That person will need a *minimum* of 70 grams of lean protein per day to support his muscles and organs. Each gram of protein accounts for 4 calories; therefore, his minimum protein requirement alone is 280 calories. If that represents 10% of his day's calories, he will eat 2800 calories per day. That's fine, but now he's supposed to eat 60% of those 2800 calories in complex carbohydrate (starches), and that comes to 1680 calories of starch. As for protein, every 4 calories of starch is 1 gram, and that means this gentleman will be eating 420 grams of carbohydrate per day. The rest of his calories come from fats, which don't alter insulin response at all.

Now, reason with me here. The man is an adult diabetic. His diabetes is the result of many years of a high insulin level. The dietary component that makes insulin rise, unrestrained by opposing hormones, is carbohydrate (starch and sugar). As little as 80 to 100 grams of starch in a day will cause a big outpouring of insulin. Does it make sense, then, for this person to consume nearly five times that amount of starch every day? Absolutely not! Should we be surprised that the consequences of his diabetes—the raised blood pressure, the weight gain, the fatigue, the risk for heart disease, the formation of cataracts—don't improve very much on that kind of diet? No! So what should he have eaten? I have outlined the proper composition of *macronutrients,* protein, carbohydrate, and fat best suited to control of insulin on page 23 of Section I. Refer to that discussion to construct a diet to maintain control of insulin. In the beginning, to bring insulin into line, you will have to restrict some carbohydrates even more vigorously. Try to divide your day's intake of protein, starch, and fat into roughly equal portions eaten 6 times a day. Limit your intake of carbohydrate from all sources to about 5 grams at each sitting (a total of 30 grams per day) until your sugar is normal (consistently under 140).

• *Soluble fiber* is the component "complex carbohydrates," which slows down the absorption of the digestible starch in the meal and the fat, too. In fruit, the soluble fiber is called pectin; in grains, it is called bran; and in vegetables, it is psyllium. Whatever the name, the function is the same.

As a diabetic, you should ultimately take in at least 50 grams of soluble fiber each day from the foods you eat and from vegetable fiber supplements, but don't go from little fiber to that amount overnight or you will suffer mightily with bloating, gas, and abdominal cramping. Recommendation: Aim for a steady daily total of at least 50 grams of soluble fiber per day. But do it slowly! Begin by eating a diet that includes fiber-rich vegetables and a little fruit (melon and berries preferred and in small quantities) with each of your 6 meals. To that base, add a commercial vegetable bulk powder (Konsyl, Metamucil, Citrucel) very gingerly. Begin with $1/4$ teaspoon in a sugar-free citrus beverage with breakfast for 1 week. Then add a second $1/4$ teaspoon dose at dinner for 1 week, and finally take $1/4$ teaspoon with each meal, 4 to 6 times a day. At weekly intervals, slowly increase the amount you take per dose to $1/2$ teaspoon 4 to 6 times a day, and then $3/4$ teaspoon, a full teaspoon, $1^1/2$ teaspoons, and finally 2 teaspoons 4 to 6 times a day. That will give you about 30 to 40 grams of soluble fiber in supplemental form to augment what you get from fiber-rich foods in your diet. It is very important that you maintain a constant level of fiber—for example, don't take 60 grams one day and 10 for three days and then 60 again. Be consistent with your intake, and you'll get the best results in sugar control.

• *Vitamin C* plays a more critical role in maintaining good health if you are a person with diabetes than with perhaps any other disorder except a major viral illness. It combats, through potent antioxidant protection, the constant assault on your tissues that high blood sugar causes, strengthens the integrity of small blood vessels (where so much of the damage of diabetes occurs), improves carbohydrate tolerance, and reduces the "bad" kind of cholesterol and triglycerides (another blood fat). Recommendation: Take an absolute minimum of 1 gram per day. I would further recommend that over a period of 4 to 6 weeks, you work your way up to a total daily intake of 4 to 6 grams per day, using ascorbic acid in crystalline form, or to your bowel tolerance level. Refer to the discussion of vitamin C in the A-to-Z Nutrient listing for a schedule of increasing dosage to this level. Note: People with diabetes suffer a defect in metabolizing ascorbic acid that can lead to breakdown products that can damage the linings of blood vessels. You can prevent this problem by taking the vitamin C along with bioflavonoids (see page 299). It is important to keep in mind that too much vitamin C and thiamine may inactivate insulin. Keep close tabs on your body's reaction to these supplements.

• *Biotin* improves the sensitivity of your tissues to insulin and helps to lower blood sugar. It may also help the numbness, pain, and tingling sensations you may experience in your legs, feet, and hands. Recommendation: Take a dose of about 50 mg biotin per day. If you take insulin or oral diabetic medications, you must check your blood sugar frequently each day, because it may fall too low on your current doses of medication. If you take insulin shots, you should enlist the aid of your personal physician in monitoring your blood sugar when you begin vitamin supplements that may alter it. With the help of your physician, adjust your medications according to the lower need for them.

• *The B vitamin group* is important, especially in preventing or relieving the neuropathy (nerve damage) that often comes as a consequence of diabetes. The members of the B group work best when taken all together. Even when you supplement additional amounts of certain members, you should take at least a minimal daily dose of the others. Recommendation: Take 100 mg B-complex daily, along with specific doses of individual B vitamins.

• *Niacin* (vitamin B_3) is a part of a substance called glucose tolerance factor (GTF), important in insulin and blood sugar regulation. In studies conducted on insulin-dependent diabetics, the use of niacin supplements enabled 66% of the people to discontinue insulin shots. Let me hasten to add that these people were adult-onset diabetics whose need for insulin had outstripped their own ability to make it and who had to take shots of yet more insulin to control their blood sugar, not juvenile diabetics who can make little or no insulin of their own. Recommendation: If you are an adult-onset diabetic currently taking insulin, take a 500 mg dose of niacin (as nicotinamide) 3 to 6 times daily (a total of 1.5 to 3 grams per day) while carefully watching blood sugar and slowly tapering insulin dose with the help of your personal physician. If you do not currently take insulin, you may improve your tolerance of carbohydrate (glucose) by taking 500 mg once or twice a day. Warning: Niacin causes flushing in some people. Please refer to the full discussion of this vitamin and familiarize yourself with its side effects and interactions.

• *Thiamine* (vitamin B_1) must be present for your body to use glucose normally. Deficiency of this vitamin can not only worsen blood sugar control, but may contribute to the numbness, pain, and tingling in the feet, legs, fingers, and hands that many diabetics experience. Recommendation: Take 100 mg to 200 mg thiamine daily for at least 2 weeks to assess your response. If you notice improved sensation and sugar control, continue at this level until your symptoms clear. Maintain on a dose of 50 mg daily.

• Levels of *vitamin B$_6$ (pyridoxine)* may fall especially low in people with diabetes who suffer from numbness and tingling sensations. Supplementation improves the symptoms of nerve damage that cause these feelings in some, but not all, people. Deficiency of pyridoxine also seems to worsen the problem of "insulin resistance," which is at the root of the problem of adult-onset diabetes. Recommendation: Take 50 mg vitamin B$_6$ (pyridoxine) 3 times daily for 4 to 6 weeks to assess your response. If your symptoms improve, continue to take the vitamin at a dose of 50 mg daily. Warning: Do not exceed the recommended dosage for this vitamin. Doses of as little as 200 mg per day over a several-year period have caused irreversible nerve damage in some people.

• *Vitamin B$_{12}$* deficiency may also contribute to the problems with numbness, tingling, and pain in your feet and hands in diabetes. In this instance, supplementation works best when given as a shot, although oral doses may also help. Recommendation: You will need to enlist the aid of your personal physician to administer or prescribe injectable cyanocobalamin (vitamin B$_{12}$) in a dose of 300 to 500 *micro*grams weekly until symptoms begin to respond, then dropping to a monthly dose of 500 *micro*grams indefinitely. In oral form, take 500 to 1000 *micro*grams in sublingual (dissolves under the tongue) form weekly for 4 to 6 weeks to assess your response. The oral route may not work as well, but it's worth a try.

• *Vitamin E,* the potent antioxidant, may prevent diabetic problems of the small blood vessels, the heart, and the eyes. Supplementation with this vitamin, while beneficial, should be undertaken with care if you take insulin shots, because the vitamin can reduce your need for insulin. It can also increase blood pressure in some people, and for both these reasons, you should cautiously increase your dose. Recommendation: Begin with a 100 IU dose of vitamin E (as alpha-tocopherol succinate). Check blood sugar and blood pressure on this dose. With the help of your personal physician, you may need to drop your insulin dose with each change in vitamin E.

Once your blood sugar regulation and insulin dose are stable—and if your blood pressure has not risen above 140/90—increase your vitamin E dose to 200 IU. Check and stabilize again for a week or two after each dose increase. If your sugar control and blood pressure remain normal, aim in a stepwise fashion for a daily dose of 600 to 800 IU per day.

• Depletion or loss of *inositol* from the muscle fibers of the blood vessels and in the nerve tissues may contribute to the development of small blood vessel damage (which contributes to high blood pressure and hardening of the arteries) and the numbness and tingling in feet, legs, and hands common in diabetes. Again, some people respond to supplementation with inositol, and others don't seem to. Recommendation: Take a dose of 500 mg of myoinositol twice a day for 2 weeks to assess your response. If your symptoms respond, continue a dose of 500 mg to 750 mg per day.

• *Chromium* is a critical component of glucose tolerance factor (GTF), which is a substance that improves the response of your tissues to insulin and promotes blood sugar control. Deficiency of chromium not only worsens sugar metabolism, it may also contribute to the development of the numbness, pain, and tingling in your feet, legs, and hands that diabetes causes. Recommendation: Take chromium (as chromium picolinate) in a dose of 400 to 600 *micro*grams per day, or 9 grams of chromium-rich brewer's yeast per day. Within 4 to 6 weeks, you should see improvement in blood sugar control, as well as lessening of the tingling sensations.

• *L-glutamine* reduces the craving for sugar. Recommendation: Take 500 mg 2 times daily.

• *Taurine* aids in the release of insulin. Recommendation: Supplement with 500 mg twice daily.

• *Quercetin* protects the membranes of the lens of the eye from the accumulation of polyols, which can ultimately damage the lens. Recommendation: Take 100 mg 3 times daily.

• *Magnesium* deficiency occurs quite commonly in adult diabetics, especially those who must take insulin. Magnesium plays a key role in regulation of blood sugar, energy production, the release of insulin from the pancreas, and as a protector and preserver of the fragile, insulin-producing cells (the beta cells) in the pancreas. When your levels of magnesium fall too low, you increase your risk for the complications of diabetes: heart disease, eye disease, kidney disease, and hypertension. Recommendation: Take 1000 mg of magnesium twice a day for 4 weeks to assess response. (Also take 1500 mg of calcium a day during this period.) You should see at least some improvement of your sugar control and blood pressure, and feel less fatigue. After that period of 4 weeks, reduce your intake to 500 mg per day, taken along with 1000 mg of calcium. Refer to the discussions of magnesium and calcium, which interact with one another, for more information about why these two minerals should be taken together.

• *Manganese* levels may fall in people with diabetes to as low as one-half the level found in nondiabetic people. Manganese is important in the breakdown and use of blood sugar, and therefore, deficiency of it can cause intolerance to sugar. Recommendation: If you take insulin or oral medications to lower blood sugar, you must enlist the aid of your personal physician to carefully watch your blood sugar and help you to adjust your medication doses accordingly. Begin with a daily dose of 5 to 10 mg. (If you take blood sugar–lowering medications or insulin, adjust the doses as your blood sugar level falls.) After 2 to 3 weeks, increase your dose to 20 mg per day (and adjust medicines again if needed) and remain there.

• *Phosphorus* deficiency, also common in diabetes, may worsen blood sugar control and contribute to fatigue. Recommendation: Take phosphorus as calcium phosphate, 1 gram, 3 times a day. (If you take this kind of calcium-phosphorus supplement, you should discontinue supplementation of other forms of calcium.)

• *Potassium* deficiency can worsen the effects of magnesium deficiency on the heart and kidneys and can interfere with the use of glucose (blood sugar) by the tissues. Recommendation: Begin by eating foods rich in potassium: broccoli, tomatoes, bananas, and citrus fruits. You can purchase a potassium-containing salt substitute, called NO SALT, at most grocery stores. Use $1/4$ to $1/2$ teaspoon of this product in cooking each day to add potassium to your diet. Warning: If you take insulin, do not supplement with extra potassium unless your physician has instructed you to do so after verifying you to be deficient. Dangerously high levels of potassium can result from taking supplemental potassium in this instance.

• *Zinc* deficiency can occur in the tissues of people with diabetes, even when the blood levels test normal. Deficiency of zinc worsens blood sugar control and changes the way your body metabolizes fats. Recommendation: Take 10 to 20 mg chelated zinc (zinc aspartate, picolinate, or gluconate) each day. Warning: Supplementation of zinc in its ionic form can create deficiencies of other minerals, such as copper, by competing with them for absorption from the intestine. Chelation of the minerals (see discussion, pages 30–31, Section I, on chelation) prevents this competition to get into the body, allowing you to fully absorb each of them.

• Diabetes affects the metabolism of the *essential fatty acids* linoleic acid (GLA) and marine (fish) oils (EPA), by altering the body's conversion of these fats into less of the "good" and more of the "bad" kind of eicosinoid messengers. (Eicosinoids, Section I, pages 24–27, fully explains the action of these hormone-like body chemicals.) Suffice it to say here that when you have diabetes, many of the problems that trouble you—high blood pressure, poor circulation, heart disease, nerve damage, cholesterol and blood fat elevations, and hardening of the arteries—occur at least in part because of an overabundance of members of the "bad" eicosinoid group. Regaining a better balance in these chemical messengers will improve your overall health. Recommendation: Remember to begin with the basic dietary framework as outlined above and in Macronutrients, Section I, page 23. To that sound base, add gamma-linoleic acid (GLA) and fish oil (EPA) in a ratio of 1:4 (GLA:EPA) 1 to 3 times daily. The EicoPro essential fatty acid product manufactured by Eicotec, Inc., of Marblehead, Massachusetts, contains ultrapure sources of linoleic acid and fish oils already combined in this ratio. If you cannot get that product, you can purchase linoleic acid in a product called evening primrose oil at most health and nutrition stores, and EPA fish oil as well. Because it is not as pure a form, the milligram dosing will be different. You can make a reasonable substitute by combining evening primrose oil capsules with fish oil capsules plus vitamin E. Take 500 mg of evening primrose oil (a source of linoleic acid in capsule form), plus 1000 mg EPA fish oil, plus 200 IU vitamin E 1 to 3 times a day. (Warning: EPA fish oil can cause blood sugar fluctuations in some diabetics. Carefully monitor your blood sugar if you use this supplemental oil and discontinue its use if your blood sugar becomes difficult to control.)

• The *bioflavonoids* prevent the abnormal metabolism of vitamin C that often occurs in diabetes. If you supplement with vitamin C (and I strongly urge you to do so), you should also supplement with bioflavonoids. Many vitamin C products available at health and nutrition stores already contain bioflavonoids in their formulation. If you supplement at higher doses using the crystalline or powdered form of vitamin C, you will want to add these substances to your regimen. Recommendation: Take the bioflavonoid rutin in a dose of 250 to 500 mg with each dose of vitamin C. A mixture of multiple bioflavonoids is also available at health and nutrition stores as bioflavonoid complex (1000 mg). Take 1 bioflavonoid complex tablet (1 gram) for each 4 gram dose of vitamin C you take.

Herbal remedies

• *Fenugreek* contains compounds that help regulate blood sugar levels. It also increases the blood levels of "good" cholesterol while lowering total cholesterol.

• *Onion* skins contain quercetin, which helps with the eye problems often associated with diabetes.

• *Bay leaves* help the body reduce insulin. In animal tests, it has also lowered blood sugar levels.

• Indian studies indicate that *gurmar* boosts insulin production. This product is just beginning to find its place on the shelves of health food stores.

• *Huckleberry* promotes insulin production.

• *Ginseng* tea is thought to lower blood sugar levels. Caution: Do not use this herb if you have high blood pressure.

As always, consult a physician before beginning any herbal remedies. Dosages vary according to duration and severity of symptoms.

What makes it worse?

• *Alcohol* may further impair your sensitivity to insulin, and it is insensitivity to insulin that is at the very root of the problem. If you are a diabetic in very good control (blood sugars less than 140 mg/dl, no numbness or tingling sensations, normal blood pressure, cholesterol and triglycerides in the normal range), then a modest amount of alcohol—on the order of 1 ounce of distilled spirits or a glass of wine or a single "lite" beer per day—probably won't worsen your problem. Heavier drinking certainly could. Recommendation: Until you have brought your diabetes under very good control, I would advise you to avoid alcohol.

• Some diabetic people develop elevations in ferritin, the protein that binds and carries *iron* in the blood. Treatment of these people with a chemical (called desferrioxamine) that chelates the iron (binds it up and allows it to be removed from the body) improved diabetic control, allowed the people to reduce or discontinue insulin and oral blood sugar–lowering medications, and even reduced their cholesterol and triglycerides. I am not able to say, from the research available to me at this point, whether your taking iron in multivitamins would lead to worse diabetic symptoms or, on the other hand, whether your reducing iron intake would make a difference in control of your diabetes. Still, the response of this particular group of people with high ferritin levels is quite impressive. Recommendation: I would certainly recommend that you ask your personal physician to check your ferritin level, and if it is elevated, to consider this treatment for you. I would further not recommend your taking any kind of supplemental iron unless you specifically suffer from iron deficiency and are anemic.

• Some recent research (1990) suggests that a protein in *cow's milk* may promote the development of juvenile-onset diabetes. Recommendation: Although the connection here is a tenuous one so far, I would recommend erring on the side of caution. If your family includes people who developed the childhood form of diabetes (insulin dependent or Type I diabetes), I would advise not feeding cow's milk to your infant or toddler.

Diarrhea

What is it?

By strict medical definition, diarrhea refers only to the passage of abnormally frequent bowel movements. In general use, however, it has come to mean loose watery stools. By either definition, the causes of diarrhea are legion. Some of them—inflammatory bowel problems and sprues (see Crohn's Disease, Ulcerative Colitis, and Celiac Sprue)—cause ongoing problems with diarrhea over many years. Other causes arise from infections by viruses (the stomach "flu"), from food or drink contaminated with bacteria (the spectrum on these runs from traveler's diarrhea, or "Montezuma's Revenge," to life-threatening cholera), and from parasites (amoebic dysentery). Some people develop diarrhea because of food allergies or sensitivities, such as milk intolerance. And finally, diarrhea can develop because of overconsumption of antibiotic medications, chemical "laxatives" such as Milk of Magnesia and fiber, and sorbitol (a sugar substitute used to sweeten diabetic candies and gum). This kind of diarrhea usually stops readily when you stop taking the medication or chemical.

The specific treatment you would need to stop the other kinds of diarrhea would depend, naturally, on what had caused it. I have discussed inflammatory bowel disorders fully under the listings given on page 301, and food allergy causes and treatments under the listings Ulcerative Colitis and Celiac Sprue. In this listing, I will briefly describe each basic type of infectious diarrhea and then, at the end, address general nutritional support during and immediately after the problem.

Viral diarrhea

Many viruses—and there are quite literally hundreds—that afflict you with sore throats, colds, rashes, and fever can also cause diarrhea. Once the virus enters your intestinal tract, it causes a sudden and dramatic increase in motility (bowel contraction) and in secretion (production of mucus and lack of water reabsorption). Those two activities result in the waves of cramping in your belly, a bloated feeling, and finally the passage of stools every 30 minutes to an hour that become progressively looser and finally watery. Fortunately, most bouts of viral diarrhea last only a few days, but it's sometimes a miserable few, and then you're left feeling wrung out and weak for several more days. If your symptoms last only a day, the best advice is to try to ride them out and not interfere with medicines to stop the diarrhea. Doing so may prolong the symptoms. However, frequent watery stools for a longer period really have to be stopped because of lost fluid, loss of electrolytes, and the risk of irritating your colon/rectum to the point of bleeding.

Bacterial diarrhea

When you eat or drink food contaminated with foreign bacteria—at home or abroad—severe symptoms can occur. Treatment depends on the bacterium involved and the severity of symptoms. Anytime you have diarrhea that fails to clear in 48 to 72 hours, you should see your personal physician.

Typical "food poisoning" caused usually by a staphylococcus bacterium results in sudden onset of both vomiting and diarrhea with severe stomach cramping, but usually with no fever or other body symptoms. The symptoms may begin as quickly as 1 hour after eating the "bad" food, although a delay of 4 to 8 hours is not uncommon. Other bacteria *(Salmonella, Shigella, E. coli, Vibrio cholerae, Clostridium botulinum)* can also cause the diarrhea, but the delay in onset of the symptoms may be from a day and a half to 3 days, and the symptoms can be much more severe and even life-threatening. The bacteria contaminating the food produce a toxic chemical that, when eaten, causes a sudden increase in motility and secretion. The bacteria themselves don't cause the symptoms, and therefore this kind of diarrhea truly is a "poisoning" and not an infection. Antibiotic medications usually are not needed in mild cases; however, let me stress a couple of points. See your doctor right away if you develop: bloody diarrhea, fever, double vision, difficulty swallowing, difficulty talking, or difficulty breathing, or if the diarrhea continues for more than 48 to 72 hours. Do not ignore or attempt self-treatment of these kinds of symptoms.

Parasitic diarrhea

Parasites are living creatures that live off of other living creatures. They can range in size from the tiny (*Amoeba* and *Giardia* are but a single cell in size) to the huge (fish tapeworms can grow up to 60 feet in length). Infestation by a parasite can cause sudden severe bloody diarrhea with fever (amoebic dysentery) or many weeks of daily diarrhea without many other symptoms (*Giardia,* roundworm, pinworm). All cases of parasitic diarrhea ultimately will require treatment with prescription medications to kill the parasite.

What helps it?

• *Diet* modification plays a crucial role to help normalize the activity of your bowel during and after any of these types of diarrhea. Coaxing your intestine back to normal requires patience—don't rush it! Let me outline some basic dietary guidelines for you to follow:

(1) Immediately stop all intake of food or drink at the onset of diarrhea (and vomiting). Take nothing by mouth for at least an hour.

(2) Begin first by melting ice chips in your mouth, but take nothing more. If you tolerate the ice chips, you may have small bites of Popsicle. Continue this regimen for several hours.

(3) Progress to small sips of cool Gatorade *Light,* which contains glucose but not sucrose and is rich in the electrolytes sodium and potassium, which you lose from diarrhea. Try to take in 8 ounces of fluid per hour in small sips. Continue this regimen throughout the first day. Keep a glass at your bedside to sip on during the night if you awaken. If you don't have Gatorade Light, use any clear liquid

without caffeine—regular Gatorade, Sprite, 7-Up, Kool-Aid, decaffeinated tea, or water.

(4) The following day, progress to clear broth (chicken or beef) and small bites of dry toast or Saltine crackers. Continue to drink ever-increasing amounts of Gatorade Light and add other *clear* liquids (clear does not refer to color, but means containing no solids— i.e., no protein and fat) without caffeine or alcohol.

(5) If you tolerated the broth and toast, later in the day, add an ounce or 2 of lean beef or skinless chicken or a couple of scrambled eggs. Continue to drink plenty of clear fluids as before.

(6) Spend the next day drinking fluids and eating bigger amounts of lean meat, chicken, or egg, dry toast, and crackers. You may add a little rice or a few noodles. If you tolerate this level of intake, you're almost healed.

(7) Finally, add milk products back to your diet, beginning with an ounce or two of yogurt or buttermilk and working up over several days to return to your normal diet.

(8) Avoid caffeine, alcohol, and spicy foods until your symptoms have completely cleared.

Anytime you advance your diet and diarrhea and cramping return, drop back to the previous level and wait another half day or day before trying to advance again.

• *Sodium* levels fall with diarrhea of large volume or many days. Low sodium makes you feel washed out, weak, dizzy with minimal activity, and nauseated. That's why it's helpful to use Gatorade and broth in addition to water and other clear beverages. Replenishing sodium will help to speed your recovery. Recommendation: Gatorade Light, as outlined above, will begin to replace sodium losses. Increase your salt intake by salting food a little more heavily and drinking a cup or two of bouillon daily for several days following recovery.

• Diarrhea also causes a loss of *potassium*, which adds to the weak, breathless, washed-out feeling that lingers after your recovery from such an illness. Using Gatorade Light to replenish your lost fluid in the early stages will help to forestall this loss of potassium; however, you may still need to supplement this important electrolyte for several days following recovery. Recommendation: You may increase your intake of the salt substitute called NO SALT, which contains potassium salts, by adding $1/2$ to 1 teaspoon per day to foods.

Or you may take 50 to 100 mg of potassium gluconate once or twice a day for several days.

• *Bismuth* subsalycilate products (such as Pepto-Bismol) help to prevent traveler's diarrhea, help to treat viral and traveler's diarrhea in children and adults, and may be helpful in other kinds of mild bacterial diarrhea as well. You should be aware that bismuth darkens the bowel movement to near black and may also blacken the coating on your tongue and lips. The black color means nothing, is not dangerous, and goes away spontaneously, but its appearance can unnerve you if you're not expecting it. Recommendation: When you travel, take bismuth liquid or tablets daily as per package directions to help stave off traveler's diarrhea. If you develop a diarrhea (traveler's or otherwise) that fails to resolve in 1 day, take liquid bismuth subsalycilate—again, following package directions for your age.

Herbal remedies

• Commission E in Germany promotes the use of *agrimony* for common diarrhea, probably due to its high tannin content. Make a tea using 2 to 3 teaspoons of leaves.

• *Apple* has long been used as a remedy for diarrhea. The pectin is useful in that it helps harden stool. It's actually amphoteric, which means it's also good for constipation because it will soften stool when necessary.

• *Blackberry and raspberry* are high in tannins. Make a tea with 2 teaspoons of either, or 1 of each.

• *Carob powder* shortens the duration of diarrhea. One study focused on 41 infants with bacterial or viral diarrhea. The placebo group had diarrhea for an average of 4 days; babies given the powder had it for just 2 days.

• *Fenugreek* seeds contain almost 50% mucilage, so they swell in the gut and relieve diarrhea. Use no more than 2 teaspoons at a time, or you may have abdominal pain.

• *Psyllium* works the same way as does fenugreek. Assess your reaction, though; many people are allergic to this herb.

Dosages may vary, depending on duration and severity of symptoms. Follow any package directions, or consult a qualified health practitioner.

What makes it worse?

• *Rushing back to food* will make your cramping and diarrhea recur almost without fail, since the toxic or infectious assault on the gastrointestinal tract leaves it temporarily weakened and unable to tolerate "normal" solid meals.

• *Dairy products* place an added burden on the system, because absorption of milk and other dairy foods requires a special enzyme (lactase) to break down the milk sugar. The "sick" bowel quits making the lactase, and it takes several days to coax it back into production. If, before your bowel is ready to cooperate, you eat some milk or cheese, you won't be able to absorb it and you'll develop diarrhea once again.

Diverticulitis

What is it?

This is a condition where the mucous membranes lining the colon become inflamed. The result is small, pouchlike areas called diverticula in the large intestine. Once formed, these never go away, and although they cause no symptoms themselves, they can become inflamed and infected if waste matter gets trapped in them.

Diverticula typically form when a person becomes constipated, and the condition can be acute or chronic. Symptoms include cramping, bloating, tenderness on the left side of the abdomen, constipation or diarrhea, nausea, and an almost constant need to eliminate. You may see blood in the stool. Although millions of Americans are affected with this disorder, many don't know it because they've come to consider their symptoms as simple indigestion.

Nutrition is key in preventing diverticulitis. Let's see how it's done.

What helps it?

• *Fiber* is key here. Fiber keeps the colon clean and allows for regular elimination of waste matter. You need at least 30 grams of fiber daily, which you can obtain through food or supplements or both. Recommendation: Eat foods high in fiber: whole grain cereals, brown rice, bran, most fresh fruit, nuts, seeds, beans, lentils, peas, and fresh raw vegetables. Unsalted, unbuttered popcorn is another excellent source of fiber. If you choose to use a supplement, try psyllium seeds, which can be mixed with liquid and consumed quickly. Metamucil contains psyllium hydrophilic muciloid and is often recommended by physicians. There are other supplements that are more natural, however, available at health food stores. Take your supplemental fiber separately from other supplements to ensure its strength and effectiveness.

• The *B vitamins* are needed for all enzyme systems and for proper digestion. Recommendation: Take 100 mg 3 times daily.

• *Garlic* aids digestion and destroys those nasty bacteria and parasites. Recommendation: Take a yeast-free formula in the dosage of 2 capsules 3 times daily.

• *L-glutamine* provides metabolic fuel for intestinal cells and maintains absorption surfaces of the gut. Recommendation: Take 500 mg twice daily on an empty stomach. Take with water or juice, but never with milk.

• A deficiency of *vitamin K* has been linked to intestinal disorders. Recommendation: Consume plenty of green leafy vegetables. Supplement with 100 *micro*grams of vitamin K daily.

• To heal and protect the lining of the colon, get a healthy supply of *vitamin A*. Recommendation: Take 25,000 IU daily. Do not exceed 8000 IU if you are pregnant.

• *Vitamin C* reduces inflammation and boosts the immune response. Recommendation: Take 3000 to 8000 mg daily in divided doses. Use a buffered form for easier assimilation.

• *Vitamin E* is an antioxidant that protects mucous membranes. Recommendation: Take up to 800 IU daily.

• On the day of an attack, take 4 *charcoal tablets* with a large glass of water. This will absorb trapped gas. Always take charcoal separately from other supplements, and don't take it for prolonged periods. Although it absorbs gas, it also takes with it beneficial nutrients.

Herbal remedies

• People with intestinal disorders often have a vitamin K deficiency. *Alfalfa* is a good source of this vitamin. It also contains chlorophyll, which aids healing.

• *Aloe* heals inflamed areas. Drink ½ cup of aloe vera juice 3 times daily.

• Other useful herbs include *cayenne, chamomile, goldenseal, red clover, and yarrow*.

Dosages may vary, depending on the duration and severity of your symptoms. Consult a qualified herbal practitioner, and talk to your doctor before beginning herbal remedies. Some remedies cannot be used in combination with conventional pharmaceuticals.

What makes it worse?

• *Certain foods* make symptoms worse. Avoid grains, seeds, and nuts (except for well-cooked brown rice). They are hard to digest and can get caught in the crevices of the colon wall. This results in bloating and gas. Other foods that can worsen the condition are dairy products, red meat, sugar products, fried foods, spices, and processed foods.

Dysmenorrhea

What is it?

Painful menstrual periods (dysmenorrhea) occur in one-third to one-half of women, but in 5% to 10% of women, the pain is severe and disabling. Although many women suffer menstrual pain without any obvious abnormality in the reproductive tract, sometimes it occurs because of pelvic infection, endometriosis, or structural differences in the womb. Because there may be such a problem, if you develop painful cycles, you should consult a gynecologist to be certain everything is normal. If there seems to be no problem, nutritional and vitamin therapy may help relieve the pain.

You usually feel the pain of dysmenorrhea low in the middle of the abdomen as a wavelike cramping ache. You may also feel the ache in your low back or down into your thighs, and you may suffer nausea, dizziness, diarrhea, headache, and flushed feelings along with the abdominal cramping. The pain occurs because of an abundance of "bad" prostaglandins that constrict the blood vessels and cause spasms of the muscular wall of the uterus (womb). Refer to eicosinoids, Section I, pages 24–27, to learn more about the prostaglandins. What can nutrition offer to stop "the cramps"? Let's see.

What helps it?

• *Essential fatty acids* may play a more crucial role than any other nutrients in control of dysmenorrhea because of their effect on the production of prostaglandins. If you have not done so, read the discussion in Section I on eicosinoids, pages 24–27, which will explain about the prostaglandins (members of the eicosinoid group) in greater detail. In a nutshell, the body takes the essential fatty acid linoleic acid (GLA) and alters it in a series of steps to produce both the "good" group of eicosinoid messengers and the "bad" group. Proper diet and fish oil (EPA) help to control the production, tipping it in favor of more of the good kind of messenger. Good, in this case, means a prostaglandin (or eicosinoid) messenger that causes the uterus to relax. Bad ones cause spasms and cramping. Recommendation: Begin with a solid macronutrient framework (see macronutrients, Section I, page 23) and to that sound base add gamma-linoleic acid to EPA fish oil in a ratio of 1:4 (GLA:EPA) 1 to 3 times daily. The EicoPro essential fatty acid product manufactured by Eicotec, Inc., of Marblehead, Massachusetts, contains ultrapure sources of linoleic acid and fish oils already combined in the proper ratio. If you cannot get this product, you can purchase linoleic acid in a product called evening primrose oil at most health and nutrition stores, and EPA fish oil as well. Because it is not as pure a form, the milligram dosing will be different. You can make a reasonable substitute by combining evening primrose oil capsules with fish oil capsules plus vitamin E. Take 500 mg of evening primrose oil (a source of linoleic acid in capsule form), plus 1000 mg EPA fish oil, plus 100 IU vitamin E 1 to 3 times a day. (Warning to diabetics: EPA fish oil can cause blood sugar fluctuations in some diabetics. Carefully monitor your blood sugar if you use this supplemental oil and discontinue its use if your blood sugar becomes difficult to control.)

• *Niacin* along with *vitamin C* and the bioflavonoid *rutin*, taken in the premenstrual week, help to prevent or lessen the symptoms of dysmenorrhea. Niacin alone can help to stop cramping once it has begun. Recommendation: Beginning 7 to 10 days before your menstrual bleeding should commence, take 100 mg of niacin, plus 300 mg vitamin C, plus 60 mg rutin each day. During a bout of severe menstrual cramping, you may take 100 mg of niacin every 2 to 3 hours.

• *Vitamin E* may act to enhance the release of your body's natural narcotic chemicals, beta-endorphins. Precisely how this occurs is unclear; however, some women can relieve their menstrual pain by using vitamin E. Recommendation: Begin supplementing about 10 days before your menstrual bleeding should begin. Take 100 IU vitamin E (as alpha-tocopherol succinate) 3 times a day and continue for 4 more days.

• *Iron* supplementation, *if you are low in iron and anemic,* may help to relieve your menstrual pain. I could find no indications in the literature that this remedy would help if you were not anemic from iron deficiency. Recommendation: If you are low in iron, take 90 to 100 mg iron as ferrous sulfate 3 times per day (or a prescription-strength iron replacement from your physician).

• *Magnesium* has a relaxing effect on the muscular wall of the uterus. Deficiency of magnesium may worsen painful cramping and low back pain during menstrual bleeding. Recommendation: Take 250 mg magnesium aspartate once or twice a day the day before and the first 2 days of your menstrual period.

Herbal remedies
• *Angelica root, cramp bark, kava kava, and red raspberry* have antispasmodic properties and help alleviate cramping.
• *Black haw and rosemary* relieve cramps and calm the nervous system.
• *Wild yam* contains natural progesterone and can alleviate cramping.

Dosages vary according to the severity of your symptoms. Consult a qualified health practitioner before beginning any herbal regimen.

What makes it worse?
• Eat fewer dairy products. They block the absorption of magnesium and increase its urinary excretion. Refined sugars also increase magnesium excretion.
• Caffeine is linked to breast tenderness.
• Sodium causes bloating. Omit salt, red meats, processed foods, and junk/fast foods from your diet for at least 1 week prior to the onset of symptoms.

Ear Infections
(see Chronic Ear Infection)

Eating Disorders
(see Binge Eating and Bulimia Nervosa)

Eczema
(see Dermatitis)

Edema

What is it?

The puffiness and swelling that makes your rings too tight and your socks leave imprints on your skin happens because of excess fluid, or "water," in the skin—a condition called edema. Such swelling can occur because of a backing up of fluid in the lower legs and lungs from weakness of the heart muscle—a condition known as congestive heart failure—which I fully discuss in its own separate listing and won't address here. But you might retain fluid for a variety of other reasons: as a consequence of salt retention; in response to excessive heat and humidity; from increased capillary fragility (tiny blood vessel weakness) that allows fluid to "leak" out into the tissues; because of allergies; from protein malnourishment; or as a response to the hormone changes that occur in the menstrual cycle. While there isn't much you can do with vitamins, minerals, and nutrients to prevent or resolve the swelling caused by heat and humidity, you can make a difference in the degree of edema caused by most of the other circumstances. Let's see how.

What helps it?

• *Vitamin B_6* (pyridoxine) helps to block the salt-retaining effect of estrogen that causes premenstrual swelling (see also Premenstrual Syndrome). Recommendation: Take 25 mg of vitamin B_6 daily. If this remedy works for you, you should respond with reduced swelling and shedding of fluid within 1 week. If your response is not adequate, you can increase the dose to 50 mg, but I would not recommend your going beyond that level, because if it has not worked at 50 mg, it's not likely to work for you. There is also a risk to nerve tissues of oversupplementing vitamin B_6; I refer you to the listing for this vitamin for more information.

• *Vitamin E* is especially helpful to block the increased swelling that occurs because of histamine release in allergies. I discuss this topic in greater detail in the Allergies listing, and I recommend you read that section if your swelling occurs for allergic reasons. Recommendation: Take a dose of 400 to 600 IU of vitamin E as alpha-tocopherol succinate for 5 to 7 days when you have retained fluid because of an allergic attack. Warning: Vitamin E can cause elevated blood pressure in some people. You should establish that you do not respond in this manner by first taking a dose of 100 IU, then 200 IU, then 400 IU, and checking your blood pressure between each increase over a period of at least a week. An average of 4 to 5 blood pressure readings should not exceed 140/90. See the Vitamin E listing for more information.

• The combination of *vitamin C plus bioflavonoids* reduces the capillary fragility or weakness that permits fluid in the bloodstream to leak out of the tiny blood vessels and into the tissues, causing swelling of especially your hands, feet, ankles, and lower legs. Recommendation: You can purchase a combined product containing the bioflavonoid complex with vitamin C. I would recommend you take this kind of product sufficient to provide you with 2 to 4 grams of vitamin C per day. If you currently supplement vitamin C alone, you may add bioflavonoid complex in a 500 to 1000 mg tablet to your daily regimen.

• *Proper dietary composition*—sufficient in protein but not excessive in starchy carbohydrates—helps to reduce fluid retention by controlling your production of the hormone insulin. Insulin acts on your kidneys to encourage them to hold on to salt (sodium), and wherever sodium goes, so goes fluid. Refer to the discussion of Macronutrients in Section I, page 23, for details on how to construct a diet that will help control insulin production. Recommendation: If you are retaining fluid now, drop your intake of total carbohydrate (starches and simple sugars, including fruit sugar) to fewer than 20 grams per day for several days. Remember to keep your intake of lean meat, fish, poultry, or egg white high enough to support your lean tissues and to drink at least 64 ounces of fluid per day. You should see a dramatic flushing out of excess body fluid and resolution of the swelling in this short period if elevated insulin levels cause your problem. After the washout, you may return to the 40% nonstarchy carbohydrate, 30% lean protein, 30% essential fat composition described earlier.

• *Salt avoidance,* in the absence of basic dietary modifications as described above, really has very little impact on fluid retention, although excessive use of salt may worsen the problem (see page 313). Recommendation: Unless you also control the body chemicals that make your kidneys hold on to sodium, you will see very little progress in shedding extra body fluid from salt restriction alone.

Herbal remedies

• *Alfalfa* supplies important minerals as well as chlorophyll, a powerful detoxifier.
• Other herbs that may be beneficial include: *butcher's broom,*

dandelion root, horsetail, juniper berries, lobelia, marshmallow, and parsley. Caution: Do not take lobelia on an ongoing basis.

As always, consult your qualified health practitioner before beginning an herbal remedy. Dosages vary according to duration and severity of symptoms.

What makes it worse?
• *Food allergies* certainly contribute to fluid swelling through the release of histamine in the skin. Identifying offending foods and removing them from your diet will help to relieve the problem. Recommendation: Refer to the discussion of Food Allergy for additional information, identifying culprits, and a systematic approach to eliminating suspected problem foods.

• *Excessive addition of salt* to your foods will increase the sodium load your kidneys have to handle and will worsen fluid retention if you already have a tendency to retain salt. Remember, too, that MSG (mono*sodium*glutamate) used in the preparation of Chinese food counts as "salt," and it can be quite a potent (and often overlooked) culprit in fluid retention. Recommendation: Don't make it your habit to add extra salt or MSG to foods for flavor.

Epilepsy

What is it?
Your brain—which is much like a cross between a complex electrical switching station and a lightning-fast computer —functions to instantaneously process billions of pieces of incoming information at an unconscious level, regulates the billions of body functions going on simultaneously, coordinates the movements of all body parts, and on a conscious level, thinks, reasons, speaks, listens, and responds to the world around you. That's quite a job, but one that most of us take for granted. In some people, the electrical relays get short-circuited or out of sync for a variety of reasons, resulting in the production of abnormal bursts of brain waves. These abnormal bursts of electrical activity cause seizures—the condition you may know better by the name epilepsy.

Epilepsy comes in various forms: the grand mal seizure type, with unconsciousness followed by large-scale, spasmodic jerking of both the arms and legs; the petit mal seizure, sometimes called an absence seizure because there is no jerking, just a temporary loss of connection with the conscious level, as though for a moment the person within was "absent"; and a peculiar form of seizure—called a temporal lobe seizure for the part of the brain in which the abnormal activity begins—in which the person appears able to walk, talk, and act, but may have impaired awareness of what is happening without actually losing "consciousness." Abnormal electrical activity in this area of the brain may cause bizarre actions, such as lip smacking, or may cause hallucinations of hearing, vision, taste, or smell. In some cases, the person suffering the temporal lobe seizure, although conscious, cannot understand what is said to him or her, may be unable to name common objects or people, or may suffer a disturbance in perception of musical notes or melodies.

Seizures can develop after a blow to the head, following severe viral illnesses involving the brain (such as meningitis or encephalitis), with high fever (especially in children), and after damage to the brain from a stroke or a tumor. In some cases, thorough testing fails to uncover any cause for the epilepsy; however, anyone who has a seizure should consult his or her personal physician or a neurologic specialist for a complete evaluation and search for a cause. In addition to presciption medications that you may need to help control seizures, can vitamin and mineral intake make a difference? In some cases, yes. Let's see how.

What helps it?

• *Ketogenic diet,* one virtually devoid of any starch or sugar and high in fat, has been used as a treatment for epilepsy in children who fail to respond to medication. (The medical literature reports the use of a diet composed of 4 grams of fat to 1 gram of protein and carbohydrate combined.) In the absence of starch or sugar, the body can burn fat as a source of fuel, with production of waste products called *ketones.* Hence, the name—ketogenic—which means "producing ketones." How the ketones act to suppress the abnormal electrical bursts that cause seizures is unclear. These chemicals do have a suppressing effect on appetite through chemical changes in the feeding center in the brain, so perhaps through some similar change in brain chemicals, the ketones reduce the tendency to electrical "short-circuiting." The main problem with this kind of a diet is that it contains too little protein to support growing bodies and too much fat for good health in the long run.

Although I cannot recommend long-term therapy with a diet this heavily weighted in fat and with so little protein, I would recommend an abbreviated period of ketosis, attained by less stringent means, followed by a return to a mildly ketotic diet as a trial. I would recommend you try this remedy only under the supervision of your personal physician. Recommendation: Begin with a fasting period of 24 hours, during which time you should take nothing by mouth except water. Then for a period of 5 to 7 days eat lean beef, chicken, fish, or egg white sufficient to provide ½ gram of protein for each pound of lean body mass. (In children, who usually have very little body fat, just use 90% of their weight in pounds as a rule of thumb for lean body mass.) Divide the intake into 6 approximately equal servings throughout the day, drinking 12 to 16 ounces of water or decaffeinated tea or coffee with each serving. With small feedings of protein, absent any starch or sugar, most people will produce ketones readily during this period. (You can check your urine for ketone production using Ketostix test strips available at most pharmacies.) If seizures have been occurring frequently, you will be able to see if their development will improve seizure control during this period. Begin to slowly advance the carbohydrate portion of the diet, adding 5 grams* per day over the next week or two until seizure activity becomes more frequent or until you reach a balance of 30% of your day's calories coming from protein; 40% from low-starch, no-sugar carbohydrates; and 30% from fats and oils. Refer to Macronutrients, Section I, page 23, for more information about this kind of balanced diet. On the balanced intake of protein and carbohydrate, you will not be in ketosis most of the time. For more information regarding the ketogenic diet, contact the Pediatric Epilepsy Center at Johns Hopkins Hospital, 600 N. Wolfe St., Baltimore, MD 21287–7247, (410) 955–9100.

• *Folic acid* may be important to you in 3 ways if you have epilepsy. The folic acid content of the brain falls after a seizure; however, the exact relationship of this vitamin to the development of seizures is unclear. Anticonvulsant medications used to control

---

*A 5 gram portion of starch would be: about ½ cup of green beans, broccoli, zucchini, cauliflower, or asparagus; 2 or 3 crackers; 1 slice of "lite" bread; ⅛ cup of rice; ½ cup sliced fresh unsweetened strawberries; ½ cup cottage cheese. Purchase a carbohydrate gram counting book at any bookstore and begin to search out portion sizes of foods you enjoy that contain approximately 5 grams or multiples thereof.

seizures also reduce folic acid levels in the blood, and there has been some speculation that depletion of the vitamin by both these means may contribute to increasing the frequency of seizures in some people. While supplementation of folic acid has proven to reduce the number of seizures in some studies, it has failed to do so in others. And finally, a number of medical studies have shown that using a folic acid solution as a mouthwash can reduce the gum overgrowth (called gingival hyperplasia) that commonly occurs in children who must take the drug Dilantin (phenytoin) to control their seizures. Recommendation: If you are an adult, take 5 mg folic acid per day. Children age 5 to 15 should take 2.5 mg per day. The mouthwash solution of folic acid, prepared by your pharmacist, contains 1 mg of folic acid per teaspoon of solution made in an aqueous base. Children should swish 1 to 2 teaspoons of the mouthwash in their mouths for 2 minutes at bedtime each day to inhibit the gum overgrowth that comes from taking Dilantin. Warnings: Folic acid supplementation can result in: a decrease in blood levels of anticonvulsive drugs (especially phenobarbital), *promotion* of seizures in some people, and a sharp reduction in the vitamin B_{12} levels of people taking anticonvulsive drugs. Do not undertake supplementation of this vitamin without the knowledge, approval, and willingness of your personal physician to adjust doses of your seizure medicines and check you for vitamin B_{12} deficiency.

• *Niacin* can increase the effectiveness of medications used to control seizures. The high amounts of anticonvulsive medications sometimes needed to stop seizure activity may make you so sleepy that you cannot function normally during the day. Supplementing with niacin may permit you to control your seizures with lower doses of medication. Recommendation: Begin with a dose of 500 mg of niacin per day. Increase that dose to twice and then three times per day. If you do not develop flushing or other uncomfortable side effects from the niacin (see its listing in A-to-Z Nutrients, Section I), you may slowly increase your dose of niacin to a maximum of 1 gram 3 times per day. During this time, you should work closely with your personal physician to begin a slow reduction in the medications you take for seizures, carefully monitoring for any change in seizure frequency as you do. Do not attempt to alter doses of these medications on your own!

• Levels of *thiamine*, like folic acid, also fall in people who have seizures. The low blood levels may be a consequence of taking anticonvulsant medications. Some medical research suggests that low levels of thiamine may provoke seizures. Recommendation: Take thiamine beginning at a dose of 50 to 100 mg per day.

• Deficiency of *vitamin B₆* (pyridoxine) is known to cause seizures and, as with folic acid and thiamine, taking anticonvulsant medications may reduce your body's pyridoxine levels. Supplementation with this vitamin helps to reduce seizure activity. Recommendation: Take 100 mg of pyridoxine per day for 2 to 4 weeks. Increase to 150 mg, and finally to 200 mg on weekly intervals if you experience no side effects from taking the 100 mg. Side effects might include numbness, tingling, or pins-and-needles sensations of the hands, feet, fingers, arms, or legs. Warning: At doses as small as 200 mg per day over a several-year period, permanent nerve damage has resulted in some people. If you develop any tingling or pins-and-needles sensations, you should immediately stop taking this vitamin.

• Supplementation with *vitamin E* appears to significantly reduce the frequency of seizures in both children and adults. As with the B vitamins, anticonvulsant medications may cause a depletion of vitamin E and therefore contribute to deficiency. Recommendation: Children over the age of 5 may take vitamin E as d-alpha-tocopherol succinate, beginning with a dose of 100 IU. Remain at that dose for a week or two. Take your blood pressure to be certain that there has been no increase, since occasionally vitamin E will elevate blood pressure. If your average blood pressure remains below 140/90, you may increase your vitamin E dose to 200 IU, remain there a week, and check pressure again. Finally, increase to 400 IU and remain there. (For children unable to swallow pills or capsules, vitamin E is available in liquid form in a strength of 11 drops of the oil providing about 240 IU of tocopherol.)

• *Magnesium* deficiency can increase your tendency to have seizures. Even with normal intake of magnesium and "normal" blood levels of the mineral, relative transient deficiencies can sometimes occur during heat stress, with fever, or after heavy physical exertion of a sufficient degree to trigger seizure activity. Recommendation: Daily supplementation of 500 mg magnesium aspartate may help to reduce seizure frequency; especially if you become ill and have a fever during extremely hot weather, or during and after a period of unaccustomed physical exertion, supplement with 500 mg of magnesium aspartate per day.

• *Taurine,* an amino acid, acts to inhibit abnormal electrical activity in the brain tissue. Areas of the brain where the seizure activity begins often test low in this amino acid in medical research studies. Supplementing taurine may decrease seizure frequency and may allow you to reduce the doses of medication needed to control your seizures. Recommendation: Begin with 250 mg taurine per day. After 2 weeks, increase to 500 mg, then 750 mg, and finally 1000 mg (if needed), remaining at the new dose for at least 2 weeks before progressing. Stop at the dose level at which you begin to experience fewer seizures. Do not advance beyond 1000 mg. Warning: Do not supplement with this amino acid or attempt to reduce your prescription anticonvulsant medications without the knowledge and approval of your personal physician. Worsening of the EEG (electroencephalogram) has occurred at higher doses of this nutrient.

Herbal remedies

• *Black cohosh, hyssop, and lobelia* aid in controlling the central nervous system. Use them on an alternating basis. Caution: Do not use black cohosh during pregnancy.

• *Alfalfa* supplies you with necessary minerals. Take in capsule or extract form.

• *Sage* should be avoided by anyone suffering from seizures.

Dosages vary depending on duration and severity of symptoms. Consult your qualified health practitioner before beginning any herbal regimen.

What makes it worse?

• *Food sensitivities* may trigger seizures in certain people. Particularly if you have a known history of food allergies and sensitivities in your own background or if these problems run strongly in your family, you might consider this possibility as a triggering stimulus for seizures. Recommendation: Pursue food allergy testing with a specialist and undertake a strict food elimination trial under his or her care.

• *Omega-6 fatty acids,* a particular kind of essential fat found in evening primrose oil, may worsen the frequency of temporal lobe seizures. Recommendation: Do not supplement with omega-6 fatty acids if you have a history of this kind of seizure.

• *Aspartame,* the nonsugar sweetener added to diet beverages, puddings, gelatins, and yogurt, and sold under the name Equal in little blue packets for sprinkling on foods, may cause seizures in some people. Because aspartame is a protein, it can promote allergic-type reactions in sensitive people, and one of those reactions could be abnormal brain electrical activity. Recommendation: If you suffer from epilepsy and have experienced an increase in seizure frequency, eliminating aspartame-containing foods and beverages from your diet may be important.

Eye Health
(see Cataract and Glaucoma)

Fatigue

What is it?

One of the most frequent complaints that brings a person to see the doctor is fatigue, under any of its names: weakness, tiredness, sluggishness, lack of energy. When doing normal activities just seems to exhaust you, you suffer from fatigue, but the fatigue can occur for a wide variety of reasons. Among these are: thyroid problems, both too much and too little thyroid hormone; heart problems, such as congestive heart failure; infections, both short-lived ones, like a cold or the flu, and those more serious viral infections that cause chronic fatigue syndrome; breathing problems, such as emphysema or sleep apnea (a condition in which people cannot breathe normally during sleep and consequently don't sleep very well); anemia; chronic diseases such as arthritis or cancer; alcoholism; and finally, psychological conditions, such as depression.

To truly treat the fatigue, you must direct your therapy at what's causing it, but there are a number of nutritional remedies that may help to relieve the symptoms while you're working on uncovering the cause. Let's look at the nutritional shelf to see what looks promising.

What helps it?

• *A properly constructed diet* as described in the Macronutrient discussion of Section I, page 23, will provide the basic framework to begin recovering your energy level. Refer to that section to construct a diet that provides you with a *minimum* of ½ gram of complete lean protein (lean meat, fish, poultry, egg white) for every pound of your lean body tissue each day. (I have provided a quick means to help you estimate your lean tissue weight in that section.)

Multiply your protein requirement in grams by 4 to arrive at the number of calories per day you should eat as lean protein. Make that number of calories 30% of your daily minimum calorie total. For example: If your lean tissue weight is 120 pounds, you would need 60 grams of protein daily. Sixty grams multiplied by 4 calories for each gram is 240 calories from protein. The 240 calories should represent 30% of your day's *minimum* total calories. That would mean that your absolute minimum base need in calories would be 800 per day, divided as 30% protein, 40% carbohydrate, 30% essential fats, or 240 calories coming from protein, 320 calories coming from complex starches, and 240 calories coming from essential fats. You may at this point be thinking that you would starve on 800 calories, and that is true! Remember, I've said this is the minimum. Most of you will eat double or even triple that amount of calories to maintain your weight, but you should keep the proportions the same: 30% lean protein, 40% low-starch carbohydrates, and 30% essential fats and oils. Also, see the discussion on page 324 about food sensitivities when constructing your diet. Recommendation: Construct a 30–40–30 diet as outlined above and in Section I. Except for rare variances, make this your daily dietary goal.

• Your need for *B vitamins* increases when you are sick, injured, or stressed emotionally or physically to enhance energy production. Under these conditions, if you do not supplement your diet with certain members of this group, fatigue commonly occurs. Recommendation: Although the entire complex works best given together in a dose of 100 mg 3 times daily, you may also need to increase your intake of specific B family members as follows.

• Supplementation with extra *folic acid* may improve fatigue associated with depression, burning sensations in the feet and hands, and "restless leg syndrome" (a condition in which people cannot keep from wanting to move their legs when they lie down to sleep). Recommendation: Take 10 mg folic acid per day. Symptoms of burning or tingling and the restless legs should subside quickly, often as early as 3 weeks. The fatigue and depression usually respond in 2 to 3 months. Warning: Even if taking 50 to 100 mg of vitamin B-complex or extra vitamin B_{12} by mouth, remember that high doses of folic acid can mask a deficiency of vitamin B_{12} that could result in severe symptoms and permanent nerve damage. You should always have your personal physician check the level of vitamin B_{12} in your blood and if needed provide you with extra supplementation of it in shot form.

• The most common symptom of deficiency of *pantothenic acid* is fatigue associated with sullenness, sleeplessness, and depression. Recommendation: Take 100 mg pantothenic acid (vitamin B_5) daily along with the 100 mg 3 times of vitamin B-complex.

• Deficiency of *vitamin B_{12}* often causes fatigue, even before it occurs to a degree sufficient to cause anemia or nerve problems. Recommendation: In addition to B-complex, take 2000 *micro*grams of vitamin B_{12} either by mouth or in the form that dissolves under the tongue once a week for a month, then monthly. You may also take the vitamin in shot form, which absorbs more completely, with the assistance of your personal physician.

• Complaints of fatigue occur more commonly in people who take in little *vitamin C* and who consequently have a "marginally" adequate intake. Most medical studies looking into this question have not been able to clearly demonstrate that supplementation with vitamin C relieves fatigue; however, it does seem to improve concentration and ability to do work in people who suffer fatigue. Recommendation: Refer to the discussion of this vitamin for recommendations on how to slowly increase your intake to a level optimal for you. If you do not currently take any extra vitamin C, begin with a 500 mg dose of time-release vitamin C twice a day. If you tolerate this dose well, but still feel impaired in your ability to do work, increase to 1000 mg twice daily. If you do not tolerate taking the vitamin in tablet form because of stomach burning or upset, you may tolerate it better in crystalline (powdered) form. You can find the instructions for taking larger doses of vitamin C in crystalline form in the listing for the vitamin in Section I on page 178.

• *Dimethylglycine* increases oxygen and energy levels in the body. Recommendation: Supplement with 50 to 100 mg daily.

• *Iron* deficiency, because it reduces red blood cell production and leads to anemia, can certainly contribute to fatigue, difficulty concentrating, and poor efficiency in work. Recommendation: *Only* supplement iron if your physician has checked your blood and has determined that your level of iron is low. If so, he or she may prescribe a stronger supplement; you can purchase ferrous sulfate at health and nutrition stores in 30 to 45 mg strengths. You should take 90 mg 3 times daily along with at least 250 to 500 mg vitamin C to help you absorb the iron better. Take iron with food if your stomach rebels.

• *Magnesium, potassium, and aspartic acid* all play key roles in energy production individually and in concert. Magnesium is needed to produce ATP, the body's basic energy form, and aspartic acid helps to get the magnesium and the potassium into the cells for use. Recommendation: In fatigue, because the 3 nutrients work together, you should supplement them together. Take 1 gram (1000 mg) each of potassium aspartate and magnesium aspartate twice daily. Note: Magnesium works in conjunction with another related mineral, calcium. For intermittent therapy with magnesium or treatment of short duration (less than 3 months), you probably don't need extra calcium when you supplement with magnesium; however, I would refer you to the discussion of these minerals in Section I for interactions.

• A sense of fatigue and lethargy may occur in people with a marginal deficiency of *zinc*. Another sign that you might be minimally deficient in zinc is the appearance of leukonychia, the white spots that appear on your fingernails. If you develop these spots (without having sustained injury to the nail) and also suffer lethargy and fatigue, you may benefit from zinc supplementation. Recommendation: Take 50 mg chelated zinc 2 to 3 times per day. Warning: Supplementation of zinc in its ionic form can create deficiencies of other minerals, such as copper, by competing with them for absorption from the intestine. Chelation of the minerals (see discussion, pages 30–31, Section I) prevents this competition to get into the body, allowing you to fully absorb each of them.

Herbal remedies

• Fatigue can be fought using *acacia, cayenne, ginkgo, guarana, and Siberian ginseng*. Caution: Do not use this ginseng if you have high blood pressure, a heart disorder, or hypoglycemia.

Consult your qualified herbal practitioner before beginning any herbal remedies to get effective dosages.

What makes it worse?

• A diet high in refined and simple *sugars* can increase fatigue and sleepiness, especially in some people. The effect probably occurs because the high intake of sugar permits a flood of tryptophan (an essential amino acid) to enter the brain quickly. Sleepiness occurs when an abundance of tryptophan enters the brain. The same phenomenon occurs in certain complex starches, such as potato starch, wheat starch, and corn starch. If you wonder if sugar and starch makes you sleepy and fatigued, you may want to conduct a simple experiment. Eat nothing after eight o'clock in the evening except water. The next morning, treat yourself to a breakfast of a large stack of pancakes or waffles with lots of syrup and butter and a big glass of orange juice. Don't eat any eggs, meat, or caffeinated coffee to blunt the response. Just the pancakes and syrup and butter. Wait about 30 minutes to an hour quietly—watch TV or read. If you become stuporous to the point of wanting to go to sleep, you'll know that carbohydrate has a fatiguing effect for you. Recommendation: Try to avoid simple sugars, such as table sugar, corn syrup, molasses, high-fructose corn syrup, and all foods made with these including sugared desserts, candy, cookies, cakes, pies, ice cream, cereals, soft drinks, and the like. Honey, although also a simple sugar, causes less of a fatigue problem because it is higher in glucose than sucrose (table sugar), but you should use even honey in small, infrequent amounts if you suffer from fatigue. Try to limit your intake of the fatiguing starches (potato, wheat, corn) and rely on the less-starchy vegetables (green leafy vegetables, green vegetables, and yellow and orange vegetables) along with oats and rice as your complex sources of carbohydrate. Reserve your intake of simple sugars for fruit and milk sugar. Eat solid fruits in quantities limited to $1/2$ fruit per serving to reduce the absolute amount of fruit sugar taken in at a sitting. Drink milk, eat yogurt or cottage cheese in amounts providing no more than 8 to 10 grams of carbohydrate at a time, and eat hard cheeses in 1- to 2-ounce portions.

• Although we think of *caffeine* in coffee as the "wake-me-up" chemical, chronic use of it may cause fatigue, headache, moodiness, and depression in some people. Because caffeine boosts energy through increasing the production of ATP, the basic unit of energy production in your body, one school of thought suggests that chronically stimulating this system may deplete it, sort of like overworking the soil in farmland. Recommendation: If you are a caffeine junkie (more than 3 cups of coffee a day) and can't get through the day without your coffee fix, you may be promoting your fatigue with caffeine and need a rest period. Go slowly with your reduction to zero caffeine to avoid developing overwhelming sleepiness and a bad headache. Begin by purchasing a tin of 50/50 caffeinated and decaffeinated blend coffee. Mix 3 parts of your regular full-strength brand with 1 part of the blend and drink that slightly weaker mixture for 1 week. Next, mix 2 parts of your regular brand with 1 part of the blend, and drink for a few days. Then mix them in equal parts for a few days. Drop down to 1 part regular and 2 parts blend for a few days. Then use 1 part regular and 3 parts blend for a few days. Now just drink the 50/50 blend. Purchase a tin of 100% decaffeinated coffee. Follow the same mixing ritual as above: 3 parts blend, 1 decaf; 2 parts blend, 1 decaf; 1 blend to 1 decaf; 1 blend to 2 decaf; 1 blend to 3 decaf. Finally you're ready to take the last plunge to a 100% decaffeinated life and should not have experienced any noticeable withdrawal from caffeine doing it this slowly. Remember that chocolate and many soft drinks also contain significant amounts of caffeine. It won't do any good to eliminate caffeine in coffee if you're getting it in other foods. Stay caffeine-free for at least 3 or 4 months before resuming drinking it. You might, however, elect to remain caffeine-free for good.

• *Iron* overload can also cause extreme and disabling fatigue, and hence the warning on page 321 not to supplement iron unless you are certain that you are deficient in it by blood testing. Recommendation: Supplement iron only for documented deficiency.

• *Food sensitivities* can cause fatigue. This problem is especially common in people who suffer allergies to the environment around them: pollens, weeds, flowers, animals, and dust. Recommendation: Begin to systematically avoid foods you think may cause the problem one at a time. If your symptoms disappear, you're home free. If they do not, however, continue your step-by-step search. Typical offenders are chocolate, strawberries, peanuts, wheat, various food dyes, and sugar, but any food is possible. You may want to seek help from an allergy specialist to help you narrow your search. You will have to undertake an elimination trial—totally abstaining from that food and anything made with it—for 3 to 4 weeks to assess your response. After the symptoms have cleared, you must prove the connection between the food and your symptoms by eating the food in a significant quantity and seeing the return of your fatigue. That may sound cruel, but you will not know with certainty that you've hit the culprit food otherwise.

Fibrocystic Breast Disease

(see Breast Disease, Benign)

Fibromyalgia

What is it?

This is a rheumatic disorder that causes chronic achy muscular pain for no obvious reason. Usually the lower back, neck, shoulders, back of the head, upper chest, and/or the thighs are affected. The pain is described as burning, throbbing, shooting, and stabbing, and is often accompanied by headaches, strange sensations in the skin, insomnia, irritable bowel syndrome, and temporomandibular joint (TMJ) syndrome. Other symptoms include painful menstrual periods, anxiety, palpitations, memory impairment, dry eyes and mouth, dizziness, impaired coordination, and the need for frequent changes in eyeglass prescription. Depression also accompanies this disorder.

We don't know what causes fibromyalgia. It seems to be related to problems with the immune system, but the relationship is not understood. Because many people affected by this disorder have a history of clinical depression, it is thought that there is a link between the condition and a disturbance in brain chemistry. Some experts believe the disorder is related to chronic fatigue syndrome.

Whatever the cause, it is apparent that malabsorption problems are common in people with fibromyalgia, so all nutrients need to be supplemented at higher than usual doses.

What helps it?

• A *properly constructed diet* is important in treating fibromyalgia. Eat lots of vegetables, fruits, whole grains, nuts and seeds, skinless turkey or chicken, and deep-water fish. These foods provide an abundance of important nutrients that energize and build immunity. Food should be eaten in 4 or 5 small meals so that your body receives a steady supply of proteins and carbohydrates necessary for muscle function.

• To flush out toxins, drink plenty of *steam-distilled water.*

• *Coenzyme Q₁₀* improves oxygenation of tissues. Recommendation: Take 75 mg daily.

• *Proteolytic enzymes* improve the absorption of foods, especially protein. Recommendation: Follow the dosage on the label, and take 6 times daily.

• *Vitamin A* protects the body's cells. Recommendation: Take

25,000 IU for 1 month, then slowly reduce to 10,000 IU daily. Warning: Do not exceed 8000 IU daily if you are pregnant.

• *Vitamin E* enhances the immune function because it is a potent antioxidant. Recommendation: Take 800 IU daily for 1 month, then reduce your daily intake to 400 IU. Use the emulsion form.

• Energize your body with *vitamin C*. Recommendation: Take a vitamin C with bioflavonoids supplement at a dosage of 5000 mg (5 grams) to 10,000 mg (10 grams) daily. Use a buffered form for easier assimilation.

• People with fibromyalgia are often deficient in *magnesium*. Recommendation: Take 1000 mg daily. Balance that with 2000 mg daily of calcium.

• *Potassium* aids in muscle function. Recommendation: Take 99 mg daily.

• *Selenium* is an important antioxidant. Recommendation: Take 200 *micro*grams daily.

• *Zinc* helps maintain the immune system. Recommendation: Take 50 mg daily in chelate form. Do not exceed this amount.

• To promote healthy sleep, look to *melatonin*. Recommendation: Start with 1 gram daily, taken 2 hours before bedtime. If this has no effect, slowly increase your dosage (1 gram at a time). Continue doing this up to 8 grams. Use a sustained-release formula.

• *L-tyrosine* relieves depression and aids in relaxing the muscles. Recommendation: Take 500 to 1000 mg daily at bedtime. Warning: Do not take this supplement if you take an MAO inhibitor drug.

• *Essential fatty acids* protect cells from damage and help reduce fatigue and pain. Recommendation: Take 4 to 6 fish oil capsules daily. The usual supplements contain between 180 and 400 mg of EPA and 120 to 300 mg of DHA.

Herbal remedies

• Remove parasites with *black walnut and garlic*. Experts don't know what causes this disorder. Some evidence points to immune system problems, other evidence points to viral infections. What is known is that infections worsen the symptoms. That's where parasites come in. The parasites that cause/carry the infections need to be wiped out.

• *Astragalus and echinacea* enhance immune function.

• Brew teas using *burdock root, dandelion, and red clover*. These

beverages will promote healing by cleansing the bloodstream and enhancing the immune system. Drink 4 to 6 cups daily.
• *Ginkgo* improves circulation and brain function.

Dosages may vary, depending on the duration and severity of your symptoms. Consult a qualified herbal practitioner, and talk to your doctor before beginning herbal remedies. Some remedies cannot be used in combination with conventional pharmaceuticals.

What makes it worse?
• *Solanine* interferes with enzymes in the muscle, which can lead to pain and discomfort. Recommendation: Limit your intake of green peppers, eggplant, tomatoes, and white potatoes.
• *Saturated fats* raise cholesterol levels and interfere with circulation. They promote the inflammatory response and increase pain. Recommendation: Limit your consumption of meat, dairy products, fried foods, processed foods, shellfish, and white flour products such as bread and pasta.
• *Caffeine, alcohol, and sugar* are not good for this disorder. Sugar in any form promotes fatigue, increases pain, and disturbs sleep. Recommendation: Eliminate these substances from your diet if possible. If they have been a regular part of your diet, your symptoms will actually get worse for a short period of time. However, soon you will notice a marked improvement in your condition.
• *Food allergies* can worsen the symptoms of fibromyalgia. Recommendation: If you notice particular foods causing you problems, eliminate them from your diet and see if there is improvement.

——— Fluid Retention ———
(see Edema)

——— Food Allergy ———
What is it?
Some people inherit a tendency to react to the world around them, the pollens, the weeds and trees, the animals, the plants, and even the foods they eat. I have discussed, under Allergies in this listing, how allergies come about, and I refer you to that discussion for this information, because food allergies develop in much the same way. You may respond to food allergy with your skin (hives, swelling, or a rash), with

your nose and sinuses (watery nasal drainage, tearing, or stopping up), with your gastrointestinal tract (cramping, diarrhea, or constipation), with your musculoskeletal system (joint pain and stiffness), or with your head (a headache, depression, agitation, sleepiness, sleeplessness, or irritability). The results vary, but the cause stays the same—something you eat or drink makes you respond in this fashion. Some food allergies are very straightforward: You eat a strawberry, you break out in hives. Simple to deduce. But more often, the problem takes time to unravel, because most of the foods we eat contain multiple ingredients—any of which could be the culprit. Recommendation: Avoid the culprit. You may want to enlist the aid of an allergy specialist to do some testing to help you narrow down the possibilities so that you can undertake a food-elimination trial. To do this, you must systematically take each potential allergy-causing food and totally eliminate it and anything made with it from your diet for a minimum of 3 to 4 weeks. During this time, your symptoms should disappear. If they do not, that food is probably not your culprit. If they do, however, you must prove the connection by eating a significant quantity of that food substance and seeing your symptoms reappear. If they do, you've found at least one cause, but since there could be others, your search should continue until all possible culprits have passed or failed the test.

What helps it?
• For other nutritional remedies that may help this kind of allergy and others, refer to Allergies.

Herbal remedies
• See entry under Allergies, page 176.

What makes it worse?
• See Allergies.

———————— Food Poisoning ————————
What is it?
Every year, more than 2 million Americans report illnesses that can be traced to foods they have eaten. The actual number of food poisoning cases is probably much higher, however, because people often mistake the symptoms for those of stomach flu.

Food poisoning is more serious than you may think. As many as 9000 deaths occur annually from all types of food poisoning. What's more, many cases lead to chronic health disorders.

There are many types of food poisoning, depending on the agent that caused it. Symptoms vary, but the most common are nausea, vomiting, diarrhea, headache, and abdominal pain. There are a number of reasons why food poisoning occurs: Animals raised in confined quarters are susceptible to bacterial infection; food processing is more centralized these days, so a single ingredient that is tainted with a contaminant can show up in a plethora of products; imported food often comes from countries with poor hygiene in food production; many Americans are simply unaware of how to properly prepare food in their own kitchens. The fact is, many cases of food poisoning are preventable. Let's see what helps in preventing and treating this disorder.

What helps it?

• *Charcoal tablets* remove toxic substances from the colon and bloodstream. Recommendation: At the first sign of illness, take 5 tablets. They can be sucked on until they disintegrate if you can't swallow them. Then take 5 tablets again in 6 hours. Take these tablets separate from other supplements, since they can absorb vital nutrients as well as toxins. The other supplements can be taken once you no longer feel the need to vomit. The supplements should not in any way upset the stomach.

• *Garlic* destroys bacteria in the colon while it detoxifies. Microbiologist David Hill found that in the presence of garlic, disease-causing microbes were eliminated. Recommendation: Take 2 capsules 3 times daily, with food.

• Diarrhea causes an imbalance in your electrolyte levels. Recommendation: Take 99 mg of *potassium* to restore that balance.

• *Vitamin C with bioflavonoids* works with *vitamin E* to detoxify the body and enhance the immune system. Recommendation: Take 8000 mg daily of vitamin C with bioflavonoids (in divided doses) along with 600 IU vitamin E.

• *L-cysteine* and *L-methionine, selenium, and superoxide dismutase* are nutrients essential in immune function. Recommendation: Take 500 mg of L-cysteine and L-methionine daily, on an empty stomach. Take 200 *micro*grams of selenium daily. Take 5000 mg of superoxide dismutase daily.

Some of the best measures of prevention are the ones that make the most sense but are often the most overlooked. To help prevent food poisoning, keep in mind these tips:

• Wash your hands before handling food and after handling raw meat or poultry.

• Use 2 cutting boards: 1 for meat, the other for vegetables. Wash them at least 3 times weekly with a solution of ¼ cup hydrogen peroxide and 2 gallons of water.

• Throw away cans that are bulging, rusted, bent, or sticky; these are warning signs of possible botulism.

• Wash kitchen towels and sponges with a solution of 1 part bleach to 20 parts water daily.

• Thaw all frozen foods, especially meats and poultry, in the refrigerator.

• Avoid these foods when eating at salad bars: chicken, fish, creamed foods, foods containing mayonnaise, undercooked foods, and soups that are not kept at near-boiling temperatures.

Herbal remedies

• *Lobelia* enemas can rid the body of poison. Add a dropperful of alcohol-free goldenseal to the enema for added strength.

• *Goldenseal* is a natural antibiotic that destroys bacteria in the colon. At the first sign of food poisoning, take a dropperful of alcohol-free goldenseal extract. Repeat every 4 hours for 24 hours.

Dosages may vary, depending on the duration and severity of your symptoms. Consult a qualified herbal practitioner, and talk to your doctor before beginning herbal remedies. Some remedies cannot be used in combination with conventional pharmaceuticals.

What makes it worse?

• *Improper home-canning techniques* are responsible for over 90% of cases of botulism in America. Recommendation: Avoid home-canned meats, fruits, and vegetables unless they have been prepared in a pressure cooker. The old "stovetop" method of home canning is NOT a reliable way to seal jar lids.

———————— **Gall Bladder Disease** ————————

What is it?

The gall bladder is nothing more than a storage bag for the bile (also called gall) that you produce in your liver. When a meal you've eaten, containing some fat, enters the small intestine, the gall bladder springs into action, squirting some bile down the bile duct and into the intestine where it combines with the dietary fat, making it easier for you to absorb. Without the bile, much of the fat would pass through and cause a fatty diarrhea. When the gall bladder functions normally, your digestion proceeds happily.

Problems occur, because sometimes the bile becomes very thick, like sludge, and won't pass down the duct as it should. Because bile contains a high amount of cholesterol, when it sits and thickens, or when the cholesterol content becomes too high in the bile, some of the cholesterol "crystals" can fall out of the solution. As these "crystals" group together, they form "stones" of cholesterol and bile salts. The stones fill up the gall bladder and impair its function. Now when the call comes for the gall bladder to spring into action, it squeezes down on a bunch of rocks and it hurts—this is gall bladder colic or a gall bladder attack. Once these stones have formed, and the gall bladder no longer can work properly, surgery usually is the only reliable cure. Fortunately, nowadays surgery can often be done using a laparoscope (a lighted flexible magnifying periscope), allowing the surgeon to operate through a tiny incision. You recover, following this kind of gall bladder surgery, in terms of days, not weeks.

But what if you just have sludge and poor gall bladder function, or if gall bladder disease runs in your family, or you are a member of the group most likely to develop gall bladder problems: overweight, female, over 40, multiple children or have taken birth control pills? Can nutrition, vitamins, or minerals help you before you develop stones? Let's see.

What helps it?

• *Proper dietary construction and total calories* sufficient to reach and maintain ideal body weight and fat percentage will reduce your risk for gall bladder disease. Refer to Macronutrients (Section I, page 23) for general information about how to construct a diet that provides adequate protein to support your lean body mass. (You will find methods of calculation of lean body mass in the section.) Begin with protein intake sufficient to provide $1/2$ gram of complete lean protein (lean meat, chicken, fish, egg whites) for each pound of lean body mass. Because each gram of protein provides 4 calories, you can determine the number of calories from protein by multiplying your gram requirement by 4. For reducing gall bladder disease risk, this number of calories should account for 25% of your day's calorie total. Another 45% of your calories should come from whole fruits, vegetables that are low in starch (broccoli, cauliflower, string beans, carrots, squashes, green peas, leafy greens), and rice and oats. The final 30% of your diet should be a mixture of dietary fats, with 20% from olive oil, canola oil, or sunflower oil and 10% from animal fat.

• *Dietary fiber* helps to reduce the cholesterol content in bile. Recommendation: Aim for a total daily fiber intake of 40 to 50 grams per day. Although choosing vegetables that are low in starch will usually mean those richer in fiber, you will still probably need to take extra fiber supplementation. I recommend that you use a vegetable bulk powdered preparation containing psyllium, such as Konsyl, Metamucil, or Citrucel, which provide about 3 to 6 grams of fiber per teaspoon depending on which brand you choose. Begin to slowly add this fiber supplement to your daily intake of fruits and vegetables. Take care not to increase your dose rapidly, because you may develop unpleasant side effects, such as bloating, cramping, and gas. Begin with just $1/4$ teaspoon in juice or a sugar-free citrus beverage at bedtime. Increase after a week to $1/4$ teaspoon morning and night. Then increase to $1/2$ teaspoon doses morning and night, then 1 teaspoon, $1 1/2$ teaspoons, and finally 2 teaspoons morning and night. At that level, you will be adding 12 to 24 extra grams of fiber a day to your food intake. You can continue to increase to a full tablespoon (3 teaspoons) at each dose, which will provide 20 to 36 grams of supplemental fiber per day. The key to success is to go slowly and to be consistent with your intake from day to day.

• *Substituting soy for milk protein* may help to reduce your risk for developing stones. Research in laboratory animals suggests a reduction in gall stone formation by removing casein (the protein of milk) from the diet and using soy products instead. Whether these results will bear out as beneficial in people is not yet clear. Recommendation: If you are at high risk for developing gall stones and like soy milk and tofu, use them in place of milk products. It *may* reduce your risk for gall bladder disease. Without clearer and more certain evidence, I would not categorically recommend substituting soy products for milk protein in everyone at risk.

• For gall stones, mix 3 tablespoons of *olive oil with the juice of one lemon* before bed and when you awake. Stones are often passed and eliminated in stool using this technique.

• *Eat your breakfast.* People who skip breakfast or only have coffee develop gall stones more frequently. Remember, as I mentioned earlier, the gall bladder only works when it senses fat in the small intestine, and since the longest period of time without food (and therefore with the gall bladder stagnant) is from one evening meal to the next breakfast, it's important to eat a morning meal. Recommendation: Eat a regular breakfast containing some protein, some fat, and some starch. That could be as simple as a serving of scrambled eggs and a piece of lightly buttered toast. It could be a little fruit and yogurt or cottage cheese. It could be a small piece of meat or a hard-boiled egg with half a bagel. A bowl of oatmeal. A bran muffin with a little butter or margarine. It doesn't have to be a major production, it just shouldn't be skipped.

• People who drink a *moderate amount of alcohol* ($\frac{1}{2}$ to 1 ounce per day of distilled spirits or 1 glass of wine or 1 "lite" beer) develop fewer gall stones than strict abstainers. Recommendation: Drink a single glass of wine with dinner. You may instead drink an ounce of distilled liquor 3 to 4 times a week or a "lite" beer 3 or 4 times a week. Please do not use this remedy if you are an alcoholic or someone with a strong history of alcoholism in your family.

• *Moderate coffee consumption* may inhibit the formation of gall stones. Recommendation: If you like coffee, a moderate intake, which means 3 or fewer cups of regular coffee per day, may reduce your gall bladder risk if you don't already have stones. See the warning on page 335 under "What makes it worse."

• *Vitamin C* deficiency may increase the tendency to form gall stones. Supplementing with the vitamin can reduce your risk. Recommendation: Refer to the discussion of this important vitamin in the A to Z Nutrient listings in Section I. You should take a minimum of 500 mg time-release vitamin C twice daily, but you may tolerate (and need) a higher dose. The listing for this vitamin describes how to take a higher dose using the crystalline (powdered) form.

• *Vitamin E* may reduce the risk of developing gall stones made purely of cholesterol (most stones contain a lot of cholesterol along with other bile salts and calcium) by reducing the levels of cholesterol in the bile. Recommendation: Begin with a small dose of vitamin E (100 IU per day) and be certain taking the vitamin does not elevate your blood pressure. If your pressure remains at 140/90 or less on average (take 5 readings on different days and average that number), you may increase your dose to 200 IU, 400 IU, 600 IU, and finally 800 IU, checking blood pressure before each increase.

• *L-glycine* is an amino acid essential for the proper biosynthesis of nucleic and bile acids. Recommendation: Take 500 mg on an empty stomach with water or juice.

• *Lecithin,* which provides dietary choline, may help to keep cholesterol in solution in the bile and prevent the formation of stones. Recommendation: Take 1 to 2 grams of soybean lecithin per day if you know you have "sludge" in your gall bladder. If you have no symptoms or documented sludge, take 500 mg lecithin a day as a means of prevention.

• People who follow a *vegetarian lifestyle* have fewer gall stones. But strict vegetarians may suffer a host of other medical maladies, and so the trade-off is probably not to your benefit in the long run. The fact that the human body cannot build, grow, or repair itself without sufficient complete protein every day makes a tough job for a true vegetarian. Although you can find all the necessary components for complete protein in the plant world, learning to match foods to make all the essential amino acids available at the same time can be tricky and takes some degree of expertise. Adding egg whites, however, solves the problem, since egg white is complete protein all by itself. With that single change, you can live very nicely on a diet of fruits, grains, vegetables, and egg whites. Each egg white contains 6 grams of complete protein, and since most adults usually need 60 to 80 grams of protein per day, you have to eat a lot of egg white to get your allotment with egg white alone. But you can do it. (For my money, unless you have philosophical objections to eating the flesh of other living creatures, some fish, shellfish, and occasional poultry rounds your diet out nicely—it's just not vegetarian.)

Herbal remedies

• The Chinese cultures have been using *beggar-lice* for centuries to treat gall bladder disease. It decreases the amount of calcium excreted in urine and increases the amount of citrate excreted. This reduces the likelihood of gall stone formation.

• *Couchgrass* is recommended by Commission E for preventing gall stones and inflammatory disorders of the urinary tract.

• *Ginger.* Make a hot compress using ginger. The compress causes superficial skin irritation, taking the mind off the more intense gall stone pain.

• *Peppermint and spearmint* can be made into tea to treat gall stones.

• Commission E also endorses *turmeric* for treating and preventing gall stones. It contains curcumin, a compound that has been tested for its effect on gall stones. It increases the solubility of bile, which prevents stone formation and increases the likelihood of eliminating any stones already formed. Add this spice to your cooking.

• *Milk thistle* contains silymarin, which protects the liver. Studies also indicate its ability to increase bile solubility, which helps prevent or alleviate gall stones.

• Make a tea using *parsley*. This herb prevents and treats gall stones.

Dosages may vary, depending on the severity and duration of your symptoms. Consult a qualified herbal practitioner. Alert your physician to your decision to use herbs; not all herbal remedies can be used in combination with conventional pharmaceuticals.

What makes it worse?

• The people of Chile and the North American Indians suffer gall stones more often than any other people. These two populations also rely on *legumes* as a major source of food. Studies conducted to try to find a connection indeed proved that a diet high in legumes may reduce the ability of the bile to hold the cholesterol in solution, allowing it to fall out as crystals that lead to stone formation. Recommendation: If you are at risk for gall bladder disease, limit your intake of legumes (dried beans, field peas, and lentils), eating them only occasionally and in small amounts.

• High intake of *sugar* causes the development of gall stones, probably because it leads to an increase in the body's production of cholesterol. Recommendation: Sharply reduce or totally eliminate your intake of sugar and all foods and beverages prepared with it.

• Development of gall stones occurs more readily on *a diet too rich in polyunsaturated fats* than one of saturated (animal) fat, although you would be best served to limit intake of all kinds of fat to no more than 35% of calories. For reasons that are unclear to me, in testing, fats that are solids at room temperature (butter, lard, margarine) provoke less spasm of the gall bladder caused by sludge (or stones) than fats that are liquid at room temperature. Recommendation: Try not to overeat fats of any kind, and try to eat foods that provide a mixture of fats and oils: butter, margarine, olive oil, canola oil, fish oil.

• When you have gall stones, drinking *coffee* can trigger a gall bladder attack. Recommendation: Don't drink more than a single cup of coffee per day if you know you have stones.

Gall Stones
(see Gall Bladder Disease)

Garlic Odor in Breath

What is it?

Just as the name implies, sometimes people develop a breath odor that smells (and sometimes tastes) like garlic. When they've not eaten any garlic, the odor may be the result of taking too much selenium.

What helps it?

• Recommendation: Stop taking selenium supplements or eating foods that contain high amounts of it. Refer to the A-to-Z Nutrient listing for a listing of the foods containing selenium. After 3 to 4 weeks without supplementation, take a dose of selenium to see if the symptom returns.

Herbal remedies

• I know of none.

What makes it worse?

• Except for continuing to take selenium supplements or foods rich in selenium, I know of no nutrient that makes the problem worse.

Gastritis
(see Heartburn and Peptic Ulcer Disease)

Gingivitis

What is it?

You may have heard of this disorder of the gums under a variety of other names, such as trench mouth (also called Vincent's infection) and periodontal disease. These two gum disorders differ in several ways.

Trench mouth occurs in young people under stress, traditionally

cropping up at examination time in high school or college, but also
brought on by severe chronic illnesses, and now often seen in young
people suffering from AIDS. The combination of two forms of bacteria (a rod-shaped one and a spiral one) working as a team bring
about a severe infection of the gums that neither bacteria alone
cause, with the sudden onset of painful swollen ulcers that may
bleed, bad breath, fever, and swollen lymph nodes in the neck. Although the cause of the disorder is infectious and not nutritional, and
the cure usually requires antibiotic medications, poor nutrition may
set the stage to predispose a person to developing the problem and
proper nutrition can help to prevent it.

Periodontal disease or periodontitis is a chronic infection of the
gums that causes—over a period of years—the gums to draw away
from the teeth, exposing the tooth root and allowing entry of the
bacteria into the deeper tissues. Once again the cause is bacterial,
and the cure very often requires surgery to scrape away diseased
gum tissue and may even lead finally to extraction of all teeth and
replacement with dentures. Poor nutrition sets the stage, and the
proper intake of nutrients can offer some protection. Let's see how.

What helps it?

• *Folic acid* taken as a supplement, but even more effectively
used topically on your gums as a *folic acid mouth rinse*, can reduce
inflammation and infection. Recommendation: Take 1 mg folic acid
per day or swish 1 teaspoon of a 1% folic acid solution in your
mouth for 1 minute twice a day. (A 1% solution contains 1 mg folic
acid per liquid teaspoon. Your pharmacist would probably need to
compound this mixture for you.) Women with gingivitis who also
take the birth control pill may need to increase their daily dose of
folic acid to 4 grams per day for a period of 60 days.

• Inadequate intake of *vitamin C,* even when not markedly deficient, may increase your risk of developing gingivitis. Because it is
required for the production of collagen (the basic protein building
block for the fibrous framework of all tissues), supplementing vitamin C strengthens the weak gum tissues and makes the gum lining
surface more resistant to penetration by bacteria. Recommendation:
Take a vitamin C supplement that also contains bioflavonoids,
which retard plaque growth. Take 4000 to 10,000 mg daily in divided doses.

• A true deficiency of *vitamin A* is known to predispose one to disease of the gums, including susceptibility to infection, changes in the bone beneath the gums, and the formation of pockets in the gum where infection can more easily set up. Recommendation: Refer to Vitamin A in Section I. If you have gum disease along with other signs of vitamin A deficiency, supplementing with vitamin A may improve your gum health. Remember that your body can store vitamin A, and that makes it possible for you to develop toxicity from taking too much of it. Refer again to the discussion of vitamin A in Section I and refresh your knowledge of the signs of vitamin A toxicity before taking any additional vitamin A. When you are ready to supplement, take 15,000 to 20,000 IU of vitamin A daily. Use the emulsion form for better assimilation and greater safety at high doses. An alternative method that has fewer side effects is to take beta-carotene, the vitamin A relative that your body turns into vitamin A as it needs it. The only remarkable side effect of beta-carotene is the development of an orange color to your palms and soles. Take 25,000 to 50,000 IU of beta-carotene (15 to 30 mg) daily.

• *Vitamin E* helps to reduce the inflammation (redness and swelling) of gum disease. Recommendation: Take vitamin E as d-alpha-tocopherol succinate in a dose of 200 IU 4 times daily. Bite open the capsule at each dose and distribute the contents over your gums and allow it to absorb undisturbed for 30 minutes. Warning: Vitamin E can cause blood pressure elevations in some people. Begin with only 1 capsule per day. Take your blood pressure after taking this dose for several days. If you see no elevation (average blood pressure remains below 140/90), you may continue to increase by 1 capsule per day, again taking your pressures after several days on the higher dose before moving on.

• Because the gums reside on a base of bone, deficiencies of *calcium and magnesium* could weaken that foundation and predispose your gums to infection, or at the least hasten the progress of the disease once it has begun. Research tests investigating this theory have not provided a clear-cut answer, but the connection makes sense. Recommendation: Take a combined calcium and magnesium supplement daily providing about 1500 mg calcium and 750 mg magnesium.

• Adding some *vitamin D* to supplementation with calcium and magnesium may further stall the loss of bone in the jaws of people with periodontal disease, especially those people who have lost their teeth because of chronic infection in their gums. Recommendation: Add vitamin D to your diet by increasing your intake of fortified dairy products, by regular outdoor activity in the sun when weather permits, and by adding approximately 350 USP units per day of vitamin D_2 (ergocalciferol) to your diet.

• *Zinc* deficiency may weaken the resistance of your gum tissues to invasion by foreign substances (bacteria). Using a *zinc mouth rinse* seems to reduce the spread of bacterial-laden plaque. Recommendation: Ask your pharmacist to compound a solution containing 1 mg zinc per milliliter of aqueous solution. Once a day, swish 1 tablespoon of the solution in your mouth for 1 to 2 minutes and then discard the solution. Failing that, dissolve a single 10 mg zinc tablet (or the contents of a capsule) in 2 tablespoons of water and swish the entire volume of the dissolved medication as a dose. To improve the taste, you could use a sugar-free, noncarbonated, fruit-flavored beverage, such as Kool-Aid or Crystal Light.

• *Coenzyme Q_{10}* levels in people with gum disease are often low. Supplementation may help to slow down the development of the pockets in the gum that bleed, swell, and create a hiding place for infection. Recommendation: Take 50 mg of coenzyme Q_{10} twice a day for at least 8 weeks to assess your response. Your dentist or periodontist can measure the depth of pockets before and after you take the supplement to verify improvement.

Herbal remedies

• *Bloodroot* contains the compound sanguinarine, which reduces the amount of plaque in the mouth quickly—in about 1 week. It is available in toothpastes and mouthwashes.

• *Chamomile* is an anti-inflammatory and an antiseptic.

• Add a dropper or two of *echinacea tincture* to your tea and mouthwash. Your tongue may tingle; this is a harmless effect.

• *Sage* tea is as effective as a sanguinarine toothpaste.

• Real *peppermint* fights tooth decay. But don't look to commercial toothpastes for this benefit; most of them are artificially flavored. Instead, make a tea using 2 teaspoons of crushed leaves. Or chew the fresh leaves.

• Mouthwashes and toothpastes that contain *stinging nettle* reduce plaque and gingivitis. For an even greater effectiveness, add juniper. You can find products made with these herbs at the health food store.

Dosages may vary, depending on the duration and severity of symptoms. Follow package directions, or consult a qualified herbal practitioner.

What makes it worse?

• Excess dietary *phosphorus,* found in meat, soft drinks, grains, and potatoes, may promote bone loss by interfering with calcium balance. In theory, the higher your phosphorus intake, the greater your tendency to leech calcium out of bones, which could weaken the bony foundation beneath your gums. Recommendation: If you suffer from chronic periodontal disease, you should limit your intake of meat by seeking protein from other sources, such as fish, seafood, poultry, egg white, and dairy products. Sharply reduce your intake of potatoes and grains, relying on whole fruits and other vegetables for your carbohydrate and fiber sources. And try not to drink carbonated soft drinks, diet or otherwise.

• *Sugar* intake hastens the development of gingivitis by directly inflaming the gum tissues, by promoting plaque formation on the teeth, and by hampering the action of body chemicals that call immune defense fighters to the area once infection begins. Although important, sugar avoidance alone does not protect you against developing chronic periodontal disease in the face of poor dental hygiene. Recommendation: Sharply reduce your intake of sugar and all foods containing sugar, corn syrup, molasses, or high-fructose corn syrup. With the connection between sugar and phosphorus as promoters of gum disease, it's easy to see why regular carbonated soft drinks, which the young people of this country drink by the tanker-truck full, are a bad dietary bargain.

• *Mercury* in silver/mercury amalgam fillings can leech out and cause toxicity, including gingivitis, bleeding gums, and a metallic taste in the mouth. Recommendation: See your dentist to have fillings checked and remove and replace any silver/mercury fillings.

Glaucoma

What is it?

About 1 to 2% of Americans over the age of 40 suffer from glaucoma—which is an elevation of pressure inside your eyes—but it goes undetected as much as 25% of the time. Without proper treatment to reduce the pressure, glaucoma leads to progressive impairment of vision and eventually blindness. When the pressure inside the eyeball increases, it continuously "squeezes" the optic nerve until it finally damages it permanently.

There are two forms of glaucoma: the "open angle" form that affects 90% of glaucoma sufferers, and the "angle-closure" form. Open-angle glaucoma occurs insidiously and painlessly over many years, while the angle-closure or narrow-angle form causes abrupt onset of marked pain and redness when something occludes the outflow port for circulation of fluids within the eye and the pressure shoots up suddenly. Although the angle-closure form can lead to blindness in a matter of a few days if not treated, it takes many years of slowly increasing pressure for open-angle glaucoma to rob you of normal vision. You are at greater risk to develop glaucoma if others in your family have it or if you are a Black American. All Americans over age 40 should visit an eye specialist for glaucoma screening every 3 years, but higher-risk Americans should do so every year. In addition to prevention through regular screening, what role does nutrition play? Let's look.

What helps it?

• Because maintenance of nerve tissues requires adequate *thiamine,* deficiency of thiamine could, in theory, promote damage to the optic nerve by the increasing pressure in glaucoma. Preliminary medical research to investigate this theory did show that giving thiamine and B-complex vitamins improved the vision of people with early stages of glaucoma. Recommendation: If you have borderline glaucoma or are at risk because of family history for it, take 100 mg thiamine per day along with 50 to 100 mg B-complex.

• Deficiency of *vitamin C* may cause an increase in eye pressures. Supplementation with extremely high doses of vitamin C (500 mg per kilogram of body weight, or a dose of 35 grams in a 150-pound adult) reduced pressures in 100% of patients tested, but this dose exceeded the bowel tolerance level (see discussion of Vitamin C in the A-to-Z Nutrient listings) for most of the people studied. Doses significantly less than that (but still large doses) reduced eye pressures in most of the participants in another medical study within 6 weeks to a level sufficient to reduce or discontinue prescription medications. Recommendation: The doses of vitamin C needed to reduce pressure in your eyes are high. Refer to the following discussion of this vitamin to learn how to slowly increase your dose to a level your bowel will tolerate. Use crystalline (powdered) vitamin C for ease of dosing and for ease on your stomach. Each teaspoon of the powder contains 4 grams of vitamin C. Begin by mixing ¼ teaspoon with citrus juice or a sugar-free citrus beverage at bedtime. (A carbonated one works particularly well to mix the powder into solution more completely.) Increase to ¼ teaspoon morning and night. Then increase each dose to ½ teaspoon, ¾ teaspoon, and then 1 teaspoon on weekly intervals. Finally, if you've not reached bowel tolerance and weigh more than 150 pounds, add an additional dose at midday, increasing it as before from ¼ teaspoon, ½ teaspoon, ¾ teaspoon, and finally 1 full teaspoon. At this point, you will be taking 12 grams per day. If you have still not reached bowel tolerance, add a fourth dose in the same manner until you maximize intake at 1 teaspoon four times per day. Work in conjunction with your eye specialist, who can check pressures as you go. Do not discontinue your prescription medications unless instructed to do so as your pressures fall.

• When you become deficient in *vitamin A,* the pressure in your eyes can increase. Supplementing with vitamin A can reduce the pressure. Refer to the discussion of this vitamin in Section I for other typical symptoms of deficiency. If you show other symptoms of deficiency of this vitamin, supplementation may help. Because your body stores vitamin A, taking too much can be dangerous. A safer alternative to vitamin A is to supplement with beta-carotene, the vitamin A relative that your body can turn into vitamin A as it needs it. Recommendation: You may take 10,000 to 20,000 IU of vitamin A daily, or take 30,000 to 45,000 IU of beta-carotene daily.

• *Zinc* is essential in activating vitamin A from the liver and has been beneficial in glaucoma therapy. Recommendation: Take 50 mg daily.

• *Glutathione* is a potent antioxidant that protects the lens and maintains the molecular integrity of the lens fiber membranes. Recommendation: Take 500 mg twice daily on an empty stomach.

• *Rutin,* one of the bioflavonoids with vitamin-like actions, also seems to reduce eye pressures in people with open-angle glaucoma. In medical studies, pressures in the eyes fell by 15% or more with supplementation. Recommendation: Take rutin 50 mg 3 times a day for a minimum of 4 weeks to assess your response.

• *Chromium* deficiency is frequently found in cells of people who suffer from open-angle glaucoma. I could find no information about studies under way to determine whether supplementing chromium will reduce the elevated pressure, but they are bound to follow this initial report, which appeared in 1991. This association would be especially important for people who also have a risk for other eye problems with diabetes. Recommendation: Take 200 *micro*grams chromium picolinate per day. Ultimately, higher doses may prove even more beneficial, but the data as yet don't justify a greater than normal degree of supplementation.

Herbal remedies

• *Jaborandi* (comes from a tree in South America) contains a standard glaucoma medicine called pilocarpine. This herb was used to treat eye disease as early as 1648. It reduces intraocular pressure. It can be found in natural health food stores.

• Although there is no scientific literature confirming it as such, *oregano* can be used to treat glaucoma. To prevent the disorder, experts recommend getting an abundance of antioxidants. Wild oregano has one of the highest concentrations of antioxidants.

• *Pansy* contains rutin, which, when combined with standard medications, contributes to lowering intraocular pressure of glaucoma. You can eat the actual pansy by mixing it in salad.

• *Bilberry* is useful for every eye ailment because it contains anthocyanosides that retard the breakdown of vitamin C, allowing the vitamin to do its job protecting your eye. I suggest making a juice cocktail using the juice of bilberries, blueberries, cranberries, and huckleberries. Each of these is high in anthocyanosides.

Dosages may vary, depending on the duration and severity of your symptoms. Consult a qualified herbal practitioner. Tell your physician of your decision to begin an herbal remedy. Some herbal remedies cannot be used in conjunction with conventional pharmaceuticals.

What makes it worse?

• Avoid *caffeine*. Tests monitoring pressure inside the eye showed significant increases following intake of caffeinated espresso, but did not show such increases with decaffeinated espresso. Recommendation: If you have or are at risk for glaucoma, avoid caffeine in coffee, chocolate, and soft drinks. Minimize your intake of *trans fatty acids*. Manufacturers take healthy polyunsaturated oils, which are unstable and prone to rancidity, and make them more shelf stable by heating them to high temperatures. At high temperatures, the chemical bonding of the carbon and hydrogen atoms in the oils shifts from the natural arrangement—called *cis*—to a form called *trans,* which is more stable, but less usable for the human metabolism. There is some evidence that fatty acids in this *trans* configuration can actually harm human tissues in a variety of ways, including elevating eye pressures in people prone to glaucoma. Recommendation: Use cold-pressed oils, such as extra-virgin or virgin olive oil and canola oil. Read the label of oils you purchase in the supermarket, and if it doesn't declare that the oil is cold-pressed—a much more expensive process, so the manufacturer usually will proclaim it on the label—call the company and inquire if heat extraction is used to make the oil in question. The naturally saturated fats, like real butter, are not heat-treated at these high temperatures. Deep-frying can also destroy "good" oils, so you should also avoid deep-frying your foods no matter what kind of oil you choose.

• A diet too high in *protein* may increase pressure inside the eye. In a study of 400 people with various eye disorders including glaucoma, excessive dietary protein (greater than 3 times the RDA of $1/2$ gram per pound of lean body weight) showed a tendency toward increased eye pressures. I could find no mention of the protein breakdown—that is, how much came from fish, poultry, red meat, organ meat, eggs, or dairy—and that information is significant since the levels of arachidonic acid, one of the "bad" prostaglandins (see eicosinoids, pages 24–27), varies according to the kind of protein. Red meats, organ meats, and egg yolk have higher levels of arachidonic acid than the others, and so in theory, a diet containing high amounts of these specific proteins might prove more damaging than one with the same amount of protein, but composed of fish, poultry, and egg white (without yolks). Recommendation: Because protein is absolutely essential to life, I would certainly advise you to be sure to get the required $1/2$ gram per pound of lean body weight per day, but based on the findings in this particular study, I would suggest that if you exceed that protein minimum, you eat more of fish, poultry, and egg white and less of red meat, organ meats, and yolks.

Gout

What is it?

Gout, which causes painful red swollen joints, occurs more commonly in middle-aged men of portly physique, but can afflict women and younger people, too. The cause of the disorder centers around a waste product of protein breakdown, called uric acid. Your body rids itself of this waste product through your kidneys; however, sometimes the kidneys fail to do the job and uric acid builds up. Uric acid resides not just in your blood, but in the fluid of your joints, where it can cause trouble in gout. If the levels of uric acid in your body increase, the levels in your joint fluids also increase, and when they become too rich in uric acid, crystals of this waste product begin to form in the fluid. The formation of these crystals incites an inflammation in the joint, which becomes red, swollen, and quite painful. The pain can be so extreme that you cannot bear the weight of a bed sheet on the gouty joint. When such symptoms occur, you suffer a "gouty" attack.

The joint where the great toe attaches to the foot is the joint most commonly afflicted with gout, but the bones of the middle of the foot, the ankle, the knee, and the elbow also are affected with fair regularity, and any joint can be affected. When the crystals of uric acid form in the soft tissues around the joint, they create a gouty tophus, a lump or bump filled with white, chalky matter. These tophi may also become red, warm, and inflamed in a gouty attack.

What does nutrition have to offer the person who suffers from gout? Let's take a look at what might help.

What helps it?

• *Vitamin B-complex* is important for proper digestion and all bodily enzyme systems. Recommendation: Take 100 mg twice daily, plus extra vitamin B_5 at a dose of 500 mg in divided doses. Gout is extremely stressful on the body, and pantothenic acid is the anti-stress vitamin. It should be supplemented at 500 mg daily, in divided doses.

• *Folic acid* aids in nucleoprotein metabolism. Recommendation: Supplement daily at a dosage of 200 *micro*grams.

• *Vitamin C with bioflavonoids* supplementation increases the removal of uric acid from the body through the kidneys, and thereby reduces the risk for gouty attacks. Recommendation: Work your way up to at least 4 grams of vitamin C per day. Refer to the discussion of vitamin C in the A-to-Z Nutrient listings for a method of slowly increasing your dose to this level using crystalline (powdered) vitamin C. If you weigh more than 150 pounds, you may need to increase your daily intake to 6 or even 8 grams per day if that does not exceed your bowel tolerance level.

Herbal remedies

• *Celery* seeds seem to help keep uric acid below critical levels. Eat celery daily (4 or 5 stalks) or take 2 to 4 tablets daily.

• Reports indicate that *devil's claw* lowers uric acid levels and has anti-inflammatory action. Other studies suggest it is useful for relieving arthritic conditions; gout is a form of arthritis. The downside of this information is that the studies used extract injections and consumers can get this herb only in capsule or tea form. I cannot comment on the effectiveness of these forms, but I believe they are certainly worth trying.

• Because *willow* is the herbal aspirin, it can help relieve pain and inflammation. Research also suggests it lowers uric acid levels. Make a tea using 2 teaspoons of bark. Caution: Do not take this herb if you are allergic to aspirin.

Dosages may vary, depending on the duration and severity of your symptoms. Consult a qualified herbal practitioner. Tell your physician of your decision to begin an herbal remedy. Some herbal remedies cannot be used in conjunction with conventional pharmaceuticals.

What makes it worse?

• Eating a diet high in *sucrose or table sugar* increases the risk of gouty attacks because it raises your insulin level, which alters the way your body handles the uric acid. Don't be fooled into thinking of sugar in terms of "sugary" desserts and the stuff you sprinkle on your food. Besides the obvious frosted cereals, glazed doughnuts, soft drinks, cookies, cakes, pies, ice cream, and candy, sugar is added in abundance to processed foods to the point that American sugar consumption has skyrocketed in this century. From an intake of about 2 pounds of sugar by each man, woman, and child per year in 1890, by the 1980s, we Americans each consumed on average greater than 120 pounds per year. No, that's not a misprint; it really is 120 pounds of sugar for each of us per year. Recommendation: Eliminate or sharply reduce your intake of sugar and foods made with sugar, corn syrup, molasses, and high-fructose corn syrup.

• Don't be tempted to think that because *fructose* is the sugar in fruit, it is automatically healthful. Particularly in gout, that may not be the case, because fructose increases the production of uric acid, which increases the risk of gouty attack. Recommendation: Avoid sweetening with fructose in place of sugar. Don't use fructose-sweetened candies, cookies, or soft drinks in a misguided effort to reduce sugar. In this case, you may be making matters worse. Eating a serving or two of raw, whole fruit daily is probably within the limit you can tolerate on fructose without increasing your risk for gout, but don't drink glass upon glass of fruit juices. And sweetening with artificial sweeteners (aspartame and saccharine) does not increase gouty risk.

• *Alcohol* has a position of long standing among the dietary promoters of gout, and with good cause. The metabolism of alcohol produces chemicals that compete with uric acid for removal from the body by the kidneys, allowing uric acid to build up to high levels. Beer, especially, triggers attacks of gout, because it contains more purines (see below) than either wine or distilled spirits. Recommendation: If you are at risk for gout, eliminate or sharply reduce your intake of all forms of alcohol. If you do imbibe, drink no more than a single ounce of distilled spirits, a single glass of wine, or a single "lite" beer per day.

• Foods such as red meat, organ meat, seafood, lentils, beans, asparagus, anchovies, mushrooms, sardines, and peas increase your risk of gouty attacks because they contain high amounts of *purines,* a chemical that your body uses to make uric acid. Recommendation: If you suffer from gout or are at risk (male, overweight especially in the abdomen, take diuretic blood pressure medications, or borderline diabetic), reduce your intake of these higher-purine foods. Dine on lean fish, skinless poultry, egg white, and low-fat diary products as sources of protein.

• Supplementing *vitamin A* can bring on gouty attacks in people known to have gout, and possibly in people at risk for gout. Recommendation: Do not take vitamin A supplements in these instances.

• *Glycine* is an amino acid that can be converted into uric acid more rapidly in people who suffer from gout.

• Adding high doses of *niacin,* such as you might take in attempts to reduce cholesterol, can provoke a gouty attack because the breakdown products of niacin compete against uric acid for removal from the body by the kidneys. This competition can lead to a rapid buildup of uric acid, which can cause the attack. Recommendation: If you suffer from gout or are at increased risk for gout, do not take doses of niacin above 50 to 100 mg per day.

• *Being overweight* can be especially harmful for people with gout. Losing weight lowers serum uric acid levels. Avoid crash diets, however. Abrupt elimination of foods or fasting for longer than 3 days can actually increase uric acid levels.

Gum Disease
(see Gingivitis)

Headache

What is it?

Few readers, I would imagine, have not at some time suffered from headache, so I needn't spend time telling you what it is. A headache is a headache, right? Actually, headache is one of the more difficult symptoms to evaluate in medicine, because so many different problems can cause the same end result—your head hurts. Viruses often cause headache, but fever from other types of infections can, too. Some women develop headaches that coincide with menstrual period cycles. Other people suffer mightily and often with "sick headaches" or "migraines" or "cluster migraines." They can occur with sinus pressure or allergies—the "sinus headache." Stress can bring them on. But so can too much caffeine—or too little. The list goes on and on, and most of the time, the cause of the headache is not serious or dangerous. Sometimes, however, headache can be a sign of dangerous blood vessel problems—an aneurysm or blood clot—or of benign tumors or cancers in the brain. Although most adults have at one time or another had a headache, and most pass without incident, you should never ignore a headache in a child, which almost always means an infection coming on, nor should you ignore one in yourself that is unusually severe, lasts more than a day or two, follows a blow to the head, or for which you have no reasonable explanation. Always seek medical help for any unexplained, sudden, or severe headache.

Although nutrient remedies may not be of much benefit for sudden headaches from trauma, blood pressure, or infection, which will have specific medical treatments, what if you suffer chronic headaches that you do know the cause of, such as headache from allergies, with menstrual periods, or from low blood sugar? Can nutrition offer help here? Let's take a look.

What helps it?

• *Magnesium* deficiency may contribute to premenstrual headaches and perhaps even to migraine headaches triggered by allergy. Recommendation: Take 1000 mg of magnesium (as the amino acid chelate) daily. (Note: Some experts recommend taking calcium along with the magnesium. I would recommend a dosage of 1500 mg calcium daily.)

• *Essential fatty acids,* through their influence on production of the "good" prostaglandins (see eicosinoids, Section I, pages 24–27) that reduce the blood vessel spasm and inflammation common in migraine, may help to decrease the frequency of your headaches. Much of the research has involved testing the essential fat in fish oil (called EPA) and has ignored the need for balance between EPA and the other essential fat, linoleic acid (GLA). EPA directs the cascade of chemical alterations that lead from the raw fatty acid to the final prostaglandin products toward the production of "good" prostaglandins by blocking the step that produces arachidonic acid, the forerunner of all the "bad" messengers. However, the production of "good" messengers requires sufficient raw material fatty acids and the proper basic diet. Gobbling fish oil capsules while eating an otherwise poorly constructed diet won't do much to help your headaches. Recommendation: To facilitate the best response from essential fatty acids, begin with the proper macronutrient framework (see Section I, macronutrients, page 23). Then to that nutritionally sound base add gamma-linoleic acid (GLA) and EPA fish oil in a ratio of 1:4 (GLA:EPA) 1 to 3 times daily. The EicoPro essential fatty acid product manufactured by Eicotec, Inc., of Marblehead, Massachusetts, contains ultrapure sources of linoleic acid and fish oils already combined in the proper ratio. If you cannot get that product, you can purchase linoleic acid in a product called evening primrose oil at most health and nutrition stores, and EPA fish oil as well. Because it is not as pure a form, the dosing will be different. You can make a reasonable substitute by combining evening primrose oil capsules with fish oil capsules plus vitamin E. Take 500 mg of evening primrose oil (a source of linoleic acid in capsule form), plus 1000 mg EPA fish oil, plus 200 IU vitamin E 1 to 3 times a day. (Warning to diabetics: EPA fish oil can cause blood sugar fluctuations in some diabetics. Carefully monitor your blood sugar if you use this supplemental oil and discontinue its use if your blood sugar becomes difficult to control.)

• *L-glutamine* works with *quercetin* to relieve cluster headaches. Recommendation: Take 500 mg of each twice daily.

• A diet reduced in the amino acid *tryptophan* may help to curb migraine in some people. Your body turns tryptophan into the chemical *serotonin*. Alterations in the balance of serotonin in the blood versus the amount in the brain may provoke migraine. Unfortunately, this means eating a protein-restricted diet, which you must approach with great care. You must be certain to meet your body's minimum protein requirement of $\frac{1}{2}$ gram of protein per pound of lean body weight (see Macronutrients, Section I, page 23), but try not to exceed that amount. You will find the tryptophan content of protein foods highest in egg white, followed by milk products, and then meats. Selecting lean poultry and freshwater fish as your primary protein sources and sticking closely to your minimum protein requirement will help.

• Paradoxically, headaches can sometimes occur because of overuse or chronic use of the very medications you use to relieve your headache: ergotamines (Cafergot), narcotic medications (codeine, hydrocodone), and even aspirin. These medicines, used frequently, deplete the brain's stores of natural painkillers. Research suggests that supplemental doses of *vitamin B_6* accompanied by a gradual "detoxification" by a slow and careful withdrawal from the offending medications can help to relieve this kind of headache. Recommendation: Working with the physician who has prescribed the medication for your migraines, develop a program to gradually stop using the drug. Reduce your dose in tiny increments of about 10% per week over a course of 10 weeks. (I cannot really provide you with precise milligram amounts because each medication varies in its milligram dosing, as does the dose that different people must take.) During your tapering program, take 50 to 100 mg of vitamin B_6 each day. Note: Although some people may require a little more B_6, do not exceed a daily intake of 200 mg per day, because nerve damage has occurred from such doses used over a several-year period.

Herbal remedies

• *Bay leaves* are particularly useful in preventing migraines.
• The *British Medical Journal* published studies claiming that

feverfew prevents migraine attacks. There are many ways to take this herb. You could can chew the leaves, but they taste awful. I recommend making a tea. Be careful not to bring the water to a boiling point, because it may break down the active compounds found in the leaves. You can also take capsules. Capsules come in many different dosages, so be sure to consult an herbal practitioner to find a dose that's right for you. Caution: Do not take this herb if you are pregnant. Studies indicate that it may trigger miscarriage. Nursing mothers should also avoid it so they do not pass the herb to their infants. Long-term users often report a sedative effect.

• Commission E recommends taking 60 to 120 mg of salicin to treat a headache. Salicin is found in *willow.* While white willow can help, other species are more potent: *Salix daphnoides, S. fragilis,* and *S. purpurea.* Caution: Don't take this herb if you are allergic to aspirin. Do not give willow to children with viral infections, as it increases their risk of developing Reye's syndrome.

• *Evening primrose* is a terrific source of phenylalanine, a pain-relieving compound. Nutritionists recommend a daily dose of 6 to 8 capsules of this oil.

• *Ginkgo* increases cerebral blood flow, making it a valuable treatment for headaches. In large amounts (higher than 240 mg), however, this herb may cause diarrhea, irritability, and restlessness.

• Capsaicin is a pain reliever found in *red pepper.* Capsaicin is especially helpful in preventing cluster headaches. Take cayenne capsules.

• If you're prone to headaches, nutritionists recommend getting 600 mg of magnesium daily. Magnesium deficiency has been found in people with frequent tension headaches and migraines. *Purslane* is high in magnesium.

Dosage may vary, depending on the duration and severity of your symptoms. Follow package directions, or consult a qualified herbal practitioner.

What makes it worse?

• Eating a diet high in simple *sugars* can trigger migraine headaches in some people by making wide swings in their blood sugar. When you eat a sugary food, your blood sugar rises quickly, sending out signals for your body to produce insulin to drive the blood sugar level back down by driving the sugar into the tissues to be used or stored. Some people have an exaggerated insulin response to a sugary food, and their overproduction of insulin drives the blood sugar down too fast and too far. The low blood sugar triggers migraine for some of these people. Recommendation: Avoid concentrated sweets. Try to sharply curtail your intake of sugar, corn syrup, molasses, or foods made with these, including cakes, pies, pastries, cookies, soft drinks, frosted cereals, jams, and ice cream, to name but a few. Also avoid large quantities of the starchy foods that your body can convert quickly to sugar, such as potatoes, wheat, and corn. Rice and oats make less dramatic changes in blood sugar and are better starch choices for you.

• Foods or supplements containing *copper* may trigger headaches in some people, because it plays a role in the metabolism of some of the brain chemicals involved in headache. Recommendation: If you suffer migraines, do not take mineral supplements containing copper. Also avoid foods rich in copper, such as chocolate, nuts, wheat germ, and shellfish.

• *Caffeine* can trigger headaches both from too much use and from too little. (The one special group of headaches that may respond to use of caffeine are migraine headaches. This benefit occurs because caffeine helps to prevent the dilation of blood vessels in the brain.) People who drink moderately heavy amounts of coffee or tea (4 to 5 cups per day) tend to suffer headache more frequently than their decaffeinated friends. And once you become a regular user of caffeine, withdrawal of the substance will almost universally trigger a bad headache. If you suffer with chronic headaches, you would do yourself a favor to become caffeine-free. Recommendation: Approach caffeine detoxification with caution. Don't stampede your way to a caffeine-free lifestyle. Here's a reduction schedule that will help you: Purchase a tin of a half and half blend of caffeinated/decaffeinated coffee. (There are several available in the supermarket.) Mix the blend with your regular full-strength coffee in a ratio of 1 part blend to 3 parts regular, and drink this slightly less caffeinated mixture for several days. Drop to 1 part blend to 2 parts regular, then 1 part of each, then 1 part regular to 2 parts blend, then 1 part regular to 3 parts blend, then all blend. At this point, you're 50% decaffeinated. Now repeat this schedule using the 50/50 blend and mixing in fully decaffeinated coffee. Start with 3 parts blend to 1 part decaf, 2 blend to 1 decaf, 1 blend to 1 decaf, 1 blend to 2 decaf, 1 blend to

3 decaf, and finally, you're fully decaffeinated. By taking it slow and easy, you avoid the sometimes severe headaches that withdrawal from caffeine can cause.

• *Aspartame,* the sugar substitute in the sweetener NutraSweet, can trigger headache in as many as 10% of migraine sufferers. Recommendation: Undertake an elimination trial of aspartame to see if it acts as a trigger in your migraines. Totally eliminate the sweetener and all products made with it from your diet for 3 to 4 weeks. If you suffer no headaches during that period, you must challenge yourself by eating or drinking products containing aspartame. If doing so brings on a headache, you'll know with certainty that this sweetener acts as a trigger for you.

• Nearly half of the sufferers of chronic headaches of all causes report that *alcohol* acted as a trigger for their symptoms, and that percent increases to nearly 60% for migraine sufferers. Beer and wine, especially red wine, seem to cause greater problems than distilled spirits, although all kinds of alcohol may be at fault. Recommendation: If you drink alcohol and suffer chronic headaches, you may want to undertake an elimination trial. Begin by eliminating all forms of alcohol from your diet for a period of 3 to 4 weeks. Then test one kind of alcoholic beverage at a time. For example, drink 2 to 3 glasses of red wine daily for 3 to 4 days. If you fail to develop a headache, red wine probably does not act as a trigger for you. Allow yourself a washout period of 3 weeks between trials, then move on to another kind of beverage—say, white wine or beer or distilled spirits. By systematic elimination, you can discover whether alcohol in general or some specific form of it triggers your headaches.

• *Nitrates/nitrites,* found in cured meats and hot dogs, may cause migraines in some people. Recommendation: An elimination trial conducted for each suspected food as described above for alcohol.

• *Red wine, aged cheese, fermented sausages, and sour cream* all contain high levels of the amino acid tyramine, which serves as a trigger for migraine in some people. Recommendation: An elimination trial for each of these substances as described above for alcohol.

• *Chocolate* contains a chemical called phenylethylamine that can trigger migraine in some people. Recommendation: An elimination trial as described above for alcohol.

• If you have a lactase deficiency and cannot tolerate *milk* and other dairy products, eating dairy products can cause headache in addition to—or in place of—the gastrointestinal distress usually seen in milk intolerance. Recommendation: If you have any history of milk intolerance, still eat other dairy products, and suffer frequent headaches, you may want to investigate the connection between the dairy products and your symptoms. Recommendation: Undertake an elimination trial of all dairy products and foods containing diary products as described on page 353 for alcohol.

Hearing Loss

What is it?

I don't expect that I need to define loss of hearing for you, but I'd like to devote this space to a brief explanation of how hearing works. The "ear" really consists of three major parts, an outer visible ear and canal, a middle ear space, and a portion deeply embedded in the bone of the skull called the inner ear. The visible ear, called the *pinna,* catches sound waves from noises around you and directs them down the ear canal, where they strike the eardrum and make it vibrate. The vibrating drum moves a series of three tiny bones attached to it that attach in turn to another drumlike membrane on the other side of the middle ear space where the bones of hearing lie. Movement of this other drum sets up waves of motion in the inner ear fluid, which move hairlike nerve endings that line the *cochlea,* the actual "organ of hearing" in the inner ear. Stimulation of these nerve endings sends nerve impulses through the nerve of hearing to your brain, and you "hear" the noise.

Hearing loss can occur for a variety of reasons: damage to the tiny bones that move with the eardrum (called a conductive hearing loss, bone deafness, or otosclerosis), or damage to the hairlike nerve fibers in the cochlea or to the nerve of hearing itself (called a sensorineural hearing loss or nerve deafness). When the problem originates in the inner ear structures, dizziness and ringing of the ears may accompany the loss of hearing—a disorder called Ménière's syndrome. Although chronic exposure to noise promotes hearing loss more than nutritional factors, certain nutrients and dietary restrictions may help to lessen the damage. Let's take a look at these.

What helps it?

• *Proper diet* to correct disorders of blood lipids—high cholesterol with too much of the low-density or "bad" cholesterol (LDL) and high triglycerides. Many people with progressive hearing loss, ringing of the ears, and dizziness (Ménière's syndrome) also suffer from being overweight, borderline diabetes or sugar intolerance, high cholesterol and triglycerides, heart disease, fluid retention, and hardening of the arteries. All are classic symptoms of insulin excess. Constructing a basic diet that helps to control the root cause of these other problems often helps the ear symptoms, dizziness, and muffled hearing. Recommendation: If you suffer from these related problems, or if they run strongly in your family, you may find your ear symptoms improve on a diet that helps keep control of insulin release. Refer to Macronutrients, Section I, page 23, to begin to construct a diet for yourself that will help to normalize your blood cholesterol and triglycerides, blood sugar, and fluid retention by controlling your production of insulin. Recommendation: After reviewing the information in the discussion, you can begin to plan a basic diet that provides a minimum of $\frac{1}{2}$ gram of lean protein for each pound of your lean body mass. Your protein requirement makes up 50% of your day's calories. To that base, add nonstarchy or at least less-starchy carbohydrates (crunchy vegetables, rice, oats, and fresh fruit) to equal 20% of your day's calories. The remaining 30% comes from fats and oils (20% polyunsaturated oils and 10% animal fats). You will not remain on this diet long, usually no longer than 2 to 4 weeks, but restricting the food substances (starches and sugars) that promote insulin release will allow the levels of insulin to fall. Once that occurs, the consequences of elevated insulin begin to disappear and you will see a gradual improvement of blood cholesterol and triglycerides, you will shed fluid, you will begin to shed fat, and you will stop retaining fluid. At that point, you may slowly increase the amount of carbohydrate in your diet and decrease the amount of protein until you return to percentages closer to those specified. Balance your intake with 35% lean protein, 35% low-starch carbohydrate fruits and vegetables, and 30% fats.

• The cochlea, where the tiny hairlike nerve endings reside, has a very high concentration of *vitamin A*, because proper functioning of these nerve fibers depends on sufficient amounts of this vitamin. In medical research on both animals and people, deficiency of vitamin A can contribute to hearing loss, and a number of studies have shown that supplementing vitamin A can sometimes improve hearing in these cases by as much as 15% to 18%. It is especially helpful in the loss of hearing and relieving the heightened sensitivity to loud noises (called presbycusis) that occurs with aging. Recommendation: Refer to the discussion of this vitamin in the A-to-Z Nutrient listings to acquaint yourself with the signs of deficiency and the signs of toxicity. If you feel you may be deficient in vitamin A, you can approach replacing it in two ways. First, you may take 15,000 IU of vitamin A per day for a week or two. Watch for any signs of toxicity to develop (dry skin and cracking at the corners of the mouth usually occur quickly). If no signs develop, continue with this level of intake for 6 to 8 weeks to assess your response. If you cannot tolerate this level of vitamin A, take 30,000 IU to 45,000 IU of beta-carotene instead. Your body will convert some of this vitamin A relative to vitamin A as it needs to, and there is little risk of your developing toxic symptoms.

• Adding *vitamin E* to your vitamin A supplementation is of particular benefit in improving the hearing loss and presbycusis of aging. Recommendation: To your vitamin A or beta-carotene dose, add 600 IU vitamin E per day. Refer to the A-to-Z Nutrient listing for this vitamin and follow the recommended schedule given there for gradually increasing your dose to guard against blood pressure increases that vitamin A sometimes can cause.

• Deficiency of *vitamin D* which contributes to your also developing deficiency of *calcium* may be important in the hearing loss that occurs in Ménière's syndrome, otosclerosis, and some kinds of nerve deafness. Recommendation: Refer to the listing for vitamin D in the A-to-Z Nutrient section and acquaint yourself with the signs of vitamin D deficiency and toxicity. The first method of increasing your vitamin D is a simple one: Expose your skin to natural sunlight for at least a half hour per day by getting outside in light clothing with arms and legs uncovered. Walk in the park, sit and read in the sun, or engage in a sport, if you like. A short span, 15 to 30 minutes a day, will usually be enough to increase your skin's conversion of vitamin D. If you are very fair, take care not to burn. If you live in an area with little sunshine or if for some other reason you cannot get outdoors to take some sun, you may want to purchase a Vita-Lite full-spectrum sunlight blub (available from Duro-Test Company, New Bergen, N.J.). The cost, although expensive for a light bulb, is really minimal—about 15 to 20 dollars for a fluorescent fixture tube that lasts 5 years. Failing that, you can take 400 to 800 IU vitamin D (such as that found in cod liver oil capsules) each day plus calcium. Your calcium dose of roughly 1000 mg should include magnesium, too, in a dose of 500 mg per day. You can purchase combinations of these two minerals at most health and nutrition stores. Take this form without the supplemental vitamin D if you get plenty of sunshine.

• *Coenzyme Q_{10}* is a powerful antioxidant whose role is crucial in getting circulation to the ears. Recommendation: Take 30 mg daily.

• *Magnesium* deficiency itself can cause damage to the inner ear structures, causing ringing of your ears, loss of hearing, and dizziness. The connection between magnesium and hearing loss has received a fair amount of attention from medical research. For example, research has shown that magnesium deficiency makes laboratory animals more susceptible to hearing loss from exposure to loud noises. And another theory suggests that the damage to hearing that certain antibiotic medications (the aminoglycosides, such as gentamicin or neomycin) cause may occur because they deplete magnesium in the hairlike nerve fibers in the cochlea. What do these studies mean to people? I'm not certain medical science has that clearly answered yet. Recommendation: Because supplementing magnesium has so little risk of toxicity, if you live or work in a noisy environment, I would certainly recommend you consider taking a calcium/magnesium supplement daily (as specified above in calcium) along with wearing proper ear protection. If you suffer from Ménière's sydrome, supplementing with these minerals is certainly worth a try.

• Deficiency of *manganese* has been linked to ear disorders. Recommendation: Supplement daily with 10 mg.

• Correcting an *iron deficiency* can improve hearing in some people with partial nerve deafness. Because you don't want to take iron if you are not truly deficient (iron overloading has its own problems), ask your personal physician to check you for this deficiency. If your iron stores are indeed low and you suffer from some hearing loss, supplementing with iron may improve your hearing to some degree. Recommendation: Take an amino acid chelate of iron (such as 10 mg iron glycinate per day), if you can find it. Refer to chelation in Section I, pages 30–31. Your stomach will tolerate the chelate much better and you will absorb the iron more fully. (If you cannot find a chelated iron supplement, contact Metagenics, Inc., San Clemente, California, a vitamin and mineral company that specializes in a line of vitamins and chelated minerals.) Failing that, take iron sulfate in a dose of 90 mg 3 times a day with food.

• *Zinc* levels decline with aging, and some research suggests that the low levels may contribute to the dizziness, continuous ringing in the ears, and progressive loss of hearing that older people suffer. Although I have not seen any research to back up the theory, it makes logical sense that this connection may also be true for that other disorder in which younger people suffer dizziness, ringing of the ears, and hearing loss—Ménière's syndrome. Recommendation: Take chelated zinc (glycinate, aspartate, or picolinate) in a dose of 20 to 40 mg per day for 3 to 6 months to assess your response. Warning: Supplementation of zinc in ionic form (zinc sulfate) can create deficiencies in other minerals, such as copper, by competing against them for absorption in the intestinal tract. Chelation of the zinc prevents this from happening. See pages 30–31, Section I, on chelation for more information.

Herbal remedies

• *Echinacea* aids poor equilibrium and reduces dizziness. It can be taken in tea or capsule form. It is recommended that the herb be taken for 6 to 8 weeks, then take a break for 1 to 4 weeks to give the immune system a rest. For hearing loss, take either 2 to 3 capsules daily, or mix 2 teaspoons of the root material with 1 cup of water or tea.

• The following herbs have decongestant properties and reduce ringing in the ears: *ephedra, eucalyptus, hyssop, mullein, and thyme.*

• To soothe inflammation and fight infection, take *mullein oil.* Put a few drops in the affected ear 3 times daily. To help improve circulation and blood flow to the ear area, use *butcher's broom, cayenne, chamomile, gingerroot, turmeric, and yarrow.*

Dosage may vary, depending on the duration and severity of your symptoms. Consult a qualified herbal practitioner. Let your physician know of your decision to use herbal remedies, as not all remedies can be used in conjunction with conventional pharmaceuticals.

What makes it worse?

• *Sugar* can cause inner ear problems (bringing on bouts of dizziness, ringing, and decreased hearing) in people with Ménière's syndrome. It may also do so in other people prone to low blood sugar (hypoglycemia). Recommendation: Eliminate or sharply curtail your intake of concentrated sugars, sugary foods and snacks, and the starchy vegetables known to quickly increase blood sugar (potatoes, wheat, corn, and foods made with these starches). See the listing on page 355 concerning constructing a proper diet.

• *Saturated fats* have received a bevy of research attention in hearing loss because people with high blood fat readings (cholesterol and triglycerides) often suffer impairment of hearing as well. The probable cause in these cases is arteriosclerosis (hardening of the arteries) in the tiny arteries that supply blood to the cochlea. With decreased blood flow, the tiny hairlike nerve fibers can't receive proper nourishment and oxygen, and they wither or die. These fats also contribute to excess production of earwax. Recommendation: If you have high cholesterol or triglycerides and you are losing your hearing, returning your blood values to normal may help.

• *Food sensitivities* may be the culprit behind hearing loss, ringing, and dizziness in some people with Ménière's syndrome. If you suffer from these symptoms and have tried drugs to combat the spinning dizziness without much success, food allergy or sensitivity is one avenue to explore. Recommendation: Consult an allergy specialist to help direct your investigation into possible food sensitivities and allergies. Using blood testing and skin testing, an allergist can narrow down the list of possible food culprits, each of which has to be checked by a systematic elimination trial. See Food Allergy in this section for more details of how to conduct such an elimination trial. If you have no access to an allergy specialist, you can use the commonsense approach. Divide foods into groups: milk products, citrus, beef, seafood, fruits, chocolate, and so on. Begin your search by eliminating whole groups of foods for 3 weeks—for example, all dairy products. If your symptoms disappear, you will at least be suspicious that something in that group caused them, but not precisely what. Then reinstitute individual dairy foods one at a time to see if symptoms recur. If they do, you'll have found a culprit. Certainly, doing this kind of systematic search takes time and effort, but if it improves a daily misery, then it's worth the trouble. Good luck with your search.

Heartburn

What is it?

Heartburn occurs when you suffer an irritation of the upper part of the stomach where it meets the esophagus (food tube). The esophagus, a muscular tube, moves food from the back of your mouth to the stomach. At its lower end, the muscle is thicker and very strong, opening to allow food to pass through, then closing tightly to keep the corrosive digestive acid found in the stomach from getting up into the esophagus where the lining is too delicate to withstand it. If something—gas forming in the stomach or a spasm of the esophageal sphincter muscle—keeps the sphincter open, the acid contents of your stomach will be able to back up—or reflux—into the esophagus and burn the lining. We call that feeling heartburn, but we ought more correctly to call it "esophagus burn." The burned lining becomes inflamed, a condition called esophagitis. Sometimes the irritation is extreme enough to cause the strong muscle wall of the esophagus to spasm over its entire length—an esophageal spasm—and the pain of that spasm takes more people to the hospital emergency room fearing they're having a heart attack than any other false alarm. If the stomach acid bath continues, the lining of the esophagus can erode and ulcerate.

When under stress you produce too much stomach acid, or if you take medications such as ibuprofen, aspirin, or prescription anti-inflammatory or arthritis drugs, you can even burn the tough lining of the stomach. This generalized stomach inflammation is called gastritis. If the burn becomes extreme, and the lining of the stomach breaks down in spots, you develop stomach ulcers.

Over-the-counter antacid preparations, such as Maalox, Mylanta, Rolaids, Pepto-Bismol, Tums, and a host of others, help to neutralize the stomach acid and reduce the production of stomach gas. A number of prescription medications have come onto the market to control the acid production (Tagamet, Zantac, Pepcid, Axid) and to coat and heal the raw lining (Carafate, Prilosec), but nutrition plays an important role in stopping the symptoms of heartburn. Let's see how.

What helps it?

• Eating a *properly composed diet* helps alleviate heartburn quickly. Along with the following specific avoidances, taking care to eat properly is your best ally in combating gastritis, esophageal reflux and spasm, and plain old-fashioned heartburn. Recommendation: Refer to Macronutrients, Section I, page 23. Construct a diet based on those recommendations that provides you with plenty of lean protein to support your lean muscles and organs and that limits your intake of concentrated starches and sweets. The specifics of this kind of diet are contained in that discussion.

• The *B vitamins* are necessary for proper digestion. Recommendation: Take a vitamin B-complex at a dosage of 50 mg 3 times daily, with meals.

Herbal remedies

• *Chamomile*'s soothing qualities make it a wonderful treatment for heartburn and stomach upset.

• Numerous studies show that licorice reduces the production of stomach acid, which also decreases heartburn. Long-term use (more than 6 weeks) or ingestion of larger amounts can have some negative side effects, such as headache, lethargy, sodium and water retention, loss of potassium, and high blood pressure. To reduce gas, take *cardamom* or *cinnamon*.

• *Dill* soothes the digestive tract. Make a tea using a few teaspoons of crushed seeds. Caution: Use moderately if you are pregnant.

Dosages may vary, depending on the duration and severity of your symptoms. Follow package directions, or consult a qualified herbal practitioner.

What makes it worse?

• A diet high in *sugar* makes heartburn worse. Sugar itself irritates the lining of the esophagus and stomach and increases stomach acid, fermentation of the sugar produces more stomach gas, and a high sugar content encourages the growth of certain stomach bacteria that recent medical studies say may cause chronic stomach ulcers. Recommendation: Eliminate or sharply curtail your intake of sugar, corn syrup, high-fructose corn syrup, molasses, and all food products made with them.

• *Alcohol* is one of the few substances directly absorbed by the stomach; the small intestine does the work of absorbing the nutrients of most foods. Alcohol, like sugar, has a directly hostile effect on the stomach lining and also stimulates increased stomach acid, but it has the added deleterious effect of weakening the muscular sphincter at the end of the esophagus, making reflux of stomach acid into the esophagus more likely. Recommendation: Eliminate or sharply curtail your intake of alcoholic beverages.

• The volatile oils in *peppermint and spearmint* also weaken the closure power of the muscular esophageal sphincter. Recommendation: Avoid foods, mints, and chewing gums flavored with these oils.

• *Chocolate,* likewise, produces an almost immediate weakening of the closure power of the muscular sphincter between the esophagus and the stomach. The caffeine-like substance in chocolate seems to be the culprit in causing the problems. Recommendation: Eliminate or sharply curtail your intake of chocolate in all forms. Substitute carob for chocolate, if possible.

• Again, through the caffeine content, *coffee and tea* may both relax the muscular sphincter and increase the output of stomach acid. Recommendation: Undertake a tapering schedule—see the one given under the coffee discussion of Headache—to rid yourself of your reliance on caffeine. Take it slow and easy so that you don't suffer the symptoms of caffeine withdrawal: sleepiness, irritability, powerful headache.

• Eating a *fatty meal* almost immediately relaxes the muscular closure power of the esophageal sphincter, allowing easy access for stomach acid into the esophagus. Recommendation: Try to limit the fat content of your foods to 30% of your total calories per day and to spread those fat calories out throughout the day.

• *Milk,* although you might intuitively think of it as a food to soothe the angry stomach, actually has only a transient neutralizing effect on stomach acid, followed later by a rise in stomach acid to an even higher level than it had been. Recommendation: Although you may indeed want to add some milk products to your diet for the high-quality protein, use it in conjunction with a full meal and not as a quickie heartburn remedy.

• *Orange juice* causes problems with the coordinated wave-like muscle motion of the esophagus that may contribute to spasm, especially if the lining of the tube is already inflamed by reflux of acid. Recommendation: Delicious as it may be, curb your intake of orange juice to small amounts (2 ounces) at a time.

• *Spicy foods,* especially those made with hot peppers or pepper powders, contain corrosive acids that directly irritate the stomach lining and contribute to heartburn. Recommendation: Especially during bouts of stomach trouble, try to avoid eating chili peppers, jalapeños, or other hot spices.

• *Tomato products,* such as juices, pastes, salsa, and sauces, may irritate the stomach and esophagus lining directly and may also disrupt the normal wave-like muscular motion of the esophagus that propels food down the tube in a coordinated fashion.

Heavy Periods

(Menorrhagia, Dysfunctional Uterine Bleeding)

What is it?

Excessively heavy bleeding during your menstrual cycle can occur for a variety of reasons: hormone imbalances, infection, miscarriage of a pregnancy, or tumors in the uterus (womb). Because the causes vary so widely, any unusually heavy or prolonged bleeding demands the attention of your personal physician. But once you're sure the bleeding is not because of infection, pregnancy, or a tumor, nutrition can offer some help.

What helps it?

• Women with heavy menstrual bleeding are often found to be slightly low in *vitamin A*. Supplementation helps to return their cycles to normal. Recommendation: Take 25,000 IU of vitamin A for no more than 15 days. If your next cycle has not returned to normal, vitamin A deficiency probably wasn't the problem. Do not continue to supplement the vitamin beyond this point. If your cycles did become normal, you may continue to take the vitamin A forerunner, beta-carotene, in a dose of 25,000 IU (15 mg) per day. Your body will slowly convert this nutrient to vitamin A as it needs it, so you don't risk vitamin A toxicity from continuing to use this vitamin in high doses.

• Even when you are not deficient enough in *iron* to develop anemia, the relative lack of it may contribute to heavy periods. The heavy bleeding improves for many such women when they supplement with iron. Recommendations: Take a chelated iron, such as iron glycinate, in a dose of approximately 30 mg per day through at least 2 menstrual cycles to assess your response. If you cannot find this form of iron supplement, you can use a combination of 45 mg ferrous sulfate along with 500 mg vitamin C twice daily. (The vitamin C "chelates" the iron and makes it easier to absorb.)

• *Manganese* deficiency may contribute to your developing heavy menstrual periods. When your manganese levels are low, you also will lose more iron, copper, and zinc in the menstrual blood. Recommendation: Take manganese aspartate (or amino acid chelated manganese) in a dose of 20 to 30 mg per day through at least 2 menstrual cycles to assess your response.

• *Vitamin C plus bioflavonoids* helps to reduce the heavy menstrual flow in some women. The action of vitamin C in improving the ability of your intestine to absorb iron from foods may account for part of this effect; however, the primary role of vitamin C in strengthening capillaries and other blood vessels probably plays the major role. Recommendation: Take 500 mg vitamin C in combination with the bioflavonoids (you can purchase them in combined tablet form) 2 to 3 times daily. If you already supplement vitamin C for other purposes, you can add a 1000 mg tablet or capsule of bioflavonoid complex to your daily dose of vitamin C.

Herbal remedies

• *Lady's mantle* lessens the severity of bleeding and can be taken as a tea made from 1 cup water mixed with 1 to 2 teaspoons of the dried herb. Take for as long as the period lasts.

What makes it worse?

I know of no nutrient that worsens this problem.

───────── Hemorrhoids ─────────

What are they?

Hemorrhoids are nothing more than varicose veins in a particularly uncomfortable spot. The blood vessels that drain blood from the tissues of the rectum form a complex network of interlacing connections called the hemorrhoidal plexus. These rectal blood vessels, like the ones in the lower leg that you usually think of as varicose veins, can weaken under prolonged pressure and become distended with blood. The prolonged pressure in the rectal vessel can come from excessive weight gain, pregnancy, or chronic constipation that causes you to strain with bowel movements. The condition occurs more commonly in people who sit a good portion of their day; therefore, if you work as a truck driver or a secretary, for example, you have a higher likelihood of developing hemorrhoids.

Just as with varicose veins in the legs, blood flow in the dilated hemorrhoidal vein can become so sluggish that a clot forms. When this occurs, the normal pain and itch of your hemorrhoidal tissues becomes suddenly excruciating. The remedy for a clotted (or thrombosed) hemorrhoid is lancing—your physician must open the hemorrhoid and remove the clot—and this quick and relatively easy office procedure will give you nearly instant relief of pain.

What can you do nutritionally to help a hemorrhoid problem? Let's take a look.

What helps it?

• Eating a diet sufficiently high in *fiber* to promote bowel regularity is one of your best defenses. Dietary fiber helps to keep water in the bowel contents and prevents constipation. Recommendation: Slowly increase the amount of fiber in your diet until you reach a level of 40 to 50 grams per day. Let me emphasize *slowly*. Don't attempt to go from the standard American intake of 15 grams a day to 50 overnight, or you will suffer abdominal cramping and bloating and wish you had never tried this remedy! Please refer to the detailed schedule for increasing fiber intake recommended in a previous discussion under Colon, Spastic. Follow this guideline to gradually meet your target fiber needs.

• Drinking plenty of water or *fluids* that mainly consist of water, such as unsweetened tea or diet soft drinks, ensures that you will not become dehydrated. When your body doesn't have enough water coming in, your colon will help conserve body water by absorbing more of it out of the bowel contents, leaving the stool hard, compact, and dry. Recommendation: Drink at least 64 ounces of *noncaloric fluid* per day. That means that regular soft drinks don't count! They actually do provide water, but they also provide about 35 grams of sugar or corn syrup along with water. What I don't want to see happen is your deciding to increase your fluid intake by drinking six or seven 12-ounce colas a day. And keep in mind that the 64 ounces is a minimum. If you work or play indoors or out in extreme heat, you may need as much as double that amount to keep up with your loss of fluid through sweating.

• *Vitamin C,* because of its clear role in strengthening blood vessel walls, may help to prevent the weakening and dilation of blood vessels everywhere—including those around the rectum. Recommendation: Take a minimum of 500 mg of vitamin C 2 to 3 times per day. Refer to the discussion of this vitamin found in Section I for more information about its importance as well as a detailed schedule for slowly increasing your daily intake to the level that which Dr. Linus Pauling (and I) feel most adult human beings should take—4 to 8 grams per day.

• *Essential fatty acids,* through their control of your body's production of the eicosinoid messengers (see eicosinoids, pages 24–27), help to normalize intestinal regularity and keep the stools soft. They also help to reduce swelling, pain, and irritation of inflamed tissues (and if you suffer with hemorrhoids, you have firsthand knowledge of what I mean by inflamed tissues!). Recommendation: To facilitate your best possible response from essential fatty acids, begin with the proper macronutrient framework (see Section I, Macronutrients, page 23). Then to that nutritionally sound base, add gamma-linoleic acid and EPA fish oil in a 1:4 (GLA:EPA) ratio 1 to 3 times daily. The EicoPro essential fatty acid product manufactured by Eicotec, Inc., of Marblehead, Massachusetts, contains ultrapure sources of linoleic acid and fish oils already combined in the proper ratio. If you cannot get that product, you can purchase linoleic acid in a product called evening primrose oil at most health and nutrition stores, and EPA fish oil as well. Because it is not as pure a form, the milligram dosing will be different. You can make a reasonable substitute by combining evening primrose oil capsules with fish oil capsules plus vitamin E. Take 500 mg of evening primrose oil (a source of linoleic acid in capsule form), plus 1000 mg EPA fish oil, plus 200 IU vitamin E 1 to 3 times a day. (Warning to diabetics: EPA fish oil can cause blood sugar fluctuations in some diabetics. Carefully monitor your blood sugar if you use this supplemental oil and discontinue its use if your blood sugar becomes difficult to control.)

Herbal remedies

• *Comfrey* is anti-inflammatory, stimulates the immune system, and aids the formation of new skin. Moisten powdered comfrey with vegetable oil and apply the paste, or pound the leaf to soften the fuzzy hairs and apply the leaf itself, topically. There's no need to wash off the residue.

• *Witch hazel* is a soothing astringent that relieves hemorrhoidal pain and itching. Make a compress using generic witch hazel (available anywhere), and use it whenever you need a bit of soothing.

• *Aloe* is astringent and heals wounds. Apply it topically to the anal area. Use the gel directly from the leaf of the plant.

• The bark of the *horse chestnut* tree contains a number of chemicals that help treat hemorrhoids. This herb strengthens blood vessel walls, which reduces the risk of developing more hemorrhoids. It also has anti-inflammatory benefits. The tannins in it, however, can cause constipation if consumed. But you could make a tea and apply it to the hemorrhoids. Or moisten powdered bark and apply the paste directly.

Dosages may vary, depending on the duration and severity of your symptoms. Follow package directions, or consult a qualified herbal practitioner.

What makes it worse?

• A diet high in refined *sugar* will worsen your hemorrhoidal problems in a number of ways: High sugar intake increases insulin and high insulin can increase your weight, your blood pressure, and your tendency to produce the "bad" eicosinoid messengers from essential fatty acids. These bad messengers promote inflammation, pain, and swelling, as well as clotting of blood. Recommendation: Eliminate or sharply reduce your intake of all refined sugars, including table sugar, corn syrup, high-fructose corn syrup, molasses, and all products made with these substances.

• *Narcotic medications,* such as codeine and hydrocodone, promote constipation, and that worsens your tendency to develop hemorrhoids. Recommendation: Of course, you should take such medications only under the direct supervision of your personal physician—who has prescribed them *for you*—and even then, you should limit the amount you take to the fewest days possible to avoid their constipating effect.

• Chronic use of *aspirin* can also cause constipation. Recommendation: If you suffer with hemorrhoids and are constipated, avoid taking aspirin on a regular basis. Two tablets once in a while for a headache won't hurt, but daily intake can cause problems. Substitute acetaminophen for minor pain when possible. If you must take aspirin for other medical conditions, you might not become as constipated if you use a buffered aspirin. These formulations contain a magnesium antacid that helps to protect the stomach but also helps to loosen the stool.

Hepatitis

What is it?

Hepatitis is a generic term, meaning infection or inflammation of the liver that causes loss of appetite, nausea, vomiting, extreme fatigue, flu-like body aches and cold symptoms, aversion to smoking and bright light, fever, dark urine, painfully enlarged liver, and yellow-tingeing of the eyes and skin. The inflammation can be from any of a number of viruses that directly infect and attack the liver tissues; from chemical toxins, such as alcohol or some anesthetic gasses used to put you to sleep for surgery; and from certain medications, most notably the anti-inflammatory arthritis medicines.

Viral infection of the liver can occur from various strains of hepatitis viruses (called A, B, C, or D) that directly destroy liver tissue, as well as the inflammation of the liver caused by the Epstein-Barr (mono) virus and others. The true hepatitis viruses also differ in their routes of transmission. Type A hepatitis occurs through eating or drinking food or water contaminated by fecal waste. Type B typically passes by sharing body fluids, and types C and D are passed through contaminated blood products.

What helps it?

• *Vitamin C* improves your body's immune defense function when it's under attack by any virus, including those that cause hepatitis. Orthomolecular physicians (those who subscribe to the use of large doses of vitamins and minerals to combat disease) have used doses of 40 to 100 grams of vitamin C—taken by mouth—to achieve remarkable resolution of symptoms in acute viral hepatitis. Recommendation: Take a minimum of 4000 mg (2 grams) per day in divided doses of 1000 mg 4 times daily. Your body may need and tolerate even more of this vitamin during severe illness. Refer to the discussion of Vitamin C in Section I for more information on its importance and for general guidelines for gradually increasing your intake of vitamin C using the crystalline (powdered) form to your own bowel tolerance level.

• Because the liver is intimately involved in your body's ability to absorb *vitamin B_{12}*, a diseased or inflamed liver may not be able to keep up with your body's demand for the vitamin under stress. Recommendation: Take 1000 *micro*grams of vitamin B_{12} in shot form weekly for 4 weeks, then monthly. You will probably have to enlist the aid of your personal physician to obtain the injectable form of this vitamin. Because the B-vitamin complex works best when all its members are present, you should also take 100 mg B-complex in tablet or capsule form daily.

• Additional supplementation with the B-complex vitamin *folic acid* along with vitamin B_{12} has shown promise in helping to reduce the number of days of hospitalization from viral hepatitis and to speed healing of the injured liver. Recommendation: Take 5 mg folic acid 2 to 3 times daily for 10 days (along with the weekly injection of B_{12}). After that time, reduce your daily intake to 5 mg per day until you have no physical symptoms of hepatitis and your blood tests have returned to normal.

• People suffering from hepatitis often are found to be deficient in *vitamin E,* and this deficiency will weaken the immune system, weaken the red blood cells, and worsen the nerve and muscle damage that can occur with hepatitis. Recommendation: Supplement with a total daily dose of 600 to 800 IU of d-alpha-tocopherol daily. Warning: These doses of vitamin E can cause blood pressure elevation in some people. Please refer to the discussion of this vitamin for specific guidelines on how to safely increase from a starting dose of 100 IU to the recommended dose.

• *Selenium* may be important in helping your immune system resist attack by the virus. Your body requires selenium to make its own, natural, potent free radical scavenger, glutathione peroxidase, that helps to fend off the tissue damage caused by infection and other physical insults. For more information about this protective effect, refer to free radicals and antioxidants found on pages 19–23. Selenium and vitamin E work together in this regard, and you can reduce your dose of vitamin E by taking selenium along with it. Recommendation: Take a combination of 100 *micro*grams selenium aspartate plus 100 IU vitamin E twice daily.

• *Lecithin* helps to heal the damaged liver in chronic active hepatitis (a condition of prolonged—6 months or more—liver inflammation that sometimes develops following infection by the hepatitis B and hepatitis C viruses). Recommendation: Take 3 grams lecithin granules per day.

What makes it worse?

• Avoid drinking *alcohol.* Refer to the discussion under the heading Alcoholism for further information about what helps and harms a liver inflamed by alcohol overuse.

• A diet high in *sugar* can worsen the inflammation to the liver from any cause; however, especially in the case of viral hepatitis, the immune-defense-system-weakening sugar becomes especially important. A weak immune system makes you more vulnerable to infection from any cause. Recommendation: Eliminate sugar from your diet by curtailing your intake of table sugar, corn syrup, high-fructose corn syrup, molasses, and all products made with these substances.

• Supplementation with large doses of *vitamin A* can actually cause inflammation of the liver; unfortunately, you may also become deficient in this vitamin when your liver has been damaged by alcohol abuse. Recommendation: Although you may need some additional vitamin A, you should supplement this vitamin only under the direct supervision of your personal physician if you have hepatitis.

Herbal remedies

• *Burdock and dandelion* cleanse the liver and bloodstream.

• Research shows *licorice* to be effective in treating viral hepatitis because it has antiviral activity. Caution: Do not use this herb for more than 7 consecutive days. Do not take it at all if you have high blood pressure.

• *Milk thistle* contains silymarin, which heals and rebuilds the liver.

• Other useful herbs include *black radish, green tea, red clover, yellow dock, and goldenseal*. Caution: Do not take goldenseal internally on a daily basis for more than 7 consecutive days. Do not use it at all during pregnancy, and use it with caution if you are allergic to ragweed.

Dosages may vary, depending on the duration and severity of your symptoms. Consult a qualified herbal practitioner. Alert your physician of your intention to use herbs. Some herbal treatments cannot be used in combination with conventional pharmaceuticals.

——————— Herpes Simplex ———————

What is it?

The virus herpes simplex rose to national prominence as a cause of the sexually transmitted disease known as "herpes" in the mid-1970s and, in the pre-AIDS era, became the scourge of the burgeoning sexual revolution in America.

The herpes simplex virus—one member of a whole group of herpes-type viruses that cause such diseases as chicken pox and mononucleosis—enters the body through broken skin, makes its way up the coverings of nerves supplying that area of skin, and sets up housekeeping in the ganglion of that nerve near the spinal cord or in the brain itself, where it "rests." When the virus enters the skin of the lips, nose, or face, it resides in the brain. When it enters skin of the body (usually the exposed genital organs), it "rests" near the spinal cord in the back. From this rest area, the virus can intermittently reactivate, cause recurrent outbreaks of blisters, and place you at risk for infecting others with herpes during these outbreaks.

There are two types of herpes simplex: type I (HSV-1) and type II (HSV-2). HSV-1 causes cold sores and skin eruptions. Between 20% and 40% of the American population has cold sores caused by HSV-1. Twice that number are infected but never have physical symptoms. In all, 40% to 80% of the population carries this virus. HSV-2 affects more than 30 million Americans, though more than half never develop serious symptoms.

The initial infection with virus may be so mild as to go unnoticed, but usually there will be a few tender blisters in the area. Once the virus establishes a home for itself in the brain or near the spinal cord, it lays in wait for *something* to stimulate its reactivation.

In herpes simplex infections on your lips, that something could be a sunburn or windburn, fever, other illness such as a cold or flu, trauma to your lips, or severe physical or emotional stress. In the herpes infections of the genital area, that something could be the monthly menstrual cycle in women, minor injury to the genitalia from vigorous sexual intercourse, infections that drain your immune defenses, or severe physical or emotional stress.

When the virus becomes active, the area of skin destined to "break out" will begin to itch, tingle, burn, ache, or in some way not feel "right." This sensation means the viruses have begun to make their way back down the nerve coverings from their rest area to the skin surface where they will produce a cluster of painful blisters that trouble you for a week or two, then heal and disappear, usually to return another day. Your physician can prescribe medication designed to kill the herpes simplex virus in the skin tissues when outbreaks occur; however, even these medications do not kill the virus in its rest area in the brain. Is there anything that nutrition can do to help? Yes.

What helps it?

• See Cold Sores.

• *Vitamin A* is important for healing and prevents the infection from spreading. Recommendation: Supplement with 50,000 IU daily. Use emulsion form for easier assimilation and greater safety at higher doses. Please read the vitamin A discussion in the A-to-Z Nutrient listings.

• In genital herpes outbreaks, a solution of zinc, applied to the skin with a cotton ball or cotton-tipped applicator, soothes the itching, burning, and stinging pain of the blisters in 2 to 3 hours. Recommendation: Ask your pharmacist to compound a 0.25% saturated solution of zinc sulfate in camphor water. Apply this solution to the genital sores hourly, beginning within 24 hours of their appearance and continuing for 3 to 6 days. Regular once-a-day application to the area that breaks out may help to prevent recurrences, as well.

Herbal remedies
• See Cold Sores.

What makes it worse?
• See Cold Sores.

• During outbreaks, eat the following in moderation: almonds, barley, cashews, grains, chicken, chocolate, corn, dairy products, meat, nuts and seeds, oats, and peanuts. These contain *L-arginine,* an amino acid that suppresses l-kysine, which retards virus growth.

─────────────── **Herpes Zoster** ───────────────

(Shingles)

What is it?
Zoster—or shingles, as you may better know it—is the second coming of the chicken pox virus, varicella. The varicella virus of the herpes family (see discussion of Herpes Simplex, page 370) probably infected you as a child, causing chicken pox—a body-wide outbreak of blistered bumps that scab over to make sores and finally heal in a week or two. As with its herpes simplex cousins, the varicella virus can enter through the broken skin of any one of the "pox" sores, make its way up the nerve coverings, and make a home in the brain or near the spinal cord. Many years later, under the proper stimulation, the virus becomes active again, but this time, instead of causing pox all over the body, the virus makes it way back down the nerve covering to cause an outbreak of clustered blisters all along the path of the nerve. In zoster, significant pain (caused by the virus inflaming the nerve) occurs in a band around one-half of the chest, abdomen, or face, preceding the outbreak of tender blisters and red-

ness. The affected nerve becomes so inflamed, sometimes, that chronic neuralgia (nerve pain) lasting many months or even years can result.

The disease is also infectious. From the onset of the pain, live varicella viruses begin to "shed" from the affected skin, and consequently, you could pass the virus to a young child, to someone who had never had chicken pox as a child, or to someone who had a beleaguered immune system, such as a person on cancer chemotherapy, a person with AIDS, or a person on drugs to suppress the body's defenses after an organ transplant. If you pass the virus to any of these people, they would not develop shingles, but rather they would develop chicken pox. In an otherwise healthy child or adult, coming down with a case of chicken pox is a nuisance; in an immunocompromised person, it could prove fatal. For this reason, if you have a case of shingles, you should not visit in the hospital or with friends who fall into these categories. Even with a normal, healthy immune system, the attack rate for chicken pox is about 80%, meaning that 8 out of 10 people exposed to the virus will catch it.

But as for you, if you have zoster, what does nutrition offer to help relieve the sometimes severe pain during and after the outbreak? Let's take a look.

What helps it?
• *Vitamin C* can promote more rapid healing of the blisters. Recommendation: At the first sign of shingles, increase your intake of vitamin C to 8 to 10 grams per day, taken at the rate of 1 gram per hour, if your bowel will tolerate that dose. Continue this dose level until the blisters dry up, then drop to your normal daily intake of C (or a minimum of 1 to 2 grams if you don't normally take C). Refer to the discussion of this vitamin to learn more about how to increase your intake to the level you can tolerate.
• The action of vitamin C improves by the addition of the *bioflavonoids* in helping to speed healing of the blistering in shingles. The combination allows you to use lower doses of vitamin C, which can be helpful if your bowel won't tolerate the higher doses. Recommendation: At the first sign of pain, begin to take 600 to 1000 mg of vitamin C and 600 to 1000 mg of bioflavonoid complex 5 times daily for 3 days.
• Many sufferers of shingles report "dramatic" improvement

from supplemental injections of *vitamin B₁₂*, with relief of pain and rapid healing of blisters beginning about 2 to 3 days after commencing therapy. Recommendation: You may need to enlist the aid of your personal physician to take the vitamin in shot form. Take 1000 *micro*grams twice daily for 6 days, then weekly for 6 weeks.

• *Vitamin E* supplementation has shown to be beneficial to people suffering from chronic nerve pain after zoster. Recommendation: Take 400 to 600 IU of vitamin E as d-alpha-tocopherol succinate 3 times daily with meals. Continue this level of supplementation for 6 months. Warning: Large doses of vitamin E can cause elevated blood pressure in some people. Refer to the listing for this vitamin and follow the guidelines there to slowly and safely increase your dose, beginning at 100 IU once daily.

Herbal remedies

• Herbalists recommend *lemon balm* to treat shingles. Make a tea using lemon balm and any other mints you may have on hand, such as spearmint, thyme, sage, self-heal, and rosemary.

• The capsaicin found in *red pepper* relieves pain by blocking pain signals from nerves just under the skin. Even the FDA recognizes the value of capsaicin and approved commerical creams containing the substance. You can buy the cream, or you can add powdered red pepper into any white skin lotion until it turns pink. Dab it on a small area of skin to test your reaction, and be sure to wash your hands immediately to avoid getting it in your eye.

• *Licorice* contains several antiviral and immune-boosting compounds. Nautropath Joseph Pizzorno, co-author of *The Encyclopedia of Natural Medicine,* claims to have seen people with shingles whose pain and inflammation cleared up within 3 days following application of a licorice ointment.

Dosages may vary, depending on the severity and duration of your symptoms. Follow package directions, or consult a qualified herbal practitioner.

What makes it worse?

• Except for nutrients that depress your immune function (see Immune System Health on page 382), I know of no substances that worsen zoster.

———————— **HIV Infection** ————————
(see AIDS/ARC)

———————————— **Hives** ————————————
(see Urticaria)

———————— **Hyperinsulinemia** ————————
(see Obesity)

———————— **Hypertension** ————————

What is it?

Hypertension, or high blood pressure, affects about 50 million Americans. The U.S. Public Health Service reports that hypertension affects more than half of all Americans over the age of 65. The percentage of African Americans with high blood pressure is one-third higher than that for whites. Most people develop a problem with blood pressure between ages 20 and 55, but a few cases begin before the age of 20; in these very early cases, there is usually some abnormality of the kidneys, their blood supply, or narrowing of the major blood vessels leading into the lower body that causes the elevation in pressure. Unless you fall into this youngest category, your high blood pressure most likely is not the result of any structural abnormality in blood vessels or the kidneys themselves. You, like 95% of Americans with high blood pressure, probably have what your physician calls "essential hypertension," which basically means high blood pressure without certain cause. That phrase is a little misleading, however, because as advances in medical technology have expanded our understanding of human biology to the microscopic and even submicroscopic level, we are now much more certain about what causes "essential" hypertension.

Some people with essential hypertension produce an overabundance of adrenaline under stress, and their blood pressure rises markedly during these times but is normal in between. Others produce too much of the body chemicals called angiotensin II that act to powerfully constrict the blood vessels, which raises the blood pressure. In some cases, the kidney, though normal to look at, cannot normally rid the body of excess sodium, and where sodium goes, so goes water. Increased body water may mean increased pressure. One reason that a seemingly normal kidney might hold on to sodium more tightly is that it is being driven to do so by a high level of insulin in the blood. This last cause may explain elevated blood pressure in the vast majority of Americans. But the list goes on as new causes come to light.

A number of external causes also contribute to your risk of developing high blood pressure: Cigarette smoking raises blood pressure; alcohol raises blood pressure; taking estrogen, vitamin E, and decongestant medications can increase blood pressure; and obesity raises blood pressure (usually because of excess insulin). Exercise helps to reduce blood pressure and so does weight loss. What does nutrition have to offer in combating hypertension? Let's take a look.

What helps it?

• Probably the single most important step in reducing high blood pressure is for you to eat a *properly constructed diet* focusing on several fundamentals: adequate in lean protein, extremely low in sugar and refined starches, reduced in fat, high in fiber, and with an increase in consumption of raw fruits and vegetables. Please refer to Macronutrients, page 23, where you will find the information necessary to calculate your adequate protein needs and guidelines for constructing a diet that meets the criteria outlined above. The diet traditionally prescribed for high blood pressure—a high-complex-carbohydrate, low-salt, low-fat diet—doesn't work; even now the current medical research literature on hypertension has begun to dub it the *"controversial* high-complex-carbohydrate, low-fat diet used in the treatment of high blood pressure."* It doesn't work, quite simply, because the vast majority of people with "essential" hypertension most likely have a problem relating to the overproduction of insulin. Force-feeding them a diet heavily weighted with starches (complex carbohydrates are nothing more than starches with added fiber) only makes their insulin problem worse, which makes their blood pressure problem worse. The diet I describe for you in the Macronutrient discussion will help to alleviate the overproduction of insulin and consequently reduce blood pressure. Please also see "What makes it worse?" on page 329 for some additional dietary information related to blood pressure.

• *Essential fatty acids,* through their ability to control the production of "good" or "bad" prostaglandin messenger production (see the Yin and Yang of Human Health, pages 24–27, for a full discussion of this topic), have a powerful influence on blood pressure.

Too many "bad" ones leads to hypertension, plenty of "good" ones to reduced blood pressure. Adding small amounts of these eicosinoid forerunners to your nutritional regimen can help direct the flow of these messengers toward the good side. Recommendation: To facilitate the best response from essential fatty acids, begin with the proper macronutrient framework (see page 23). Then to that nutritionally sound base, add gamma-linoleic acid (GLA) and fish oil (EPA) in a 1:4 (GLA:EPA) ratio. The EicoPro essential fatty acid product manufactured by Eicotec, Inc., of Marblehead, Massachusetts, contains ultrapure sources of linoleic acid and fish oils already combined in the proper ratio. If you cannot get that product, you can purchase linoleic acid in a product called evening primrose oil at most health and nutrition stores and EPA fish oil as well. Because it is not as pure a form, the milligram dosing will be different from the EicoPro product, but you can make a reasonable substitute by combining 500 mg of evening primrose oil (a source of linoleic acid in capsule form), plus 1000 mg EPA fish oil, plus 200 IU vitamin E 1 to 3 times a day. (Warning to diabetics: EPA fish oil can cause blood sugar fluctuations in some diabetics. Carefully monitor your blood sugar if you use this supplemental oil and discontinue its use if your blood sugar becomes difficult to control.)

• *Vitamin A* deficiency may contribute to hypertension. Because your body stores vitamin A and it could build up and cause problems itself, you should not supplement additional vitamin A for this condition, unless your personal physician confirms on blood testing that you have a deficiency. You can, however, safely add the vitamin A forerunner, beta-carotene, to your diet without risk of problems. You body converts beta-carotene to vitamin A as you need it. Recommendation: Take 25,000 IU (15 mg) beta-carotene per day.

• *Vitamin C* deficiency may contribute to the development of hypertension, and supplementation may help to slightly reduce the pressure. Vitamin C also reduces blood-clotting tendencies. Recommendation: Take 3000 to 6000 mg time-release vitamin C in divided doses, daily. Refer to the discussion of this important vitamin for information about its many health benefits and how to determine your own tolerance level for the vitamin.

• *Vitamin D* assists in the absorption of calcium, which has been shown to reduce blood pressure. Recommendation: Because your body can store vitamin D, regular supplementation can result in a buildup and possible health problems. Your body can make plenty of vitamin D as long as your skin gets some exposure to sunlight. As little as 30 minutes a day will probably be enough. In addition, dairy manufacturers routinely fortify their products with vitamin D. From either of these sources, you can get enough vitamin D to prevent deficiency that could impair your ability to absorb calcium.

• If your intake of *calcium* is low (under 700 mg per day from all sources), you increase your risk for developing high blood pressure. Supplementation of extra calcium helps to reduce the pressure in these instances. It is also important to keep the calcium and its mineral partner, phosphorus, in the proper ratio of 2 parts of calcium for 1 part of phosphorus. Recommendation: Take 1000 to 2000 mg of calcium per day along with 500 to 1000 mg phosphorus for 2 months, regularly checking your pressure to assess your response to this regimen.

• *Magnesium* has the ability to relax the blood vessels and allow them to open more widely. This relaxing effect reduces blood pressure. Deficiency of magnesium alters the balance of calcium flowing into the smooth muscle of the walls of the blood vessels; the vessels constrict or spasm, and the blood pressure goes up in a fashion similar to what happens when you put a nozzle on a water hose. When you reduce the size of the opening, the pressure of the stream of water coming out shoots up. Recommendation: Take 500 to 1000 mg daily ($\frac{1}{2}$ the dosage of whatever calcium supplement you are taking).

• *Coenzyme Q_{10}* lowers blood pressure. Recommendation: Supplement with 100 mg daily.

• A deficiency of *selenium* has been linked to heart disease. Recommendation: Take 200 *micro*grams daily.

• Low *potassium* can contribute to high blood pressure, but the effect is especially magnified when calcium and magnesium levels are deficient. If you have high blood pressure and take diuretic medications (fluid or water pills) such as hydrochlorothiazide, Lasix, or Bumex, you are at higher risk to develop potassium deficiency because these medicines make you lose potassium in your urine. Recommendation: If your physician has prescribed diuretics that require extra potassium, he or she will usually have given you a prescription for the drug. However, even if you don't take water pills and do have high blood pressure, your potassium may become low. Eat foods rich in potassium, such as broccoli, tomatoes, citrus fruits, and bananas. You can purchase a product in the salt section of your local market called NO SALT that is nothing more than potassium salts. Use it to sprinkle on foods in cooking to add extra potassium. You can also take 99 mg potassium gluconate daily to help raise your potassium levels. Warning: Some blood pressure medicines—Zestril, Capoten, Capozide, Zestoretic, or any other member of the group of blood pressure medications called ACE inhibitors—help your kidney conserve or hang on to potassium, and if you take these medications for blood pressure, you should not supplement extra potassium unless your personal physician advises you to do so.

Herbal remedies

• High blood pressure can be improved with the use of *cayenne, chamomile, fennel, hawthorn berries, parsley, and rosemary.* Caution: Do not use chamomile on an ongoing basis or you may develop a ragweed allergy.

• *Angelica* reduces blood pressure levels.

• *Garlic* is effective in lowering blood pressure. Recommendation: Take 2 300 mg capsules 3 times daily.

• *Valerian root* calms the nerves.

Dosages may vary, depending on the duration and severity of your symptoms. Consult a qualified herbal practitioner. Alert your physician of your intention to use herbs. Some herbal treatments cannot be used in combination with conventional pharmaceuticals.

What makes it worse?

• Drinking *alcohol* in more than very modest amounts causes an elevation in blood pressure. When you stop drinking, your blood pressure falls rapidly, usually within a week, sometimes as quickly as within 24 hours. Recommendation: Sharply curtail your alcohol intake to no more than $2/3$ ounce of distilled spirits, 4 ounces of wine, or 1 "lite" beer per day.

• Because *caffeine* does increase blood pressure briefly, especially in men prone to high blood pressure, you should avoid excessive consumption of caffeinated coffee, tea, and chocolate. The blood pressure rise that comes after drinking caffeine doesn't last long, with pressure soon returning to its usual level. An occasional cup of caffeinated coffee or tea is not going to cause a problem; however, if you measure your coffee in pots and not cups, you would do well to cut it back. According to *The New England Journal of Medicine,* coffee, when consumed in large quantities, can elevate blood cholesterol levels and more than double the risk of heart disease. Recommendation: Drink no more than 1 to 2 cups of caffeinated coffee or tea per day. If you currently drink coffee or tea heavily, you will need to reduce your intake slowly to avoid the headache and sleepiness that accompany caffeine withdrawal. Please refer to the caffeine listing under the heading Breast Disease (Benign) for a guideline to help you taper your caffeine intake without misery.

• If you are taking an MAO inhibitor (a drug prescribed to lower blood pressure and counter depression), avoid the chemical *tyramine* and its precursor, tyrosine. Tyramine-containing foods include almonds, avocados, bananas, beef or chicken liver, beer, cheese, chocolate, fava beans, herring, meat tenderizer, peanuts, pickles, pineapples, pumpkin seeds, raisins, sausage, sesame seeds, sour cream, soy sauce, wine, yeast extracts, and yogurt.

• For years, physicians told their patients with high blood pressure to restrict their intake of *sodium (salt).* Recent medical data suggests that simply restricting salt has very little effect on hypertension unless you also correct imbalances in calcium, magnesium, and potassium. Once these nutrients are back in line, sodium intake ceases to be a factor influencing blood pressure as long as the kidneys are "normal." Recommendation: Don't be misled into thinking that all you have to do is eat a diet low in salt to reduce blood pressure. While I would not recommend that you bury your food in salt, neither would I advise your going to great lengths to purchase special foods low in salt unless you have a severe kidney problem and your physician has advised you to. Or you may be one of the 80 million Americans who have an increased sensitivity to dietary sodium; you need to assess your needs based on your circumstances. Adding a dash of it will not adversely affect your pressure if you take care of the basics in diet as outlined above.

• Avoid *obesity.* Although the association is not 100%, many overweight people also suffer from high blood pressure, probably because the high insulin that promotes fat storage also promotes their hypertension. The two problems, then, are both just different symptoms of another bigger problem: hyperinsulinemia or Syndrome X. Please refer to the discussion of this problem under the heading Obesity for more information. Recommendation: Begin now to reduce your weight and body fat to normal levels. Refer to the discussion of Macronutrients on page 23 to construct a basic diet for yourself that will help you to begin to slowly reduce your weight. The fundamentals of this kind of diet are: 45% lean protein (mostly chicken, fish, veal, and egg white); 35% nonstarchy carbohydrate (mainly from green vegetables and a little fruit); 20% monounsaturated fats, such as olive oil, canola oil, and 10% animal fat. Your diet should contain no sugar, corn syrup, high-fructose corn syrup, or products made with these substances, and no refined starches or meals or products made with these.

• Limit your intake of *red meat and egg yolk* because both these foods contain high amounts of arachidonic acid, a forerunner of the "bad" prostaglandins that cause constriction of blood vessels and increase blood pressure. Recommendation: Eat red meat no more than once a week, and limit egg yolk to 1 a day (white of the egg is all protein and therefore contains no arachidonic acid).

Hypoglycemia
(Low Blood Sugar)

What is it?

When you eat starch, sugar, or protein, your body breaks down and absorbs the nutrients in the food, and your blood sugar rises. This rise in blood sugar signals your pancreas to produce and release insulin, the hormone that acts to return your blood sugar to normal by driving it into the tissues to be used or stored. In some people, the rise in blood sugar stimulates the release of too much insulin, which drives too much blood sugar into the tissues, leaving the level in the blood too low. In medicine, we call this condition hypoglycemia. When the blood sugar swings wildly, first hurtling upward then plummeting too low, you may suffer symptoms of nausea, clammy sweats, dizziness, muscle cramping, and even fainting. We refer to these unpleasant symptoms accompanying the falling blood sugar level as "reactive" hypoglycemia. Symptoms come not from the low level itself but from the rapid change. A stable low blood sugar— one that's low but is always about the same degree of low—rarely causes symptoms. People with overactive insulin and reactive hypoglycemia often develop adult-onset diabetes mellitus. I would ask you to refer to the discussion of that disorder in this text for additional information about the side of the hypoglycemia coin. The nutritional remedies of these two disorders—although they seem opposites—are actually virtually identical, and there would be no value in simply repeating the recommendations here.

What helps it?
- See Diabetes Mellitus.

Herbal remedies
- See Diabetes Mellitus.

What makes it worse?
- See Diabetes Mellitus.

─── Immune System Health ───

What is it?
Your immune system is the line of defense that protects you from attack by anything that is "not you." That broad category includes bacteria, fungi, viruses, and anything your body's immune system watchdogs declare to be a "foreign" substance, which could mean a transplanted kidney or heart, a dose of penicillin or some other medication, or a grain of dust or plant pollen. In some cases, "foreign" turns out to be your own body's cells that have gone haywire and lost their normal "you" characteristics. Your immune system vigilantly patrols on the lookout for these potential cancer-causing rogue cells. Anytime the immune defenders come across something foreign, they call for an array of immune defense troops to charge in and destroy the invader. We're all assaulted every day by invaders from the world around us—we breathe them in, eat them, get them on our skin—and from the world within us, as cells age, go haywire, and must be removed before cancers can form. We depend on a healthy immune system, working around the clock, to defend us from the world. Without a healthy immune system, capable of destroying our enemies, we would—like the boy who lived in the plastic bubble—quickly die. In that light, it's easy to see that one of your most important goals in maintaining optimum health has to be proper nourishment of your immune system. What does that entail? Let's take a look.

What helps it?
- Inadequate *dietary protein* cripples the immune system. Deficiency of this nutrient alone accounts for the greater susceptibility

to disease seen in impoverished nations, where complete protein (one containing all the essential amino acid building blocks of protein) is often a luxury. Complete proteins are readily available in this country in lean meat, fish, poultry, egg white, and dairy products. Recommendation: Your body must have a minimum of ½ gram of complete protein for every pound of your lean muscle tissue every day to build and repair the tissues and to maintain a healthy immune system. You can refer to Macronutrients, page 23, to learn how to calculate your lean body weight and protein needs.

• Your body takes *essential fatty acids* from your diet and through a series of alterations produces the "good" and the "bad" prostaglandin messengers. (See the Yin and Yang of Human Health, pages 24–27, for complete discussion of these messengers.) The "good" prostaglandins act to stimulate immune function, but more important is a balance between the "good" and "bad." Recommendation: To facilitate the best response from essential fatty acids, begin with the proper macronutrient framework (see Section I, Macronutrients, page 23). Then to that nutritionally sound base add gamma-linoleic acid to EPA fish oil in a ratio of 1:4 (GLA:EPA) 1 to 3 times daily. The EicoPro essential fatty acid product manufactured by Eicotec, Inc., of Marblehead, Massachusetts, contains ultrapure sources of linoleic acid and fish oils already combined in this ratio. If you cannot get that product, you can purchase linoleic acid in a product called evening primrose oil at most health and nutrition stores, and EPA fish oil as well. Because it is not as pure a form, the milligram dosing will be different. You can make a reasonable substitute by combining evening primrose oil capsules with fish oil capsules plus vitamin E. Take 500 mg of evening primrose oil (a source of linoleic acid in capsule form), plus 1000 mg EPA fish oil, plus 200 IU vitamin E 1 to 3 times a day. (Warning to diabetics: EPA fish oil can cause blood sugar fluctuations in some diabetics. Carefully monitor your blood sugar if you use this supplemental oil and discontinue its use if your blood sugar becomes difficult to control.)

• Deficiency of *vitamin A* reduces the vigilance of your immune defenders against invaders and supplementation improves their response. Because your body stores vitamin A, supplementation can sometimes result in toxic side effects building up. Your body, however, can make vitamin A from its forerunner, *beta-carotene,* as it needs to; therefore, by supplementing with this relative to vitamin A, you can avoid toxicity problems. Your personal physician can perform a blood test to check for vitamin deficiency, and if your levels are truly low, you may need to supplement with vitamin A itself to quickly bring your levels up to normal. Recommendation: If you are deficient in vitamin A, take 25,000 IU of vitamin A daily for 1 week, then switch to beta-carotene. Take 15,000 to 25,000 IU beta-carotene per day to maintain adequate raw materials for your body to turn into vitamin A.

• The *vitamins of the B-complex* help to stimulate your immune defenses in the face of physical stress, such as following surgery or trauma. When the levels of these vitamins fall too low, your body's ability to make antibodies to fight infection declines markedly and you fall victim to frequent infections. Recommendation: Take 100 mg vitamin B-complex per day. Also, several specific vitamins in the complex serve important immune stimulating functions as well.

• Deficiency of *folic acid* decreases the ability of your immune defenders to respond readily to invaders. Recommendation: Take a minimum of 1 gram of folic acid each day.

• Deficiencies of both *pantothenic acid* and *riboflavin* (vitamin B_2) reduce your production of antibodies to fight infection. Recommendation: Take 100 mg pantothenic acid and 50 mg riboflavin daily.

• Your body must have adequate *vitamin B_6* (pyridoxine) to build new immune fighters when the call goes out that an invader has attacked. The templates for these fighters reside in the lymph nodes, the bone marrow, and the blood itself. When you need to be defended, these templates duplicate themselves rapidly, turning out identical copies to swell the ranks of defenders against the foreign invader. Vitamin B_6 assists in copying the encoded genetic message that must pass from one immune cell to its copy. Recommendation: Take 50 mg of vitamin B_6 3 times per day.

• Deficiency of *vitamin B_{12}* reduces the vigor of response of your immune defenders and slightly reduces their killing power. Recommendation: Take B_{12} in oral or sublingual form in a dose of 1000 to 2000 *micro*grams daily.

• *Manganese* is necessary for proper immune function, and it works with the B vitamins to provide a general feeling of well-being. Recommendation: Supplement with 2 mg daily.

• *Coenzyme Q_{10}* protects the cells and heart function by enhancing oxygen. Recommendation: Boost your immune system with 100 mg daily.

• Deficiency of *vitamin C* can impair your immune defense system in several ways: It prevents some immune fighters from responding as readily to the distress signal sent out to attract them to the area of invasion by bacteria, viruses, and the like; it reduces the production of antibodies to fight against infection; and it may even impair the killing power of the immune defenders. Recommendation: Supplement daily with a minimum of 500 mg time-release vitamin C twice daily. Research experts in this area feel (and I agree with them) that a total daily adult dose should be more in the neighborhood of 4 to 8 grams per day, but I would encourage you to at least meet the 1 gram minimum. You may wish to reread the discussion in Section I concerning this important vitamin, its uses, and how to determine your own body's tolerance level for it.

• Deficiency of *vitamin E* depresses the ability of your immune system to defend you. Supplementation of this vitamin improves resistance to disease in all age groups; however, it is especially beneficial for older people. Recommendation: Adults should take vitamin E, as d-alpha-tocopherol succinate, in a minimum dose of 200 to 400 IU per day, with older men and women needing as much as 600 to 800 IU per day. Warning: Vitamin E can cause elevation of your blood pressure. Please refer to the discussion of this vitamin in the A-to-Z Nutrient listings for information on how to safely increase your dose of vitamin E.

• *Selenium* deficiency weakens your immune system in several ways: It hinders your production of antibodies to fight infection, it reduces the killing power of certain defenders, and it reduces the numbers of the cells that send out the "call to arms" signals to attract killing immune defenders to the area under attack. Your body also requires selenium to produce its own natural antioxidant and free radical scavenger, glutathione peroxidase, which protects your own tissues from being damaged by the killing chemicals released against the invaders by your immune defenders. Recommendation: Take 100 to 200 *micro*grams of selenium picolinate or selenium aspartate each day. Warning: Do not overuse selenium, because some medical research has suggested that excessive intake of this mineral might actually *impair* the immune system.

• Deficiency of *iron* impairs the killing power of some of your immune defenders as well as the ability of certain others to copy and propagate themselves to increase their ranks in time of need. Recommendation: If you are deficient in iron (discovered by blood testing through your personal physician), you should take 20 mg iron glycinate twice a day, or if you cannot find this chelated form of the mineral, take a combination of 90 mg ferrous sulfate plus 500 mg vitamin C 3 times daily. If you are not iron deficient, do not supplement with additional iron, but do keep your body's iron stores up by eating foods rich in iron regularly.

• In all ages, but especially in the sagging immunity frequently seen as we age, *zinc* deficiency clearly plays an important role. But even when there is no true deficiency, supplementation with extra zinc can improve the responsiveness of your immune defense system to attack. Recommendation: Take zinc in chelated form, such as zinc picolinate or zinc aspartate, in a dose of 50 to 80 mg per day. To balance the zinc, take 3 mg of *copper* daily. Warning: Supplementation of zinc in its ionic form can create deficiencies of other minerals, such as copper, by competing with them for absorption from the intestine. Chelation of the minerals (see pages 30–31, Section I, on chelation) prevents this competition among minerals to get into the body, allowing you to fully absorb each of them.

Herbal remedies

• *Suma* enhances the immune system and helps the body adapt to stress.

• *Astragalus* boosts the immune system and generates anticancer cells in the body. Caution: Do not take this herb if you have a fever.

• *Bayberry, fenugreek, hawthorn, horehound, licorice root, and red clover* enhance the immune response. Caution: If used on a long-term basis (more than 6 weeks), licorice can elevate blood pressure and cause water and sodium retention. Do not take it if you have high blood pressure, and no one should take it on a daily basis for more than 7 consecutive days.

• One of the most popular immune boosters is *echinacea*.

• *Goldenseal* also strengthens the immune system while it cleanses the body. Caution: Do not take internally on a daily basis for more than 1 week at a time. Use with caution if you have a ragweed allergy.

Dosages may vary, depending on the duration and severity of your symptoms. Consult a qualified herbal practitioner, and tell your physician of your decision to treat herbally. Some herbal remedies cannot be used in combination with conventional pharmaceuticals.

What makes it worse?

• A diet high in refined *sugar* debilitates your immune defense system by impairing your body's ability to produce antibodies to fight infection and by reducing the killing power of certain types of immune defenders. In medical studies, researchers could detect measurable drops in antibody production after people consumed as little as 18 grams of sugar—that's about the sugar or corn syrup content found in half of a regular canned soft drink! Recommendation: Sharply reduce your intake of sugar, corn syrup, high-fructose corn syrup, molasses, and all products made with these substances.

• Some early research (done in 1972) showed that *coffee* (specifically the caffeine in coffee) *may* suppress your ability to produce antibodies against infection. More recent studies have suggested that while coffee intake of greater that 5 cups per day slowed the response of immune defenders to mount an attack against foreign invasion by 30%, it also seemed to stimulate the production of natural killer cells, the white blood cells designed to do the actual job of destroying the invader. So what does that mean to your coffee habit? Recommendation: Since the research seems to point in both directions, I would recommend taking the middle ground. If you are currently in good health and trying to stay that way, keep your caffeinated coffee intake to a cup or two a day. If you suffer from frequent infections and your immune system needs all the help it can get, eliminate caffeinated coffee, tea, and chocolate from your diet. Do this slowly if you're much of a caffeine junkie, or risk a several-day stint of the powerful caffeine-withdrawal headache. Refer to Breast Disease, Benign, where I have outlined a regimen for slow withdrawal of caffeine that should prevent your misery as you decaffeinate.

Impotence

What is it?

Impotence refers to the inability to achieve or maintain an erection firm enough to engage in satisfactory sexual intercourse. The problem usually develops gradually and may be a consequence of other medical conditions, such as arteriosclerosis, high blood pressure, diabetes, or multiple sclerosis. Or it may develop because of abuse of alcohol, drugs, or tobacco; following trauma to the spinal cord; or from zinc deficiency. Impotence can also occur as an unpleasant side effect from taking certain medications, including narcotic pain medications, estrogen hormones, and disulfiram, also called Antabuse, a drug used to help alcoholics stop drinking by making alcohol poisonous to them.

Because of the wide variety of causes, you should always consult a urologic specialist if you become impotent, because only then will you uncover the cause. If you discover your impotence to be a consequence of diabetes, high blood pressure, arteriosclerosis, multiple sclerosis, or alcohol abuse, you should turn to the discussions of those conditions in this text and follow the recommended nutritional guidelines. Improving the causative disorder will quite often improve the impotence. Let's look at what nutrition has to offer otherwise.

What helps it?

• *Zinc* deficiency has been identified as a contributing cause to the development of impotence in some people. If your physician can find no specific cause for your impotence, zinc deficiency may be the culprit. Refer to the discussion of this mineral in the nutrient listings to reacquaint yourself with other signs or symptoms of deficiency of zinc. If you think you may be deficient in this mineral, supplementation may do the trick. Recommendation: Take a chelated zinc, such as zinc aspartate, in a dose of approximately 80 mg daily. Continue this dose level for a minimum of 4 to 6 weeks to assess your response. Warning: Supplementation of zinc in its ionic form can create deficiencies of other minerals, such as copper, by competing with them for absorption from the intestine. Chelation of the minerals (see discussion on pages 30–31, Section I, on chelation) prevents this competition among minerals to get into the body, allowing you to fully absorb each of them.

• *Octacosanol* is a natural source of vitamin E and improves hormone production. Recommendation: Take 1000 to 2000 *micro*grams 3 times weekly.

Also see Alcoholism, Atherosclerosis, Diabetes Mellitus, Hypertension, and Multiple Sclerosis.

Herbal remedies

• *Ginkgo* is best known for improving blood flow to the brain. However, it seems to increase blood flow to the penis. Research has continued have had very good results with 60 to 240 mg daily of a standardized extract. Don't use a higher dose than this, or you may experience diarrhea, irritability, and restlessness.

• *Yohimbe* is an African herb that improves impotence due to psychological as well as physical problems. It does, unfortunately, bring on some unpleasant side effects, such as anxiety, increased heart rate, elevated blood pressure, hallucinations, and headache. Although I usually recommend the natural herb to a commercial derivative, this is an exception to the rule. The pharmaceutical causes fewer side effects, so check with your doctor as to whether you can get a prescription.

• *Ginger* increases sperm motility and quantity.

• *Ginseng* is the most popular aphrodisiac in America, and I'm not sure why. Animal studies show that it increases their sexual activity, but it's iffy at best with humans. Still, it won't hurt you, so go ahead and try it.

• *Guarana* is the herb of choice in Brazil when it comes to treating impotence. If it works, it's probably due to the high caffeine content. You could try it by making a tea from a few teaspoons. Then again, you could drink coffee or Mountain Dew and perhaps get the same results.

Dosages may vary, depending on the duration and severity of your symptoms. Follow package directions or consult a qualified herbal practitioner.

What makes it worse?

• Research conducted at Chicago Medical School indicates that drinking *alcohol* may cause the hormonal equivalent of menopause in men.

• Boston University published a study showing that men who smoked 1 pack of cigarettes daily for 5 years were 15% more likely to develop clogging in the arteries that serve the penis. Heavy *smoking* also decreases sexual capability because it damages the blood vessels in the penis. Use of marijuana and cocaine may also result in impotence.

See Alcoholism, Atherosclerosis, Diabetes Mellitus, Hypertension, and Multiple Sclerosis.

Infections, Frequent

(see Immune System Health)

———————————— Infertility, Men ————————————

What is it?

Infertility (the inability to impregnate a woman) usually occurs in men for one of two reasons: production of too few sperm cells, or production of sperm cells that cannot "swim" vigorously or at all, a condition referred to as poor motility of sperm. Whether too few in numbers or too weak in vigor, the likelihood of fertilizing the female egg is reduced in these disorders. In couples having difficulty trying to conceive a child, male infertility is the cause about 40% of the time. To determine what kind of problem is preventing conception, you should consult a specialist in fertility. The evaluation in men usually begins with an examination of a sample of semen to check the sperm count and the vigor with which the sperm move. If, after such evaluation, your physician discovers you have a low sperm count or poor motility of sperm, are there specific nutrients that may help or worsen this problem of male infertility? Let's look.

What helps it?

• Supplementation of *vitamin B_{12}* helps both a low sperm count as well as the sluggish sperm with weak swimming motion. Recommendation: Take sublingual (under the tongue) vitamin B_{12} in a dose of 500 to 1000 *micro*grams weekly for 12 weeks to assess your response. Since these disorders are uncovered by a laboratory examination of a sperm sample—or by your spouse/partner's becoming pregnant—you may want to ask your personal physician to repeat the examination of your sperm sample to assess response.

• *Vitamin C,* in its role as an antioxidant, helps to protect sperm from oxidative damage in the relatively hostile environment of the female reproductive tract. It also helps, by a means not entirely clear, to boost sperm counts and improve their vigor. In a 1987 study, 20 of 30 healthy but infertile men studied were treated with supplementation of vitamin C for 3 months, by which time all 20 (100% of the men who took the vitamin C) had impregnated their mates. None of the 10 untreated men had done so. Recommendation: Take 2000 to 6000 mg in divided doses daily for at least 3 months to assess response.

• Low levels of *selenium* in the semen seem to contribute to male infertility, perhaps, as one theory suggests, by reducing levels of the antioxidant glutathione peroxidase, which your body cannot make without a sufficient amount of selenium. Glutathione peroxidase helps to fend off the oxidative damage from the hostile environment of the female reproductive tract through which the sperm must travel. Research has shown that a deficiency in selenium leads to a reduced sperm count, and it has been linked to male sterility. Recommendation: Take selenium aspartate in a dose of 200 to 400 *micro*grams per day.

• Deficiency of *zinc* can contribute to infertility by reducing your sperm count, decreasing the motility of the sperm, and even by reducing your production of the male hormone, testosterone. Recommendation: Take a chelated form of zinc, such as zinc aspartate or zinc picolinate, in a dose of 50 mg once or twice a day. Foods high in zinc include nuts, seeds, whole grains, and brewer's yeast. Warning: Supplementation of zinc in its ionic form can create deficiencies of other minerals, such as copper, by competing with them for absorption from the intestine. Chelation of the minerals (see discussion on pages 30–31, Section I, on chelation) prevents this competition among minerals to get into the body, allowing you to fully absorb each of them.

• Researchers have noted deficiency of *l-arginine,* one of the amino acid building blocks of protein, in some men with low sperm count and sperm motility problems. The researchers could cause men with normal sperm counts and normal sperm motility to develop sperm count and motility problems just by feeding them a diet low in l-arginine and could restore their counts and sperm motility to normal by adding the amino acid back into their diets. Recommendation: Take 4 grams of l-arginine daily for at least 3 months to assess your response.

• *Vitamin E* carries oxygen to the sex organs. It also seems to improve the quality of sperm, improving its ability to impregnate. Recommendation: Supplement with 200 IU daily, and increase gradually to 400 to 1000 IU daily. Eat foods high in vitamin E, such as whole grains, uncooked nuts, and wheat germ.

• Studies have shown that *L-carnitine,* in addition to being important for the heart muscle, also increases motility of sperm. Recommendation: Take 3000 mg of oral L-carnitine daily for 4 months and assess your response.

Herbal remedies

• *Ginger* increases sperm motility and quantity.
• For centuries, Asians have used *ginseng* for its ability to

enhance male potency. Animal research shows that it increases sexual activity.

• Arginine is an amino acid that increases sperm count. Herbs rich in this nutrient include *sunflower, fenugreek, carob, and white lupines*.

• *Oat* is said to enhance male fertility. I'd buy oatmeal; it's less expensive than oat extracts.

Dosages may vary, depending on the duration and severity of your symptoms. Follow package directions, or consult a qualified herbal practitioner.

What makes it worse?

• *Alcohol* is toxic to the male reproductive system. Chronic abuse of alcohol, or intermittent binges of high alcohol intake, can damage the system. The amount of damage wrought depends on the amount of alcohol you consume and the length of time you engage in abusing this substance. Recommendation: If you are infertile because of low sperm count or poor sperm motility, avoid alcohol. Abstinence from alcohol will improve your chances of recovering normal reproductive function. You should also refer to the listing on Alcoholism for more information on how nutrition can help you overcome dependence on this substance.

—————— Infertility, Women ——————

What is it?

A couple who has wholeheartedly attempted to conceive a pregnancy for greater than one year without results is considered infertile. About 17% of couples have difficulty conceiving a child. Although the causes of infertility in men are fairly straightforward, such is not the case in women, who can have difficulty conceiving for causes ranging from reproductive tract damage from previous pelvic infections, to ovarian cysts or tumors, to endometriosis, to hormonal imbalances. And because the causes vary so widely, the evaluation of infertility in women is often a much more extensive (and expensive) proposition. In addition to the medical remedies that may be necessary to help overcome structural or hormonal abnormalities that contribute to your infertility, what can you do nutritionally that may help? Let's take a look.

What helps it?

• Deficiency of *folic acid* can contribute to your difficulty conceiving. If you have symptoms of folic acid deficiency, ask your physician to check your blood for indications of low folic acid (large red blood cells and low folate levels in serum and in red blood cells). If this evaluation proves you to be deficient in this vitamin, supplementation with folic acid may help you conceive. Recommendation: If you are deficient, take 5 mg of folic acid 3 times daily until your blood tests return to normal, then continue to supplement 5 mg per day for 3 months to 1 year. The vitamins of the B-complex work best when all members of the group are present, so you should also take 50 mg vitamin B-complex with each dose of folic acid. Please read the discussion of this vitamin in the A-to-Z Nutrient listings, especially regarding the need to monitor your levels of vitamin B_{12} when you supplement more than $1/2$ mg of folic acid per day.

• Supplementation with *vitamin B_6* may help to increase your levels of progesterone, one of the major female reproductive hormones. Recommendation: Take 100 to 150 mg of vitamin B_6 (pyridoxine) daily for 6 months to assess your response. Some women require higher doses (sometimes as much as 800 mg per day), but doses above 200 mg per day have caused permanent nerve damage in some people when taken for prolonged periods. If you supplement above the 150 mg dose, you should only do so under the direct supervision of your personal physician. And even at lower doses, if you should develop numbness, tingling, pins-and-needles sensations, or painful sensations in your hands or arms, feet, or legs, you should immediately stop the vitamin.

• If you are low in *iron* by blood testing, that deficiency may contribute to your difficulty conceiving. Recommendation: If you are found deficient in iron, take chelated iron (iron glycinate) in a dose of 10 mg twice daily, or if you cannot find a chelated iron replacement, take a combination of 90 mg ferrous sulfate plus 500 mg vitamin C 2 to 3 times daily until you build your iron level back up to normal.

• If you have a deficiency of *vitamin B_{12}* significant enough to cause pernicious anemia, which in and of itself is a rarity in childbearing years, that usually leads to an infertility problem that you can correct by supplementing the vitamin. Recommendation: If you have pernicious anemia, take vitamin B_{12} in a dose of 500 to 1000 *micro*grams per week until your anemia responds, then continue the injection once monthly for 6 months to a year.

• *Proper body composition,* by which I mean the right amount of body fat on a normally muscled frame, is important to your ability to conceive. In medical research examining the problem of infertility in women, over half the women seeking help in trying to conceive had ceased to have menstrual periods following weight loss. Having a body weight less than 85% of the ideal weight for your height increases your risk of infertility by nearly 5 times. Having a body weight more than 120% above ideal for your height more than doubles your risk of infertility. Recommendation: Refer to the Macronutrient discussion found on page 23. Here you will find guidelines for calculating your lean body weight and instructions on how to construct a healthy diet. (If you are underweight, you should eat a number of grams of protein that will support the weight of muscle you want to build to, not the amount you currently weigh.)

• *Para-aminobenzoic acid* (PABA) stimulates the pituitary gland and restores fertility to some women. Recommendation: Take 50 mg daily.

Herbal remedies

• The following herbs are useful for treating infertility in women: *damiana, dong quai, false unicorn root, ginseng, gotu kola, licorice root, and wild yam.* Caution: Do not use ginseng or licorice if you have high blood pressure.

Dosages may vary, depending on the duration and severity of your symptoms. Follow package directions, or consult a qualified herbal practitioner. If you are taking fertility drugs, consult your physician before starting herbal remedies. Some herbal remedies cannot be taken in conjunction with conventional pharmaceuticals.

What makes it worse?

• Abuse of *alcohol* can cause your brain to release more of the hormone prolactin (the hormone that normally causes milk production during and after pregnancy), and this may interfere with your ability to conceive. Recommendation: If you are having trouble conceiving, I would suggest that you avoid alcoholic beverages entirely; however, a single glass of wine, a single "lite" beer, or a half-ounce of distilled spirits once or twice a week probably won't be enough to cause this problem.

• Explore the possibility of *heavy metal poisoning,* which may affect ovulation. Heavy metal poisoning is job hazard for some people who work daily with high concentrations of lead, aluminum, mercury, or cadmium. Also, if a person is subjected to these metals on a regular basis, say, lead in water, poisoning can result. A hair analysis can reveal intoxication.

--------------- **Inflammation** ---------------

What is it?

Inflammation results when your body responds to injury or when it mounts a localized attack against a foreign invader, such as a bacterium, fungus, or chemical. The inflammatory response causes the 4 classic signs of inflammation: redness, heat, pain, and swelling. Whether the inflammation occurs in a knee you've overused skiing, in your toe when gouty arthritis (see Gout) flares up, in your jaw with TMJ (temporomandibular joint) syndrome, or at the site of a mosquito bite on your arm, inflammation is the same. The redness and warmth occur because your body releases chemicals—when it's hurt or protecting you from invasion—that open up blood vessels to bring more blood into the affected area. Release of other body chemicals attracts immune defenders (white blood cells) into the area in such numbers that the sheer volume of them makes the area swell. This swelling stretches the tiny nerve endings in the area, contributing to the pain you feel. And the localized war that rages between your body's defenders and the invaders leaves the battlefield strewn with toxic chemicals that also contribute to the pain.

When inflammation strikes, what can nutrition offer to help alleviate your discomfort and promote healing? Let's see.

What helps it?

• *Essential fatty acids,* the raw materials from which your body produces the prostaglandin messengers (both good and bad), probably play a more important role in controlling inflammation than any other nutrients. Refer to the Yin and Yang of Human Health, pages 24–27, to learn more about these messengers. In a nutshell, however, the "good" prostaglandins help to reduce inflammation and its pain, and the "bad" ones promote it. Obviously, if when you suffer with inflammation from any cause you could encourage your body to make more of the good prostaglandins, you would feel better and heal more quickly. How can you best achieve that goal?

Recommendation: Begin with a solid macronutrient framework (see Macronutrients, Section I, page 23, and to that sound base add gamma-linoleic acid (GLA) and EPA fish oil in a ratio of approximately 1:4 (GLA:EPA). The EicoPro essential fatty acid product manufactured by Eicotec, Inc., of Marblehead, Massachusetts, contains ultrapure sources of linoleic acid and fish oils already combined in this ratio. Take 2 capsules of this product 1 to 3 times daily. If you cannot get this product, you can purchase linoleic acid in a product called evening primrose oil at most health and nutrition stores, and EPA fish oil as well. Because it is not as pure a form, the milligram dosing will be different. You can make a reasonable substitute by combining evening primrose oil capsules with fish oil capsules plus vitamin E. Take 500 mg of evening primrose oil (a source of linoleic acid in capsule form), plus 1000 mg EPA fish oil, plus 200 IU vitamin E 1 to 3 times a day. (Warning to diabetics: EPA fish oil can cause blood sugar fluctuations in some diabetics. Carefully monitor your blood sugar if you use this supplemental oil and discontinue its use if your blood sugar becomes difficult to control.)

• *Vitamin B_{12}*, by a means not entirely clear to me, helps to reduce inflammation and pain. Recommendation: Take vitamin B_{12} in the sublingual (dissolves under your tongue) form in a dose of 500 *micro*grams per day for 1 week, then the same dose 3 times the next week, twice the next, then weekly for 2 to 3 weeks. If you are going to respond, you should expect to see noticeable (not complete) relief after the first week.

• Your body's need for *vitamin C* increases under the stress of injury or infection, both of which can cause a marked inflammatory response. This extra need is not surprising when you recall that vitamin C is a potent antioxidant and that a part of the inflammatory response of your body is a horde of immune cells rushing to the area to dump their cargo of toxic (and very oxidizing) chemicals designed to kill the invader. Vitamin C helps to contain and minimize the damage of these free radical–generating toxins. For more information about oxidation, free radicals, and antioxidants, please refer to the discussion beginning on page 18 concerning them.

• *Vitamin C* has proven in animal studies to be more potent than both aspirin and phenylbutazone (Butazolidin, a prescription antiinflammatory drug) in relieving the swelling and pain of inflammation. Recommendation: Take a minimum of 500 mg of extra vitamin

C (above the amount you normally take) 4 times a day when you suffer from inflammation of any cause.

• The *bioflavonoids* enhance the action of vitamin C in preventing swelling with inflammation, and they may also help to control (reduce) the production of the "bad" group of prostaglandins your body makes (see discussion on page 395 on essential fatty acids). Recommendation: Add 250 mg bioflavonoid complex to each dose of vitamin C. You can also purchase vitamin C already containing bioflavonoids. Base your intake of these combination products on the recommended amount of vitamin C listed above.

• *Vitamin E* may also help to reduce inflammation because of its antioxidant capabilities. Recommendation: Take a minimum of 400 IU vitamin E as d-alpha-tocopherol succinate each day. Warning: Vitamin E can cause elevation of your blood pressure. Please refer to the discussion of this vitamin in the A-to-Z Nutrient listings for information on how to safely increase your dose of vitamin E.

• Your body must have adequate amounts of both *copper and zinc* to produce the body's own very potent scavenger of free radicals called superoxide dismutase (SOD). Your body's immune defenders dumping their chemical toxins into the area under attack produces a swarm of free radicals that can further damage and inflame normal tissues around them. Superoxide dismutase helps to curb their damaging effects. Deficiencies of copper and zinc can occur when you supplement either or both of them in your diet in ionic form. The minerals compete with each other for entry into the body. Chelation of the minerals prevents this competition and assures that you will be able to absorb both of them fully. Please read about chelation on pages 30–31 for more information. Recommendation: Always take supplemental zinc and copper in chelated form. An adequate daily dose would be 20 mg zinc aspartate and 2 mg copper amino acid chelate.

• *Fresh pineapple* is one of the best remedies for swelling and inflammation because it contains bromelain, which has anti-inflammatory activity. It also breaks down fibrin, which forms around the inflamed area and blocks the blood vessels. This, in turn, leads to swelling. Recommendation: Eat half a fresh pineapple daily. It should reduce pain and swelling within 2 to 6 days.

Herbal remedies

• *Bilberry* contains flavonoids that reduce inflammation.
• *Echinacea, goldenseal, red clover, and yucca* are good for

inflammation. Caution: Do not take goldenseal internally on a daily basis for more than 1 week. Do not use it during pregnancy, and use it with caution if you are allergic to ragweed.

• Combine *fenugreek, flaxseed, and slippery elm* to make a poultice, and apply directly to the affected area.

Dosages may vary, depending on the duration and severity of your symptoms. Follow package directions, or consult a qualified herbal practitioner.

What makes it worse?

• *Red meat and egg yolk* both contain fairly high amounts of arachidonic acid, the forerunner that your body alters to produce the "bad" group of prostaglandin messengers. Please refer to the Yin and Yang of Human Health on pages 24–27, for more information about prostaglandin messengers and their influence on inflammation. Recommendation: During times when inflammation of joints, tendons, or bursae trouble you, reduce your consumption of these two foods to help reduce the number of "bad" prostaglandins you can produce.

-------------------- **Influenza** --------------------

What is it?

Old-fashioned "flu" occurs from infection with one of a particular group of influenza viruses, called in the broadest sense types A, B, and C. In its mildest form (usually type C), influenza resembles nothing more than a cold, but when you come down with a case of type A or B influenza virus, you know it. These viruses cause you to suffer an abrupt onset of high fever, shaking chills, muscle aches, cough, watery nose and eyes, and a feeling that you just can't get out of bed. Abrupt onset can mean over the course of a day or in the space of a few minutes. Flu victims can often pinpoint the onset of their symptoms with incredible precision: I was sitting at the stop light when I came down with this.

Flu viruses strike more commonly in cold weather ("flu season") when temperatures drive us indoors into close quarters. Because you can predict that flu will sweep through, you can take precautions ahead of time—get your annual flu shot—to help reduce your likelihood of becoming infected. If you do become infected, what does nutrition have to offer? Again, the virus's assault and therefore, the burden of healing you, falls on your immune system. Doing everything you can to nourish your immune system will help you recover more quickly.

What helps it?
• See listings for Immune System Health.
• Prevent dehydration by consuming plenty of *fluids*. Concentrate on fresh fruit juices, herbal teas, and quality water.

Herbal remedies
• See listings for Immune System Health.

What makes it worse?
• See listings for Immune System Health.
• *Aspirin* only irritates a sore throat. Do not chew aspirin gum or use aspirin gargles. Warning: It is especially dangerous to give aspirin to a child. The combination of aspirin and a viral illness has been linked to the development of Reye's syndrome, a potentially dangerous complication.

—————— Inner Ear Dysfunction ——————
(Labyrinthitis, Ménière's Syndrome)

What is it?
The "ear" really consists of three major parts: an outer visible ear and canal, a middle ear space, and a portion deeply embedded in the bone of the skull called the inner ear. When your doctor looks into your ear with a light, he or she is looking down the canal leading to the eardrum. The middle ear space lies on the other side of the eardrum and houses the bones of hearing (see Hearing Loss); it is this space that fills with infected fluid when children (or adults, for that matter) develop an ear infection. Another thin membrane over a "window" in the bone separates this middle ear space from the inner ear deeper in the skull. Your physician cannot see the inner ear when looking into your ear.

The inner ear serves two basic functions: hearing and balance. I have discussed the hearing portion of the inner ear under Hearing Loss in this section; therefore, in this space, we will examine only the balance center of the inner ear.

The balance center—or labyrinth—consists of three hollow half-circle canals oriented clover-leaf fashion in three directions. Tiny hair-like nerve endings line the canals, each of which contains a precise amount of fluid (called endolymph) and a tiny pebble. When you move, the pebble in each of the three canals on each side of your head rolls over the hair-like nerve fibers, stimulating them. This stimulation causes the signals to travel to the brain, which averages all the signals from the six canals and translates them into a proper sense of what's happening. In effect, the brain reads the signals and tells you, "Okay, now you're standing up, now you're moving right, now you're bending down," so that your body can balance. As long as this simple system functions normally, all is literally "right" with the world. But what happens if a viral infection or something else causes too much fluid to build up in one or more of the canals, or pressure from infection in the middle ear space presses inward on the membrane of the inner ear? The pebble can't roll at the set speed and it sends haywire signals. The poor brain doesn't know what to believe: The signals from this canal say I'm moving to the right, but the ones from that one say I'm lying down, and the ones from this other one tell me I'm bending over. The brain can't integrate these different signals, and so it doesn't. The upshot is your balance goes out the window, and you feel like you're spinning around or that the world is spinning around. You become "seasick" on dry land.

What helps it?

• *Proper diet* to correct disorders of blood lipids—high cholesterol with too much of the low-density or "bad" cholesterol (LDL) and high triglycerides. Many people with progressive hearing loss, ringing of their ears, and dizziness (Ménière's syndrome) also suffer from overweight, borderline diabetes or sugar intolerance, high cholesterol and triglycerides, heart disease, fluid retention, and hardening of the arteries. All are classic symptoms of insulin excess. Constructing a basic diet that helps to control the root cause of these other problems often helps the ear symptoms, dizziness, and muffled hearing. Recommendation: If you suffer from these related problems, or if they run strongly in your family, you may find your ear symptoms improve on a diet that helps keep control of insulin release. Refer to Macronutrients in Section I, page 23, to begin to construct a diet for yourself that will help to normalize your blood cholestrol and triglycerides, blood sugar, and fluid retention by controlling your production of insulin. Recommendation: After reviewing the information in the discussion, you can begin to plan a basic diet that provides a minimum of ½ gram of lean protein for each pound of your lean body mass. Your protein requirement makes up 50% of your day's calories. To that base, add nonstarchy or at least less-starchy carbohydrates (crunchy vegetables, rice, oats, fresh fruit) to equal 20% of your day's calories. The remaining 30% comes from fats and oils (20% polyunsaturated oils and 10% animal fats). You will not remain on this diet long, usually no longer than 2 to 4 weeks, but restricting the food substances (starches and sugars) that promote insulin release will allow the levels of insulin to fall. Once that occurs, the consequences of elevated insulin will begin to disappear, and you will see a gradual improvement of blood cholesterol and triglycerides, you will shed fluid, you will begin to shed fat, and you will stop retaining fluid. At that point, you may slowly increase the amount of carbohydrate in your diet and decrease the amount of protein until you return to percentages closer to those specified in the discussion in Section I. Balance your intake with 35% lean protein, 35% low-starch carbohydrate fruits and vegetables, and 30% fats.

• If you suffer from Ménière's syndrome, try a hypoglycemic diet for 2 weeks. Experts believe this disorder is the result of a metabolic problem caused by a disturbed carbohydrate metabolism like that associated with hypoglycemia. If your condition improves, stay on the diet.

• Deficiency of *vitamin D,* which contributes to also developing a deficiency of *calcium,* may be important in the hearing loss that occurs in Ménière's syndrome, otosclerosis, and some kinds of nerve deafness. Recommendation: Refer to Vitamin D in the A-to-Z Nutrient listings, and acquaint yourself with the signs of vitamin D deficiency and toxicity. The first method of increasing your vitamin D is a simple one: Expose your skin to natural sunlight for at least a half-hour per day by getting outside in light clothing with arms and legs uncovered. Walk in the park, sit and read in the sun, or engage in a sport if you like. If you live in an area with little sunshine, or if for some other reason you cannot get outdoors to take some sun, you may want to purchase a Vita-Lite full-spectrum sunlight bulb (available from Duro-Test Company, New Bergen, N. J.). The cost, although expensive for a lightbulb, is really minimal. Failing that, you can take 400 to 800 IU vitamin D (such as that found in cod liver oil capsules) each day plus calcium. Your calcium dose of roughly 1000 mg should also include magnesium in a dose of 500 mg per day. You can purchase combinations of these two minerals at most health and nutrition stores. Take this form without the supplemental vitamin D if you get plenty of sunshine.

• *Chromium picolinate* helps control blood sugar levels, which are often high in those with inner ear disorders. Recommendation: Supplement with 200 *micro*grams daily.

• *Magnesium* deficiency itself can cause damage to the inner ear structures, causing ringing of your ears, loss of hearing, and dizziness. The connection between magnesium and hearing loss has received a fair amount of attention from medical research. For example, research has shown that magnesium deficiency makes laboratory animals more susceptible to hearing loss from exposure to loud noises. And another theory suggests that the damage to hearing certain antibiotic medications cause (the aminoglycosides, such as Gentamicin or Neomycin) may occur because they deplete magnesium in the hair-like nerve fibers in the cochlea. What do these studies mean to people? I'm not certain medical science has clearly answered that yet. Recommendation: Because supplementing magnesium has so little risk of toxicity, if you live or work in noisy environment, I would certainly recommend you consider taking a calcium/magnesium supplement daily (as specified on page 401 for calcium) along with wearing proper ear protection. If you suffer from Ménière's syndrome, supplementing with these minerals is certainly worth a try.

• A *manganese* deficiency may actually be the cause of Ménière's syndrome. Recommendation: Take 5 mg daily, separate from calcium.

• *Zinc* levels decline with aging, and some research suggests that the low levels may contribute to the dizziness, continuous ringing in the ears, and progressive loss of hearing that older people suffer. Although I have not seen any research to back up the theory, it makes logical sense that this connection may also be true for that other disorder in which younger people suffer dizziness, ringing of the ears, and hearing loss—Ménière's syndrome. Recommendation: Take chelated zinc (aspartate or picolinate) in a dose of 20 to 40 mg per day for 3 to 6 months to assess your response. Warning: Supplementation of zinc in ionic form (zinc sulfate) can create deficiencies in other minerals, such as copper, by competing against them for absorption in the intestinal tract. Chelation of the zinc prevents this from happening. See discussion on pages 30–31 in Section I on chelation for more information.

Herbal remedies

• *Butcher's broom* combats fluid retention and improves circulation.

• *Ginkgo* increases circulation to the brain when taken in tablet or extract form.

Dosage may vary, depending on the duration and severity of your symptoms. Consult a qualified herbal practitioner. Alert your physician to your decision to use herbs. Some herbal remedies cannot be used in combination with conventional pharmaceuticals.

What makes it worse?

• *Sugar* can cause inner ear problems (bringing on bouts of dizziness, ringing, and decreased hearing) in people with Ménière's syndrome. It may also do so in other people prone to low blood sugar (hypoglycemia). Recommendation: Eliminate or sharply curtail your intake of concentrated sugars, sugary foods and snacks, and the starchy vegetables known to quickly increase blood sugar (potatoes, wheat, corn, and foods made with these starches). See the listing on page 400 concerning constructing a proper diet.

• *Food sensitivities* may be the culprit behind hearing loss, ringing, and dizziness in some people with Ménière's syndrome. If you suffer from these symptoms and have tried drugs to combat the spinning dizziness without much success, food allergy or sensitivity is one avenue to explore. Recommendation: Consult an allergy specialist to help direct your investigation into possible food sensitivities and allergies. Using blood testing and skin testing, an allergist can narrow down the list of possible food culprits, each of which has to be checked by a systematic elimination trial. See Allergies for more details of how to conduct such an elimination trial. If you have no access to an allergy specialist, you can use the commonsense approach. Divide foods into groups: milk products, citrus, beef, seafood, fruits, chocolate, and so on. Begin your search by eliminating whole groups of foods for 3 weeks; for example, all dairy products. If your symptoms disappear, you will at least be suspicious that something in that group cause them, but not precisely what. Then reinstitute individual dairy foods one at a time to see if symptoms recur. If they do, you'll have found a culprit. Doing this kind of systematic search certainly takes time and effort, but if it improves a daily misery, then it's worth the trouble. Good luck with your search.

Insomnia

What is it?

Insomnia occurs when you have difficulty falling asleep, difficulty staying asleep, wake often during the night, wake very early in the morning, or any combination of these problems. It's a common disorder; an estimated 15 to 17 percent of the population suffers from insomnia at any given time. The causes can be many, and if you have a prolonged problem with sleeping, you should think about an evaluation by a sleep disorders specialist. Many hospitals nowadays run clinical centers devoted to determining the cause of sleeplessness because of its great impact on productivity and driver safety. But if you are troubled by a short period of sleepless nights—for example, while you are under stress—what can you do nutritionally to help to improve your chances of a good night's sleep? The "don'ts" outnumber the "dos" in this instance, but let's take a look.

What helps it?

• *Proper diet composition* will, over time—no instant cure here—lead you toward your ideal body weight and fat percentage and will help you to sleep. Markedly overweight people may sleep fitfully because they suffer periods of apnea (no breathing) during sleep. When they've gone too long without adequate breathing (as long as 2 minutes), their brain wakes them to a lighter level of sleep, they snore and sputter, and they get a good breath and try to sleep again. People suffering from apnea may awaken to some degree as many as 200 times throughout the night. They may never wake totally, but flop and snore and generally don't rest well all night long, wake tired, and want to fall asleep during the day. Weight loss will improve their sleep very quickly. Recommendation: Refer to Macronutrients on page 23 to discover how to compose a proper diet to begin the process of losing weight, if you are overweight, as well as maintaining proper weight if you are not. See also Obesity and the recommendations there.

• A bedtime *carbohydrate* snack helps to increase your brain's supply of serotonin, a brain chemical that makes you sleepy. Recommendation: At bedtime, you may want to drink a 6-ounce mug of warm milk sweetened with sugar substitute or a teaspoon of honey, or a slice or two of "lite" bread toasted, lightly buttered, and sprinkled with cinnamon and a sugar substitute, and a cup of decaffeinated tea sweetened with a teaspoon of honey. The idea is a *small,* warm snack that contains 10 to 15 grams of carbohydrate, but not sugar, corn syrup, or molasses. Heavy intake of food just prior to bedtime will often make your insomnia worse.

• *Inositol* enhances REM sleep. Recommendation: Take 100 mg daily, at bedtime.

• *Tryptophan* promotes sleep and can be found in turkey, bananas, figs, dates, yogurt, milk, tuna, and whole grain crackers. Eat something from this menu some time during the evening.

• *Melatonin* is a natural hormone that promotes sound sleep. Recommendation: Start with 1.5 mg daily, taken 2 hours or less before bedtime. If this doesn't help, gradually increase the dosage until you reach an effective level. You can take as much as 5 mg daily.

• *Regular exercise* improves sleep quality if it is not undertaken too close to bedtime.

Herbal remedies

• *Valerian* taken shortly before bedtime does wonders to calm nerves and promote sleepiness. It does not taste good, no matter what form you use, though capsule and tincture are the least offensive.

• *Lavender* is promoted as a sleep inducer by Commission E. British hospitals use lavender oil to help patients sleep at night. Unlike some oils, lavender goes directly to the cell membranes, which makes its effect last longer. It can also reduce irritability. It is important to remember that not all lavender is tranquilizing. Some actually stimulate. I suggest buying from an aromatherapist and stress that you want a tranquilizing effect. Don't ingest any essential oils.

• *Chamomile* has a sedative effect. Drink a cup of chamomile tea shortly before bedtime.

• Although we think of *catnip* as the herb that drives felines crazy, it actually has the reverse effect on many people. This herb works in ways similar to valerian, and it tastes much better. Make a cup of tea using catnip and drink it within an hour before bedtime.

Dosages may vary, depending on the duration and severity of your symptoms. Follow package directions, or consult a qualified herbal practitioner.

What makes it worse?

• *Caffeine,* because it is a stimulant, causes a decrease in total time your brain keeps you asleep. Some people tolerate larger amounts of caffeine even late at night (some true caffeine junkies, which unfortunately describes me, can drink coffee or tea just before bedtime without worry), and others will stare wide-eyed at the walls if they have a cup of real coffee after noon. Recommendation: If you have trouble sleeping, decaffeinate yourself. I have provided a regimen of slow decaffeination under Breast Disease, Benign, which you can follow to kick your coffee habit without the misery of caffeine withdrawal.

• *Alcohol* disrupts your normal sleep cycle, preventing dream sleep in the early part of the night and increasing it later, causing vivid dreams and frequent awakening. Recommendation: Contrary to the old wives' remedy of a "hot toddy" for sleep, you should avoid alcohol if you are experiencing insomnia.

• Research psychologist Dr. James Penland believes that many women suffer from *copper and iron* deficiencies, and that these deficiencies cause insomnia. If you suspect you may be one of these women, have a hair analysis done.

• *Tyramine* increases the release of norepinephrine, which stimulates the brain. Avoid foods that contain tyramine: bacon, cheese, chocolate, eggplant, ham, potatoes, sauerkraut, sugar, sausage, spinach, tomatoes, and wine. If you must eat them, do so in the morning or early afternoon.

Irritable Bowel Syndrome

(see Colon, Spastic)

Kidney Stone

What is it?

Kidney stones develop when minerals in the urine form crystallized deposits that gradually increase in size. The stones may be tiny bits of smooth gravel that can pass down the urine tubes and out in the urine without medical intervention (but usually with excruciating pain) or grow to jagged, rock-like mineral clumps an inch or more in size that cannot possibly pass down the urine tubes. These bigger stones once had to be removed by a major surgery, but no more. A new technique—using a machine called the lithotripter—allows us to shoot sound waves at the stones, breaking them into tiny bits that can flush down the ureter (the tube leading from your kidney to your bladder).

Apart from these advances in medical technology that make treating a kidney stone a little less barbaric, nutrition can offer some benefit in preventing their formation in the first place. Prevention is key, as there is a 20 to 50% risk of recurrence once a person has formed a stone. That risk gets even higher after the second recurrence.

What helps it?

• Keeping your intake of water and *fluid* high helps to continually flush your kidneys. Recommendation: Drink 2 to 2.5 liters of fluid per day (1 liter is about a quart, so this means a little more than $1/2$ gallon of fluid as a daily minimum). Your fluid intake doesn't have to come as eight 8-ounce glasses of water, but neither should all 64 ounces be regular soft drinks, beer, or coffee.

• *Dietary fiber* reduces your ability to absorb calcium, and because this mineral is responsible for 80% of kidney stones, reducing the amount of it helps to reduce stone formation. Recommendation: Aim for an intake of dietary fiber in the range of 40 to 50 grams per day. Please refer to the discussion of fiber under Colon, Spastic, for a guideline of how to slowly increase from your current intake of fiber to this higher level without suffering from the abdominal bloating, cramping, and gas that will occur if you try to accomplish the increase overnight. You should also increase your intake of high-fiber foods rich in phytic acid, such as whole grain wheat, corn, rye, barley, and beans, because these foods help to bind up the excess calcium in your diet and prevent your absorbing too much.

• Deficiency of *vitamin B_6*, necessary for your body to break down oxalic acid (another major component of most kidney stones), promotes the formation of mineral deposits in the kidney. Recommendation: Take 50 to 100 mg of vitamin B_6 (pyridoxine) daily. Do not increase your intake above this level, because doses of 200 mg per day over several years have caused permanent nerve damage.

• In laboratory animals, researchers can produce kidney stones simply by making the animals deficient in *magnesium*. People who tend to form kidney stones may have low levels of magnesium, and this may contribute to their forming the commonest kind of kidney stone—one made from calcium oxalate. Recommendation: Take magnesium glycinate or aspartate in a dose of 250 mg twice a day for 18 to 24 months. Then reduce your intake to 100 mg per day.

• One of the consequences of low *potassium* is that it causes your urine to be more alkaline (less acid), a condition that favors the development of kidney stones. Supplementing potassium or eating foods rich in potassium helps to minimize the high levels of calcium in the urine caused by eating a high meat/animal protein diet. Recommendation: Take 99 mg potassium citrate per day; eat more foods rich in potassium, such as broccoli, tomatoes, oranges, and bananas; and sprinkle $1/4$ to $1/2$ teaspoon of the potassium-containing salt substitute NO SALT into foods when cooking to add more potassium.

• People who live in communities where the tap water is "soft" have kidney stones more commonly than in communities with *hard water.* The hardness of water relates to its mineral content—the higher the mineral content, the harder the water. Many communities or individual homes "soften" their hard water for various reasons. Recommendation: If you live in a community where the water is soft, drink bottled mineral water.

• *Vitamin A* promotes healing of the urinary tract lining, which is often damaged by stones. Recommendation: Take 25,000 IU daily. If you are pregnant, use a natural carotenoid complex such as Betatene in place of vitamin A.

• *Zinc* inhibits crystallization, which can lead to stone formation. Recommendation: Take 50 to 80 mg of zinc gluconate daily. Do not exceed this amount, as it tends to depress immunity.

Herbal remedies

• The juice of the *aloe vera* plant is useful in preventing stone formation. It can also reduce the size of stones during an attack. Drink $1/2$ cup of aloe juice 3 times daily.

• *Ginkgo and goldenseal* are potent antioxidants that aid circulation to the kidneys and have anti-inflammatory properties. Use in extract form.

• Mix 3 to 4 drops of *lobelia* tincture and 15 drops of *wild yam* tincture in a glass of warm water to relieve pain and hasten the passing of stones. Sip this mixture throughout the day.

• *Uva ursi* relieves pain and bloating.

Dosages may vary, depending on the duration and severity of your symptoms. Follow package directions, or consult a qualified herbal practitioner.

What makes it worse?

• A diet that contains a high amount of *animal protein* (meat, chicken, or fish) promotes the loss of calcium through the kidney, which means an increased amount of calcium in the urine, which could favor the development of calcium-containing kidney stones. The effect is partially offset by making sure your diet contains plenty of potassium and vitamin B_6. Your body requires complete protein every day in an amount equal to $1/2$ gram of protein for every pound of your lean tissue weight (see Macronutrients, page 23). If you have a tendency to develop kidney stones, you should be certain to meet this minimum, but you should exercise restraint in not going over that amount. No one food from the plant kingdom contains all the essential amino acids, although soy protein comes close. If you choose to adopt a vegetarian lifestyle—and if you are troubled with recurrent kidney stones, you may wish to—you should become well versed in how to match vegetable proteins to ensure you have all the essential amino acids daily.

• A high *sodium* (salt) intake can cause your kidneys to lose calcium. Higher levels of calcium in your urine can promote the formation of calcium-containing kidney stones. Recommendation: If you suffer from recurrent kidney stones, do not add extra salt to your foods and avoid heavy consumption of salty foods such as chips, pretzels, salt-cured meat and fish, pickles, and sauerkraut.

• Foods rich in the chemical *oxalate* can result in higher levels of oxalate in your urine. This chemical combines with calcium to form solid deposits—stones. Recommendation: Limit your intake of beans, cocoa, instant coffee, parsley, rhubarb, spinach, tea, beet tops, carrots, celery, chocolate, cucumber, grapefruit, kale, peanuts, pepper, and sweet potatoes, all rich in oxalate.

• A diet high in *sugar* (table sugar, corn syrup, high-fructose corn syrup, or molasses) may also cause you to have higher levels of calcium in your urine, which can foster the development of calcium-containing kidney stones in people prone to forming them. Sugar intake also promotes higher levels of oxalate and uric acid (a component of yet another type of stone). Recommendation: If you have had a kidney stone, you should eliminate or sharply reduce your intake of the sugars listed above and all products made with them.

• Researchers have noted that people who develop kidney stones drink on average twice as much *alcohol,* especially beer, as those who do not develop stones. Recommendation: Restrict your consumption of alcohol to no greater than a single "lite" beer, glass of wine, or ounce of distilled liquor once or twice a week if you have recurrent kidney stones.

• *Caffeine* increases your loss of calcium in urine, increasing your chances of developing a calcium-containing kidney stone. This effect seems to be most prominent in women taking estrogen, but it occurs in men and women not on estrogen replacement as well.

• Because the breakdown of *vitamin C* by your body produces oxalic acid or oxalate, in theory, at least, high levels of vitamin C could promote formation of calcium oxalate kidney stones. In reality, however, the evidence that this actually happens is quite sketchy, and research has shown that urine levels of oxalate don't increase significantly until supplementation exceeds 6 grams per day, and even then it probably poses a risk only to those people with a tendency to form stones. Recommendation: To err on the safe side, if you have a history of a previous calcium oxalate kidney stone or have recurrent kidney stones, you should restrict your intake of supplemental vitamin C to 500 to 1000 mg 4 times a day (or 2 to 4 grams per day). If you must take higher doses for a specific condition, you can offset the increased levels of urine oxalate by taking vitamin B_6 in a dose of 25 mg 4 times per day along with the vitamin C.

Labyrinthitis
(see Inner Ear Dysfunction)

"Liver" Spots
(see Age Spots)

Low Blood Sugar
(see Hypoglycemia)

Lung Cancer

What is it?

Approximately 180,000 new cases of lung cancer arise yearly making this disease the leading cause of cancer death in the Unite States. Ironically, it is also the most preventable form of cancer. Ye lung cancer is responsible for 32% of cancer deaths in men and 25%

in women. The ratio of men to women suffering from lung cancer is 10 to 7.

Lung cancers develop, as do all cancers, when the normal cells of an organ (in this case, the lung) become damaged, go haywire, lose their normal characteristics, and cease responding to the body's controls. These rogue cells begin to divide and grow and infiltrate the normal tissue from which they came, choking it out. The cancerous cells can enter the bloodstream, travel to distant areas of the body, and take root there as well, forming what we call metastases.

There are approximately 20 different kinds of lung tumors, but fully one-third of them are of two types—squamous cell carcinoma and adenocarcinoma—with about another one-quarter of the small cell (or oat cell) carcinoma type. The names generally indicate what kind of lung cell went haywire—for example, squamous cell carcinoma means a cancer that arose from the cells that line the bronchial tubes (the squamous epithelial cells). Adenocarcinoma refers to a cancer that developed from mucus-producing cells, and so on.

Although other factors, such as asbestos, radiation, heavy metals, air pollution, and severe lung scarring from infection can be contributors to cell damage and the development of cancers, *the biggest and most important cause of lung cancer is cigarette smoking*. My mother died from lung cancer at the ripe old age of 55. She began smoking at about age 5 behind the garage, and she stopped smoking the day she died. I watched her try to rise from her intensive care unit bed to go down the hall to a smoking area the day following surgery to remove most of one lung. I implore you—if you currently smoke, stop! All the good nutrition and vitamins on earth won't matter if you continue to assault your lungs daily with tobacco smoke. Other carcinogens that are avoidable include marijuana smoke, secondhand smoke, heavy metals, asbestos, and air pollutants. But in addition to avoiding these risk factors, what does nutrition offer you? Let's take a look.

What helps it?

• In studies that examined lung cancer development in men, those men who had the highest intakes of *vitamin A* from *beta-carotene,* found in dark green and yellow vegetables, developed fewer lung cancers. Eating a diet rich in especially the dark yellow-orange vegetables seemed to be more protective than any other vitamin A–containing food group. Recommendation: Increase your intake of the yellow-orange and dark green vegetables as well as the yellow and orange fruits. Other foods that help include broccoli, cauliflower, cabbage, and Brussels sprouts. Make it your goal to eat a couple of servings of foods from these groups every day—not an apple a day, but in this case, a carrot a day! You should also take 50,000 IU (30 mg) beta-carotene per day.

• Taking supplemental *vitamin B$_{12}$* and *folic acid* may help to reverse the early changes in the cells lining the bronchial tree (called bronchial metaplasia) that precede the development of cancer. Recommendation: Take 5 grams of folic acid and 1000 *micro*grams of sublingual (under the tongue) vitamin B$_{12}$ each day.

• *Coenzyme Q$_{10}$* improves cellular oxygenation and reduces free radical damage. Recommendation: Supplement with 90 mg daily.

• *Garlic* enhances immune function. Recommendation: Take 2 300 mg capsules 3 times daily.

• *Vitamin C,* because it is a powerful antioxidant (see Oxidation and Free Radicals beginning on page 18) helps to protect your body against the damaging effect of toxic substances in tobacco smoke. If you continue to smoke—and I can't urge you strongly enough to quit—your need for vitamin C will be quite high. If you live with a smoker or work in a smoky environment, you need to supplement high levels of vitamin C in self-defense. Recommendation: People not exposed to smoke should take a minimum of 1000 mg time-release or crystalline (powdered) vitamin C 4 times every day; smokers or those exposed regularly to smoke should take double that amount if their bowel will tolerate it. Please refer to the discussion of vitamin C for more information on how to increase your daily intake to your bowel tolerance level. If you occasionally go into a smoky environment—and you can predict that you will be doing so—take an extra 2 to 4 grams of vitamin C prior to exposing yourself to this noxious substance. For more information on taking vitamin C, see Section I, page 178.

• Because *vitamin E* is also an antioxidant, it helps to minimize the damage to tissues caused by cigarette smoke and other cancer-causing forces (asbestos, radiation, etc.). Recommendation: Take 400 to 800 IU of vitamin E as d-alpha-tocopherol succinate daily. Warning Vitamin E can cause elevation of your blood pressure. Please refer to the discussion of this vitamin in the A to Z Nutrient listings for information on how to safely increase your dose of vitamin E.

• Even a mild deficiency in *zinc* can cause some depression of your immune defense system's ability to protect you against your own cells that have gone haywire. Some research has shown that people who develop certain lung cancers have lower levels of zinc, lose more zinc in their urine, and have weakened defenses. Recommendation: Take a chelated zinc supplement, such as zinc aspartate or zinc picolinate, in a dose of 50 mg 3 times daily for 6 weeks, then drop to 20 to 50 mg per day. Warning: Supplementation of zinc in ionic form (zinc sulfate) can create deficiencies in other minerals, such as copper, by competing against them for absorption in the intestinal tract. Chelation of the zinc prevents this from happening. See discussion page 30 in Section I on chelation of Minerals for more information.

• *Essential fatty acids,* taken properly, help to strengthen your immune function by making your body produce more of the "good" prostaglandins and fewer of the "bad" ones. Please refer to the Yin and Yang of Human Health on pages 24–27 for more information on this subject. Recommendation: Begin with a solid macronutrient framework (see Macronutrients, Section I, page 23), and to that sound base add gamma-linoleic acid (GLA) and EPA fish oil in a ratio of approximately 1:4 (GLA:EPA). The EicoPro essential fatty acid product manufactured by Eicotec, Inc., of Marblehead, Massachusetts, contains ultrapure sources of linoleic acid and fish oils already combined in this ratio. Take 2 capsules of this product 1 to 3 times daily. If you cannot get this product, you can purchase linoleic acid in a product called evening primrose oil at most health and nutrition stores, and EPA fish oil as well. Because it is not as pure a form, the milligram dosing will be different. You can make a reasonable substitute by combining evening primrose oil capsules with fish oil capsules plus vitamin E. Take 500 mg of evening primrose oil (a source of linoleic acid in capsule form), plus 1000 mg EPA fish oil, plus 200 IU vitamin E 1 to 3 times a day. (Warning to diabetics: EPA fish oil can cause blood sugar fluctuations in some diabetics. Carefully monitor your blood sugar if you use this supplemental oil and discontinue its use if your blood sugar becomes difficult to control.)

• A German study showed that vegetarians had twice the amount of immune cells (natural killer cells) that meat eaters did. It is important to stress that if you choose a vegetarian diet, you must be well informed about which foods provide which nutrients and then be sure to get a healthy balance.

Herbal remedies

See Breast Cancer.

What makes it worse?

• A *diet high in fat* may contribute to the development of lung cancer, although how it does so is not clear. Studies have shown that people who ate the lowest amount of dietary saturated fat had the fewest lung cancers. Recommendation: Follow the macronutrient guidelines as mentioned earlier to construct a diet that contains no more than 30% total fat, and try to keep saturated (animal) fat calories to 10% of your day's intake.

• Drinking more than a modest amount of *alcohol,* especially beer, increases your risk for lung cancer. Recommendation: Reduce your alcohol consumption to no more than a single "lite" beer, a single 4- to 6-ounce glass of wine, or a single ounce of distilled spirits once or twice a week.

Lupus Erythematosus

What is it?

Systemic lupus erythematosus (called SLE or simply lupus) affects about 1 in 2000 people, but overwhelmingly strikes women (85% of cases are women between the ages of 10 and 50) and occurs in Blacks more frequently than other races. The disorder occurs because your body's immune defenses become confused and attack your tissues as though they were foreign. I have discussed in detail how this mistaken identity occurs under Autoimmune Disorders. Please read that discussion for more information about this process.

A long list of drugs can stimulate the development of a lupus-like illness that in most (but not all) cases disappears when you stop taking the drug. The most common definite offenders are: chlorpromazine, a drug used in mental illness and to stop vomiting; hydralazine, a blood pressure drug; isoniazid, a drug used to treat tuberculosis; methyldopa, a drug used in the treatment of Parkinson's disease; and procainamide and quinidine, two heart rhythm drugs. An even longer list of possible offenders includes such commonly used drugs as sulfa antibiotics and propranolol (Inderal).

The attack on the body in lupus can affect the skin, the kidneys, the blood vessels, the eyes, the lungs, the heart, the nervous system, and the joints—virtually every "system" of the body, and hence the name systemic lupus. But although this widespread involvement can occur, the disease may be quite mild in some cases. What can you do nutritionally to help? Let's look.

What helps it?

• *Essential fatty acids* play a more significant role in alleviating the symptoms of autoimmune disorders, such as lupus, than perhaps any other nutrient. I refer you again to the eicosinoids (Section I, pages 24–27) for details about how essential fats reduce inflammation and pain. Nutritional help for your symptoms begins here. Recommendation: Begin with the proper basic dietary framework to pave the way for best results. To that sound base add 240 mg of gamma-linoleic acid to 960 mg of EPA fish oil—a ratio of 1:4 (GLA:EPA)—2 to 6 times daily. The EicoPro essential fatty acid product manufactured by Eicotec, Inc., of Marblehead, Massachusetts, contains ultrapure sources of linoleic acid and fish oils already combined in this ratio. If you cannot get that product, you can purchase linoleic acid in a product called evening primrose oil at most health and nutrition stores and EPA fish oil as well. Because it is not as pure a form, the milligram dosing will be different. You can make a reasonable substitute by combining evening primrose oil capsules with fish oil capsules plus vitamin E. Take 500 mg of evening primrose oil (a source of linoleic acid in capsule form), plus 1000 mg EPA fish oil, plus 200 IU vitamin E 1 to 3 times a day. (Warning to diabetics: EPA fish oil can cause blood sugar fluctuations in some diabetics. Carefully monitor your blood sugar if you use this supplemental oil and discontinue its use if your blood sugar becomes difficult to control.)

• The B family vitamins—*niacin, pantothenic acid,* and *vitamin B_{12}*—may help to relieve the skin rashes of lupus. Recommendation: Take 20 mg niacin (as niacinamide) and 250 mg of panthothenic acid daily, and 1000 *micro*grams of sublingual (under the tongue) vitamin B_{12} once a week for 4 to 6 weeks to assess your response. If the combination helps to reduce your rashes, continue this dose indefinitely.

• Deficiency of *vitamin A* may worsen the symptoms of lupus; however, excessive amounts of vitamin A can be harmful. This is a vitamin necessary for tissue healing, though, so it is important. Recommendation: Take the vitamin A forerunner, beta-carotene, in a dose of 25,000 to 50,000 IU (15 to 30 mg) per day. Your body converts this vitamin A relative into active vitamin A as you need it.

• *Vitamin E* in supplemental form helps to clear the rash in lupus.

Recommendation: Take 800 to 1200 IU of vitamin E as d-alpha-tocopherol succinate per day. Smaller doses may not be of benefit. Warning: Vitamin E can cause elevation of your blood pressure. Please refer to the discussion of this vitamin in the A-to-Z Nutrient listings for information on how to safely increase your dose of vitamin E. You can also use vitamin E oil (from the capsules or from a bottle) to apply to the rash topically.

• *Selenium* works with vitamin E in helping your body produce its own potent scavenger of free radicals, glutathione peroxidase. Some research suggests that people who develop lupus may be deficient in this natural substance and that their symptoms may improve from increasing it. Recommendation: Add 100 to 200 *micro*grams selenium (as selenium aspartate) per day.

• *L-cysteine and L-methionine* work together to assist in cellular protection. They are important in skin formation and white blood cell activity. Recommendation: Take 500 to 1000 mg of each daily, on an empty stomach. Take with water or juice, but not with milk.

Herbal remedies

• *Alfalfa* provides minerals necessary for healing.

• *Goldenseal* extract is good for mouth sores or inflammation. Use the alcohol-free extract, and place a few drops on a small piece of gauze before bedtime. Leave it on overnight. Caution: Do not take goldenseal internally on a daily basis for more than 1 week. Do not use if you are pregnant, and use with caution if you have a ragweed allergy.

• *Yucca* improves arthritis-type conditions.

• *Milk thistle* cleanses and protects the liver.

• Other herbs that help treat lupus include: *feverfew, echinacea, and red clover.*

Dosage may vary, depending on the duration and severity of your symptoms. Consult a qualified herbal practitioner. Alert your physician to your decision to use herbs. Some herbal remedies cannot be used in combination with conventional pharmaceuticals.

What makes it worse?

• A diet high in *saturated fat* may hasten the onset of such disorders and worsen the symptoms. Recommendation: The basic guidelines you should follow are to eat 30% of your daily calories as lean protein, 40% of your calories as low-glycemic carbohydrate, 20% of your calories as polyunsaturated fats, and limit your intake of saturated fats to 10% of your total calories per day. Please refer again to the discussion in Section I, Macronutrients, on page 23 for more complete instructions on how to compose this kind of eating program.

• *Food allergies and sensitivities* may play a role in the development of lupus or in triggering flare-ups. Uncovering the culprit in food allergies is sometimes quite tedious, because so many substances could be responsible. You may want to consult an allergy specialist to do some skin and blood testing to help narrow down your search. Once you have a list of suspected foods, you must undertake what's called an elimination trial to be sure. Take each suspect in its turn, completely eliminate it and all foods containing it from your diet for a minimum of 3 weeks. If your symptoms disappear or improve, that's great. To be certain it wasn't just a coincidence, however, you must challenge yourself by eating or drinking the suspect to see if symptoms return. If they do, you've found at least one culprit that you can say with certainty makes your disorder worse. Avoid it from then on and move on to test the next suspect on your list in like manner. You can easily see how time-consuming and tedious such a search can be, but if a food allergy is making your life miserable, it's worth the effort to find out.

Macular Degeneration

What is it?

The back of your eyeball is lined with a layer of special cells, called the retina, that function sort of like a projection screen. When light strikes them, these cells respond with a series of chemical changes that make electrical nerve signals your brain can interpret as an "image." The small portion of the retina most directly in the line of incoming light is called the macula, which contains the most sensitive (sharply seeing) part of the eye. With aging, the macula can begin to wear out, a condition we call macular degeneration. As this wearing out occurs—steadily with each decade of age past 50—sharpness of vision declines. By age 75, 30% of people have some degree of macular degeneration. This disorder is the leading cause of severe visual loss in the U.S. and Europe in people over 55 years of age. The problem occurs more commonly in Caucasians, slightly more often in women, and seems to run in the family. Cigarette smoking hastens its development.

Since this disorder is one of aging, it stands to reason that nutrients that help to combat the damaging effects of age might help. And indeed, they seem to. Let's see how.

What helps it?

• Deficiency of *vitamin A* in animals leads to degeneration of the retina and macula. In people, those who ate diets rich in vitamin A and beta-carotene developed macular degeneration less often than those who ate little. Recommendation: Eat foods rich in vitamin A and beta-carotene, and supplement your diet with 25,000 IU (15 mg) of beta-carotene per day.

• In its role as a powerful antioxidant, *vitamin C* helps to protect the retinal tissues from aging. However, one study has shown that excessive supplementation of vitamin C plus excessive exposure to high-energy light (ultraviolet light) in nearsighted people who don't correct their nearsightedness with glasses or contact lenses may accelerate the development of macular degeneration. Recommendation: Because vitamin C is so important to general health as well as eye health, the best course of action is to have your eyes checked to correct nearsightedness with glasses or contact lenses, and to always wear sunglasses that screen out 100% of damaging ultraviolet rays when you are outdoors in the sunlight. Take 500 to 1000 mg vitamin C at least 2 to 4 times daily. Refer also to the listing for this vitamin for more information on its importance to your health.

• Deficiency of the antioxidant *vitamin E* may increase your risk of developing macular degeneration. Recommendation: Take 600 to 800 IU of vitamin E as d-alpha-tocopherol succinate each day. Warning: Vitamin E can cause blood pressure elevations in some people. Please refer to the listing for this vitamin in this text and follow the guidelines given there to slowly and safely increase your dose to the recommended level.

• The concentration of *zinc* in the human retina is higher than in any other organ. Important chemical reactions in the retina require zinc, and without enough of it, these reactions cannot occur. Deficiency of zinc also impairs the ability of your retina to use vitamin A, a vitamin also important to retinal health. A study reported in the *Archives of Ophthalmology* indicated that opthalmologists at Louisiana State University Medical School tested the effects of zinc on people suffering from macular degeneration. Half the group was given a 100 mg tablet twice a day; the other half received a placebo.

After 12 to 24 months, the zinc group showed significantly less deterioration than the placebo group. Recommendation: Take a chelated zinc supplement, such as zinc aspartate or zinc picolinate, in a dose of 45 to 80 mg per day. Do not supplement at dosages higher than this without the supervision of a health professional. Warning: Supplementation of zinc in its ionic form can create deficiencies of other minerals, such as copper, by competing with them for absorption from the intestine. Chelation of the minerals (see discussion, pages 30–31, Section I) prevents this competition to get into the body, allowing you to fully absorb each of them. Because the retina also requires copper for good health, it is important that you take the zinc in chelated form.

• Your body must have *selenium* along with vitamin E to make its natural free radical scavenger, glutathione peroxidase. This potent natural scavenger helps to protect your tissues (in this case, the retina) from the effects of aging. Recommendation: Take 400 *micro*grams of selenium aspartate daily.

Herbal remedies

• *Bilberry* and its relatives (blueberry, cranberry, huckleberry, blackberry, grape, plum, and wild cherry) contain anthocyanosides, which are powerful antioxidants. Bilberry anthocyanosides strengthen capillaries in the retina, which helps slow macular degeneration. Make a tea using bilberries and any of its relatives. Drink up to 4 cups daily.

• *Ginkgo* maintains good blood flow to the retina. Some research suggests ginkgo may even reverse damage to the retina. Since ginkgo leaves contain very little of the active compounds, your best bet is to take a 50:1 preparation. This means 50 pounds of leaves were used to make 1 pound of extract. Do not take more than 240 mg daily or you may experience diarrhea, irritability, and restlessness.

• Studies show that *clove* oil prevents the breakdown of a substance in the retina that preserves vision in old age. Add a drop or two to mint teas, and enjoy up to 4 cups daily.

Dosage may vary, depending on the duration and severity of your symptoms. Consult a qualified herbal practitioner. Alert your physician to your decision to use herbs. Some herbal remedies cannot be used in combination with conventional pharmaceuticals.

What makes it worse?

• A high intake of *sugar* can promote aging of tissues by irreversibly attaching to and thereby changing body proteins. The cells of the retina are no exception to this phenomenon and may even be more susceptible to damage. Recommendation: Eliminate or sharply reduce your intake of sugar, corn syrup, high-fructose corn syrup, molasses, and all products made from these substances.

Ménière's Syndrome

(see Hearing Loss and Inner Ear Dysfunction)

Menopause

What is it?

When a woman's reproductive life comes to a close and her ovaries begin to reduce their output of female hormones, she enters a phase of life called the *climacteric*. Menstrual cycles begin to change, becoming heavier in some women, lighter in others, more frequent for some, widely spaced for others, but steadily more infrequent until they finally stop altogether. At the point that menstrual cycling ceases, you reach the *menopause*. But the waning of estrogen production may bring on more than erratic menstrual periods for some women. Emotional swings, moodiness, hot flashes, depression, weight gain, and fluid retention can all accompany the close of your reproductive years. Although many women will benefit from hormone replacement therapy, can nutrition offer some relief? Let's take a look.

What helps it?

• *Vitamin C* and the *bioflavonoids* work together to help relieve fluid retention and hot flashes that accompany menopause. Recommendation: Take 1000 mg vitamin C plus 1000 mg bioflavonoid complex 2 to 3 times daily.

• *Vitamin E* may help reduce menopausal headache, hot flashes, and fatigue by a mechanism that is not entirely clear. In fact, scientific literature does not offer hard evidence that this is true. But since low doses of vitamin E can offer other benefits, it can't hurt to try. Recommendation: Take 400 to 600 IU of vitamin E, as d-alpha-tocopherol succinate per day. Warning: Vitamin E can cause blood pressure elevation in some people. Please refer to the listing for this vitamin and follow the guidelines there for slowly and safely increasing your dose to the recommended level.

• *Lecithin* is an emulsifier for vitamin E. Recommendation: Take 1200 mg 3 times daily, before meals.

• There's much talk these days about the benefits of *phytoestrogens* (plant estrogens). These estrogen-like compounds are found in foods such as soybeans, tofu, miso, flaxseeds, dates, and pomegranates. Once digested, these substances act like estrogen. An article in the British medical journal *The Lancet* reported that Japanese women experience far fewer symptoms of menopause than do Western women, and credit was cautiously given to phytoestrogens. Recommendation: Try to include the foods mentioned above in your diet. Doing so can only improve your condition.

Herbal remedies

• *Black cohosh* contains estrogenic substances that relieve discomforts associated with menopause, especially hot flashes.

• *Alfalfa* has estrogenic activity. Make a tea from the leaves. Caution: Do not use this herb if you have lupus or a family history of lupus. Alfalfa may trigger the disorder.

• *Angelica* has been used for years as a women's tonic that relieves hot flashes and vaginal dryness and irritation. I have seen no scientific evidence to back up these claims, but would it be used for centuries if it didn't work? You decide.

• *Red clover* contains 1 to 2.5% isoflavones, which enhance estrogen levels. This herb makes a nice tea.

Dosage may vary, depending on the duration and severity of your symptoms. Consult a qualified herbal practitioner. Alert your physician to your decision to use herbs. Some herbal remedies cannot be used in combination with conventional pharmaceuticals.

Phytoestrogens and Menopause: Hope for the Hormones?

Phytoestrogens are naturally occurring compounds in specific plants, herbs, and seeds. After being converted by bacteria in the digestive system, these compounds produce estrogen-like effects. There are two major types of phytoestrogens, the isoflavones and the lignans.

Isoflavones

These are the most widely researched phytoestrogens. The only sources of isoflavones are soy, garbanzo beans, alfalfa, and clover. Of course, soy is available in many forms and products. Alfalfa is eaten as sprouts, and some sprouts are made from clover.

How do isoflavones work? Isoflavones bind with the dominant estrogen receptor in the body. Their activity is weak compared to the activity of human estrogen, and so they act more like antiestrogens by displacing human estrogen from the receptors. Because of their weak estrogen-like effects, isoflavones may reduce menopausal symptoms. More than one study has shown a 40 to 45% reduction in hot flashes over a 3-week period. There appears, however, to be a strong placebo effect involved in an overwhelming number of studies related to menopause. This suggests a mind-body connection that needs to be heeded.

We don't know for certain that isoflavones are effective for everyone. Studies have produced conflicting results, and experts suggest the possibility that isoflavones are effective in some women, but not in all.

Lignans

Almost all cereals and vegetables contain lignans. The highest concentration is found in oil seeds, especially flaxseed. Lignans act like estrogen and have antioxidant properties as well. They have been shown to influence sex hormone metabolism and biological activity and, more recently, to influence the enzymes in the body's cells, protein sythesis, growth factor action, cancer cell reproduction, and differentiation. What all this means is that these phytochemicals may well be natural cancer-protective compounds.

Choices during menopause are very personal; it all boils down to what you are interested in and willing to try. With no side effects, it's certainly worth trying out the phytoestrogens. These, taken in combination with a well-balanced diet, could very well improve your comfort, health, and sense of well-being during menopause. Always consult a physician before trying any therapy or treatment.

What makes it worse?

• Dairy products and meat promote hot flashes and contribute to a loss of calcium from the bones. Limit your intake of them. Avoid alcohol, caffeine, sugar, spicy foods, and hot soups and drinks. These substances can trigger hot flashes and make mood swings worse. They also make the blood more acidic, which causes bones to release precious calcium.

Menstrual Irregularities

(see Dysmenorrhea and Heavy Periods)

Migraine Headache

(see Headache)

Mitral Valve Prolapse

What is it?

Your heart is divided into four chambers: two small upper chambers, called the right and left atria; and two larger, more muscular, lower chambers, called the right and left ventricles. Between the atria and the ventricles are one-way valves that allow blood to flow from the atrium down into the ventricle, but not the other way. The valve dividing the left chambers is called the mitral valve. As many as 10% of the American population has a mitral valve that is either overly large or overly lax and billows out as it opens and shuts. This condition, called mitral valve prolapse, usually causes a click or a click and a murmur *whoosh* that your physician can hear with a stethoscope. You may have no symptoms from the "floppy" mitral valve, or you may have occasions of heart-fluttering sensations, skipped beats, breathlessness, and fatigue, especially with exercise. Sometimes your physician may prescribe medications to control rhythm problems, such as rapid heartbeat, but nutrition can help. Let's see how.

What helps it?

• Low levels of red blood cell *magnesium* occur in many people with mitral valve prolapse. There is a strong suggestion in the medical research that the deficiency of magnesium may be a contributing factor to the development of unpleasant symptoms in some people with floppy valves, while others remain happily symptom-free. Recommendation: Take a chelated magnesium, such as magnesium aspartate, in a dose of 250 mg twice a day for a minimum of 8 weeks to assess your response. Be certain to take the chelated form of magnesium, or to take a combined calcium and magnesium supplement to prevent competition for entry into your body by these two very similar minerals.

• *L-carnitine* has proven effective in treating the symptoms of mitral valve prolapse in some people. Recommendation: Take 1 gram of l-carnitine 3 times daily for 6 to 8 weeks to assess your response. If your symptoms improve, continue the dose for 4 months.

• In two scientific studies, *coenzyme Q_{10}* proved to relieve the symptoms of mitral valve prolapse in children without side effects. When the study participants stopped taking the nutrient before 18 months, their symptoms returned. Those children who continued to take the drug did not have a relapse. Although the researchers did the study on children, the same strategy should be valid for adults as well. Recommendation: Take coenzyme Q_{10} in a dose of 2 to 3 mg per kilogram of body weight per day. Remember that 1 kilogram equals 2.2 pounds, so divide your weight in pounds by 2.2 to calculate your weight in kilograms. Then multiply the number of kilograms by 2 or 3 mg to get your daily dose. (In this particular instance, you can simply take a dose equal to about 1 mg per pound of your body weight and it will be very close.)

Herbal remedies

• *Purslane* contains an abundance of magnesium. You can cook purslane like spinach and eat it several times daily. It's good raw in salads, too.

• Other good sources of magnesium are *poppy seeds, oats, cowpeas, and spinach.*

What makes it worse?

• *Caffeine* is a stimulant to the heart and will cause fluttering and racing in some people. If you feel that you notice more skipping and fluttering when you drink too much caffeine, you may want to decaffeinate your life. Recommendation: To kick the caffeine habit and avoid the terrible headache and sleepiness that often accompany caffeine withdrawal, follow the gradual reduction regimen I have outlined for you under Breast Disease, Benign. By taking it slow and easy, you should be able to wean yourself off caffeine without misery.

———— Mononucleosis ————

What is it?

Although mononucleosis once gained fame as the "kissing disease" of teenagers, the Epstein-Barr virus that causes the disease knows no age limits. In my general practice, I have seen the illness in young children and in adults as old as 56 years, but the average age of occurence for mononucleosis is 10 to 35 years. The Epstein-Barr virus, a member of the herpes virus family (human herpes virus type 4), spreads from one person to the next through saliva contact—hence the easy route of spread by kissing in teenagers. The symptoms typically include headache, sore throat, fever, swollen lymph nodes, fatigue that may be extreme, and, sometimes, a measles-like red rash.

Once you become infected, a fierce battle ensues between the virus and your immune system that can last for weeks or months. The energy required to wage this war leaves you drained and exhausted and in poor shape to withstand assault by other infections. In the throes of battling mononucleosis, people become vulnerable to strep throat, bronchitis, sinus infections, and urinary tract infections. Because there are as yet no specific medications that can kill the Epstein-Barr virus, the job of healing you falls completely on your beleaguered immune system, and therefore, your best medicine is to do everything you can nutritionally to support it.

What helps it?
• See Immune System Health.

Herbal remedies
• See Immune System Health.

What makes it worse?
• See Immune System Health.

—— Morning Sickness of Pregnancy ——

What is it?

During the first few months of pregnancy, your body produces elevated amounts of the reproductive hormones needed to support the developing baby and its environment. Unfortunately, during these early months, especially with your first child, these high hormone levels may also bring on bouts of dizziness, nausea, and vomiting. I need not elaborate further in describing these symptoms for any woman who has suffered through them. And indeed, many women experience nausea and vomiting between the sixth and twelfth weeks of pregnancy: about 50%! Although we usually speak of morning sickness, the waves of queasiness can strike in the morning, evening, or both, triggered by smells, motion, or a hot shower.

With safety concerns about using standard prescription medications to stop the nausea and vomiting when there's a developing baby in the picture, what does nutrition have to offer to help calm your queasiness?

What helps it?

• Deficiency of *vitamin B$_6$* (pyridoxine) may contribute to the nausea and vomiting seen in early pregnancy. Supplementing the vitamin helps to relieve the symptom. You must take care, however, to supplement the higher doses of vitamin B$_6$ only in the first 4 to 5 months when nausea is a problem, because doses of about 20 mg a day can reduce milk production and can acclimate the baby to higher levels of pyridoxine than he or she can get in a commercial formula. Recommendation: If you suffer severe nausea and vomiting, take 20 to 50 mg of vitamin B$_6$ daily no longer than through month 4 or 5 if needed in addition to your complete prenatal nutritional vitamin as prescribed by your obstetrician.

• *L-methionine* is effective in preventing nausea, and doctors use it to prevent toxemia in pregnancy. Recommendation: Take 1000 mg daily.

Herbal remedies

• Although there's no hard-core scientific evidence that it helps morning sickness, pregnant women claim that *ginger* eases their discomfort and nausea. Who can argue with experience? Drink 2 cups of ginger tea daily.

• *Peppermint* is a stomach soother, but if you're going to use it, make a moderately weak tea and consume no more than 1 cup daily. It may trigger miscarriage in large amounts.

• Tea made from *raspberry leaves* curbs the nausea of morning sickness. The leaf is reputed to contain a constituent that is readily extracted with hot water. Ingesting it relaxes the smooth muscle of the uterus. Drink up to 3 cups daily.

Dosage may vary, depending on the duration and severity of your symptoms. Follow package directions, or consult a qualified herbal practitioner.

What makes it worse?

• Each woman will have specific foods, tastes, and smells that trigger her morning sickness, but there are no nutrients that consistently cause a worsening of the problem.

———————— **Multiple Sclerosis** ————————

What is it?

Multiple sclerosis (MS), a common disorder of the nervous system, *usually* strikes young adults (but can occur later in life as well), causing episodes of weakness, numbness, tingling, unsteadiness, spastic or jerky weakness of the arms or legs, double vision, even sudden blindness, and loss of control of bowels or bladder. No one knows for certain what causes multiple sclerosis; however, there is some strong speculation that the disorder is another of the autoimmune problems in which the body turns on itself. What is certain, though, is that the insulation covering the nerves begins to deteriorate in spots—a lot like the bare wires exposed when the vinyl wrapping disintegrates on an electric extension cord. The exposed areas of the brain and nerves misfire and short-circuit, causing the symptoms, until the body finally reacts to lay down nerve scar tissue over the raw areas.

What helps it?

• All the early work (in the 1930s and 1940s) with *thiamine* (vitamin B_1) to help alleviate the symptoms of people with MS used the vitamin in shot form, into the vein or even into the spinal canal. And by this route, the improvements realized were described in the medical literature as "dramatic though transient." It makes perfect medical sense that thiamine should help, since, after all, the vitamin is absolutely essential to the proper functioning of the nervous system, and MS is a nervous system problem. But after these very promising early results, I found no further mention of researchers continuing to use this remedy, and that may be because the injectable (shot) form of this vitamin can cause some significant (even fatal) allergic problems. However, since thiamine absorbs very well when you take it by mouth, and is quite safe even in large doses this way, why risk taking it by shot? Based on the early dramatic results, it would seem reasonable to supplement this nutrient. Recommendation: Take 50 mg thiamine twice daily along with a 50 mg B-complex supplement. (The B vitamin group is quite interdependent and works best when you take all its members.)

• There has been some speculation in the medical literature that exposure to high carbon monoxide levels may increase your risk for developing MS, based on two pieces of intriguing information: the fact that there are more cases of MS in localities where carbon monoxide is high, and the more common occurrence of a similar degenerating nervous system disease in survivors of carbon monoxide poisoning. *Vitamin B_6* needs increase with exposure to carbon monoxide, leading to the theory that this vitamin may offer some protection against the development or progression of MS. Recommendation: Take 50 mg of vitamin B_6 along with a 50 mg dose of B-complex each day. Warning: Do not take amounts of vitamin B_6 exceeding 150 mg per day, because doses of 200 mg have caused permanent nerve damage in some people.

• *Vitamin C* has also proven to be of benefit in helping your body overcome the toxic effects of carbon monoxide. Recommendation: Take 3000 to 5000 mg of time-release vitamin C daily, in divided doses, for this condition.

• Sometimes deficiency of *vitamin B_{12}*, pernicious anemia, masquerades as MS, since both disorders cause similar nerve damage both in physical symptoms and in specialized X-ray testing. A trial of vitamin B_{12} by injection can't hurt in either case and will cure the nerve problems caused by a deficiency of B_{12}. Recommendation: With the assistance of your physician, take vitamin B_{12} as either cyanocobalamin or hydroxocobalamin in a dose of 1000 *micro*grams daily for 1 week, weekly for 6 weeks, then monthly for at least 6 months to assess your response. If you respond, continue to take injections on at least an every 3-month basis.

• Researchers have also speculated that people who live in areas where the soil is low in *selenium* may develop MS more frequently. Studies have also shown that many people with MS have low activity of glutathione peroxidase, the body's natural antioxidant and free radical scavenger (see oxidation and free radicals beginning on page 18). Deficiency of this mineral may lead to deficiency of the scavenger, which may leave the body vulnerable to damage by toxic substances, such as carbon monoxide. Studies have shown that a combination of vitamin C, selenium, and vitamin E work well together to raise the body's level of glutathione peroxidase as much as 5 times. Recommendation: Take a combination of 200 *micro*grams of selenium, plus 2 grams of vitamin C, plus 400 IU of vitamin E as d-alpha-tocopherol succinate for 4 weeks, then increase the dose to twice daily for 6 months to assess your response. Warning: Vitamin E can cause elevation of blood pressure in some people. Please refer to the discussion of this vitamin for information on how to slowly and safely increase your dose to the recommended level. In this combination remedy, I would recommend that you first begin the combi nation using only 100 IU, then gradually increase that component of the combination, leaving the others the same.

• The role of the "good" prostaglandins (see the Yin and Yang of Human Health, and Eicosinoids, pages 24–27, for more information) your body makes from dietary *essential fatty acids* in maintaining a healthy immune system, in relieving pain and inflammation, and in promoting healing of tissues is clear. Research also points to the fact that people with MS seem to be relatively deficient in the raw material fatty acid linoleic acid or GLA to make plenty of these "good" messengers. Recommendation: To facilitate the best response from essential fatty acids, begin with the proper macronutrient framework (see Section I, Macronutrients, page 23). The only variation from this plan that I would suggest is that you further curtail your intake of saturated fats from the 10% recommended to less than 5%. Then to that nutritionally sound base add gamma-linoleic acid (GLA) and EPA fish oil in a ratio of 1:4 (GLA:EPA) 1 to 3 times daily. The EicoPro essential fatty acid product manufactured by Eicotec, Inc., of Marblehead, Massachusetts, contains ultrapure sources of linoleic acid and fish oils already combined in the proper ratio. If you cannot get that product, you can purchase linoleic acid in a product called evening primrose oil at most health and nutrition stores, and EPA fish oil as well. Because it is not as pure a form, the milligram dosing will be different. You can make a reasonable substitute by combining evening primrose oil capsules with fish oil capsules plus vitamin E. Take 500 mg of evening primrose oil (a source of linoleic acid in capsule form), plus 1000 mg EPA fish oil, plus 200 IU vitamin E 1 to 3 times a day. (Warning to diabetics: EPA fish oil can cause blood sugar fluctuations in some diabetics. Carefully monitor your blood sugar if you use this supplemental oil and discontinue its use if your blood sugar becomes difficult to control.)

• Another research team has reported that a combination of *calcium, magnesium,* and *vitamin D* taken over a period of 1 to 2 years reduced the number of symptom relapses in people with MS by more than half. Their regimen used dolomite powder in an amount sufficient to provide calcium (7 mg per pound of body weight per day) and magnesium (4.5 mg per pound of body weight per day) plus cod liver oil to provide 5000 IU per day of vitamin D. Recommendation: Because your body can store vitamin D, I hesitate to recommend so high a dose for such a long period, unless your personal physician is willing to directly supervise your care while on this regimen. However, you can safely scale the doses down to use 1 teaspoon of dolomite 3 times daily with 1 teaspoon of cod liver oil without risk.

• *Coenzyme Q_{10}* improves circulation and tissue oxygenation while strengthening the immune system. Recommendation: Take 90 to 200 mg daily.

• *Choline* and *inositol* stimulate the central nervous system and help protect the myelin sheaths from damage. Recommendation: Supplement with 1000 mg each on a daily basis.

• *Garlic* is an excellent source of sulfur. Recommendation: 2 300 mg capsules 3 times daily.

• *L-glycine* supports the myelin sheaths. Recommendation: 500 mg twice daily, on an empty stomach.

• *Vitamin K* helps prevent nausea and vomiting. Recommendation: Increase your intake of dark leafy greens, and supplement with 200 *micro*grams of vitamin K 3 times daily.

Herbal remedies

• *Stinging nettle* contains a number of potentially beneficial substances. Take a fresh plant (covered with tiny stingers) and slap it against your exposed skin. This practice, as archaic as it sounds, provides microinjections of those substances.

• Dr. Andrew Weil, the popular herbal advocate, strongly recommends gamma-linolenic acid (GLA) to treat autoimmune disorders. *Black currant* oil contains GLA, which has anti-inflammatory action. Weil recommends taking 500 mg of black currant oil twice daily. Improvement can be expected after 8 weeks. Evening primrose oil is also a good source of GLA.

• *Purslane* is high in magnesium, a mineral helpful in treating MS. Steam purslane like spinach, or eat it raw in salads.

Dosages may vary, depending on the duration and severity of your symptoms. Consult a qualified herbal practitioner, and let your physician know you've decided to try herbs. Some herbal remedies cannot be used in combination with conventional pharmaceuticals.

What makes it worse?

• People with MS who markedly reduce their intake of *saturated fats* (those animal and vegetable fats that are solid at room temperature, such as lard, butter, shortening, coconut and other tropical oils) often experience relief of their symptoms. Please refer to the discussion of essential fatty acids on page 429, and replace the saturated fats in your diet with these polyunsaturated and monounsaturated oils: olive oil, canola oil, sunflower oil, safflower oil, or dietary linseed oil.

• High levels of *carbon monoxide* may trigger the development of MS. Although automobile exhaust emissions contain carbon monoxide, there is a source even closer to home: cigarette smoke. If you have MS, I urge you to give up smoking in the interest of your health. There is very little value to you in sucking carbon monoxide gasses into your lungs. Recommendation: Stop smoking.

Muscle Cramps

What are they?

Each of your muscles contains millions of individual muscle fibers that interconnect with each other in a particular fashion, allowing them to spread apart (as the muscle relaxes) or to tighten their ranks (as the muscle contracts). The spreading and tightening occur because of the ebb and flow of certain mineral ions into and out of the individual cells of the fibers. When something—such as a deficiency of calcium—disrupts the normal flow of mineral ions in and out of these special cells, their action can become confused and they can all suddenly tighten at once, causing a muscle spasm or a cramp.

Overuse and fatigue of the muscle can cause cramping, but so can mineral deficiencies, low sodium or potassium, severe anxiety with hyperventilation, low blood sugar, pregnancy, poisonings, low thyroid, high thyroid, diabetes, and this list keeps on going. With all these many causes, what can nutrition offer to help? Let's examine the possibilities.

What helps them?

• *Proper dietary construction* will help those cramps brought about by wild swings in blood sugar, such as would occur with diabetes Type II and hypoglycemia. Many people with chronic leg cramps have good relief of their symptoms by eating a diet sufficient in protein and free of sugar. Recommendation: Refer to Macronutrients, page 23, and from those guidelines construct a diet for yourself that provides you with at least ½ gram of complete protein for each pound of your lean body tissue (methods for calculation are given in that discussion), which should constitute approximately 30% of your day's calories. Another 40% should come from nonstarch vegetables and some whole fruits, and the final 30% from fats and oils, as described in that discussion. You should try to totally eliminate sugar, corn syrup, high-fructose corn syrup, molasses, and all products made with these substances from your diet.

• Supplementing *riboflavin* (vitamin B_2) helps to reduce the tendency for muscles to spasm. Recommendation: Take 20 mg riboflavin plus 50 mg B-complex (because the B-family likes to work together) daily.

• *Vitamin B_1* (thiamine) enhances circulation and may aid in maintaining proper muscle tone. Recommendation: Supplement 50 mg 3 times daily, with meals.

• *Vitamin B_6* (pyridoxine) has proven to be helpful in relieving the muscular cramping of carpal tunnel syndrome (see the listing for this disorder in this section). Many carpal tunnel sufferers also complain of nighttime cramping in their legs, and vitamin B_6 may offer some relief for these cramps as well. Recommendation: Take 50 mg of vitamin B_6 daily for 4 to 6 weeks to assess your response. If your symptoms improve, you should continue to take 25 to 50 mg per day thereafter. Warning: Do not take doses of this vitamin exceeding 150 mg per day, because permanent nerve injury has occurred in some people on doses of 200 mg per day over a several-year period.

• *Vitamin E* has proven effective in relieving nighttime leg and foot cramps, as well as neck and low back cramps in many people. Recommendation: Take 400 IU 2 to 3 times per day for a minimum of 6 weeks to assess your response. Once your symptoms have improved, you may reduce your dose to 400 IU at bedtime to maintain the benefits. Lower doses do not seem to help this condition. Warning: Vitamin E can cause elevation of blood pressure in some people. Please refer to the discussion of this vitamin for guidelines on how to slowly and safely increase your dose to the recommended level.

• Deficiencies of *calcium* and its nutrient partner *magnesium* can lead to muscle cramping. Imbalance of these two minerals is the most common cause of muscle cramping. Recommendation: Take 2 mg of calcium for each 1 mg of magnesium. Most adults will require 1500 mg calcium and 750 mg magnesium daily. Use chelate or citrate forms.

• *Vitamin D* is needed for calcium uptake. Recommendation: Take 400 IU daily.

• A deficiency in *potassium* can cause muscle cramping and

weakness. This deficiency could occur from taking fluid pills (diuretics), from exercising in extreme heat, from a bout of the stomach flu, or with dieting. Recommendation: Take 99 mg potassium gluconate daily.

• Low levels of *sodium,* which might occur for many of the same reasons listed above for its fellow electrolyte potassium, can also be a cause of nighttime leg cramping. Recommendation: At bedtime, drink a cup or two of bouillon, a glass of Gatorade Light, or if you prefer, you could take 1 or 2 pressed tablets of sodium chloride (the "salt tablets" used to replace lost salt in competitive athletes). Or if you don't mind the briny taste, simply mix a teaspoon of salt into a glass of water and drink it down.

Herbal remedies
• Rub *lobelia* on the affected area to relieve spasms.
• Relax your muscles at bedtime by taking *valerian root.*
• To improve circulation, take *alfalfa, elderberry, dong quai, ginkgo, horsetail,* and *saffron.*

Dosages may vary, depending on the duration and severity of your symptoms. Follow package directions, or consult a qualified herbal practitioner.

What makes them worse?
• Because increased intake of *phosphorus* can deplete your body of calcium, in theory at least, it could also contribute to the development of muscle cramping. Although a diet high in protein can cause some loss of calcium in your urine, carbonated soft drinks probably account for more of the phosphorus intake in the diet of most Americans than any other single source. Recommendation: Eliminate or sharply curb your intake of carbonated beverages. Turn instead to water, mineral water, tea without sugar, and noncarbonated sugar-free fruit-flavored drinks (Kool-Aid, Crystal Light) and leave the soft drinks alone.

Muscle Weakness
(Myopathy)

What is it?
Muscle weakness can occur with inherited disorders, such as the muscular dystrophies just described, with nerve problems, such as

multiple sclerosis (see listing) or polio, with defects in the ability of the mitochondria (little energy powerhouses inside each cell) to generate energy, or from any of a number of other medical causes. Because the reasons for weakness are so many, and some of them may be quite serious, anytime you develop consistent weakness of a muscle or a group of muscles, you should consult your personal physician for a thorough evaluation. If the cause isn't readily apparent after a full examination, nutrition may offer you some help. Let's see what the vitamin and mineral shelf has that may help you.

What helps it?

• Supplementation with *riboflavin,* vitamin B_2, has shown some benefit in relieving muscle weakness brought on by poor energy production within the cells. Recommendation: Take 50 mg of riboflavin per day, along with 50 mg of B-complex (the B vitamins work best together).

• The addition of a combination of *vitamin C* plus *vitamin K* to the diet helps some people with muscle weakness because of poor energy production within the cells. Recommendation: Take 2 grams (2000 mg) vitamin C (as crystalline powder containing 4 grams per teaspoon) plus 20 mg of vitamin K_3 (menadione) twice daily.

• Deficiency of *vitamin E* causes muscle weakness in laboratory animals, although the reason is unclear. Deficiency of the vitamin may contribute to muscle weakness from some causes in people as well. Recommendation: Take 400 to 800 IU of vitamin E as d-alpha-tocopherol succinate daily. Warning: Vitamin E can cause elevation of blood pressure in some people. Please refer to the listing for this vitamin and follow the guidelines you will find there to slowly and safely increase your dose to the recommended level.

• Deficiency of *magnesium* can cause muscle weakness that rapidly improves with supplementation. Recommendation: Take 250 mg of magnesium aspartate daily for a period of 2 to 3 weeks. Take the magnesium without calcium in this instance, although I usually recommend that you supplement them together.

• In some people, a deficiency of *carnitine* causes malfunction of the mitochondrial powerhouses inside the cells, limiting their ability to burn blood fats for energy. When this deficiency occurs, you will usually have an increase in fat storage in the muscle tissue accompanied by an elevation of triglycerides in your blood. Recommendation: Take 250 to 500 mg of l-carnitine 2 to 3 times daily with meals.

Herbal remedies

• To supplement the probable magnesium deficiency, use *purslane.* Steam the leaves and eat as you would spinach, or mix them in with a salad.

Dosages may vary, depending on the duration and severity of your symptoms. Follow package directions, or consult a qualified herbal practitioner.

What makes it worse?

• Some people who are sensitive to the wheat protein *gluten* develop muscle weakness related to the condition. Please refer to the in-depth discussion of gluten sensitivity under Celiac Sprue and follow the recommendations you will find there.

--------- **Muscular Dystrophy** ---------

What is it?

The muscular dystrophies are a group of at least seven inherited disorders that cause progressive muscle weakness and then wasting. Some forms begin in early childhood, others in middle to late adult life. Advances in genetic testing now allow physicians to diagnose at least two of these dystrophies before birth.

Although genetic defects passed from one generation to another cause these disorders, nutrition can help reduce their impact on health and relieve some of the unpleasant symptoms. Let's see how.

What helps it?

• Researchers in 1945 believed that deficiency of *vitamin E* caused muscular dystrophy, which we now recognize is not the case. However, many people with muscular dystrophy do have low blood levels of this vitamin, and supplementation with vitamin E has shown benefit in relieving their symptoms. A study conducted in Scandinavia showed a correlation between low selenium levels and the incidence of severe muscular dystrophy. Finnish researchers studied elderly patients and gave them large doses of selenium and vitamin E for 1 year. After just 2 months, there was obvious improvement in the patients' mental well-being, including less fatigue,

depression, and anxiety. Recommendation: Adults should take vitamin E as d-alpha-tocopherol succinate in a dose of 600 to 800 IU
per day. Children may take 50 to 100 IU per day. Warning: Vitamin
E can cause elevation of blood pressure in some people. Please refer
to the discussion of this vitamin for a guideline to slowly and safely
increase your daily dose to the recommended level.

• A combination of *selenium* and vitamin E has shown potential
benefit in improving the strength of people with muscular dystrophy. Recommendation: Adults should take 200 *micro*grams of selenium aspartate plus 200 IU vitamin E as d-alpha-tocopherol
succinate. Children should take 100 *micro*grams of selenium and
100 IU of vitamin E. Continue the regimen for at least 6 months to
assess your response in improved muscle strength and mobility. If
your symptoms improve, continue this regimen indefinitely.

• Supplementation with phosphatidyl choline, contained in
lecithin, may help to slow the progressive wasting of muscle fibers
in some people with muscular dystrophy. Recommendation: Take 20
grams soy lecithin per day for a minimum of 4 to 6 weeks to assess
response. If your weakness improves even slightly, you should continue to supplement this nutrient.

• The strength, endurance, and sense of well-being of some people with muscular dystrophy improves on supplementation with
coenzyme Q$_{10}$. Recommendation: Take 30 to 50 mg of coenzyme
Q$_{10}$ daily.

What makes it worse?

• To my knowledge, no hard science suggests that any specific
nutrient worsens this disorder.

─────────────── **Nail Health** ───────────────

What is it?

While I'm certain you're aware that healthy nails are strong,
smooth, and translucent in color, you may be unaware of the variety
of physical conditions that can undermine nail health. Severe illness,
chemical toxins, prescription medications, fungal infections, heart
disease, lung disease, and nutritional deficiencies may change the
shape, smoothness, growth rate, and color of your nails. Since this
book's focus is on nutrition, let's take a moment to examine what nutrients may lead to healthier nails.

What helps it?

• Deficiency of *calcium* can cause brittle nails. Recommendation: Take 1000 to 1500 mg calcium per day along with 500 to 750 mg magnesium per day (since the two should be taken together for best results). Continue this level of supplementation of 4 to 6 weeks, then reduce your daily intake to 100 mg calcium and 500 mg magnesium daily.

• Deficiency of *iron* can also cause brittle nails. You should supplement iron only if your personal physician has examined your blood and found you to be deficient, because overloading on iron can cause problems as well. Recommendation: Take a chelated form of iron if you can find it, such as iron glycinate, 10 to 20 mg per day. If you cannot find a chelated iron supplement, take 90 mg ferrous sulfate 3 times per day along with 500 mg time-release vitamin C at each dose. (Please refer to chelation, pages 30–31, for more information.)

• Deficiency of *zinc* also can cause brittle nails. Recommendation: Take a chelated zinc supplement, such as zinc aspartate or zinc picolinate, in a dose of 20 to 50 mg per day. Warning: Supplementation of zinc in its ionic form can create deficiencies of other minerals, such as copper, by competing with them for absorption from the intestine. Chelation of the minerals (see pages 30–31, Section I, on chelation) prevents this competition to get into the body, allowing you to fully absorb each of them. Because the retina also requires copper for good health, it is important that you take the zinc in chelated form.

• Deficient dietary amounts of the *essential fatty acids,* linoleic acid (GLA) and its modulating partner, fish oil (EPA), can make your nails brittle and reedy or ridged. Recommendation: To facilitate the best response from essential fatty acids, begin with the proper macronutrient framework (see Section I, Macronutrients, page 23). Then to that nutritionally sound base add gamma-linoleic acid (GLA) and EPA fish oil in a ratio of 1:4 (GLA:EPA) 1 to 3 times daily. The EicoPro essential fatty acid product manufactured by Eicotec, Inc., of Marblehead, Massachusetts, contains ultrapure sources of linoleic acid and fish oils already combined in the proper ratio. If you cannot get that product, you can purchase linoleic acid in a product called evening primrose oil at most health and nutrition stores, and EPA fish oil as well. Because it is not as pure a form, the milligram dosing will be different. You can make a reasonable substitute by combining evening primrose oil capsules with fish oil capsules plus vitamin E. Take 500 mg of evening primrose oil (a source of linoleic acid in capsule form), plus 1000 mg EPA fish oil, plus 200 IU vitamin E 1 to 3 times a day. (Warning to diabetics: EPA fish oil can cause blood sugar fluctuations in some diabetics. Carefully monitor your blood sugar if you use this supplemental oil and discontinue its use if your blood sugar becomes difficult to control.)

Herbal remedies

• Look to herbs rich in minerals and B vitamins, such as *alfalfa, black cohosh, burdock root, dandelion, yellow dock, horsetail, and oat straw.* Caution: Avoid black cohosh if you are pregnant.

• Essential fatty acids can be found in *borage seed, flaxseed, lemongrass, parsley, primrose, pumpkinseed, and sage.* Caution: Do not use sage if you suffer from seizures.

• *Silica* is an herb that supplies silicon, which is needed for strong hair, bones, and nails. Recommendation: Visit your local natural foods store and buy silica (or horsetail or oat straw, both of which contain silica). Follow the directions on the label.

• Herbs that improve circulation, thereby nourishing the nails, include *butcher's broom, chamomile, ginkgo, rosemary, sassafras, and turmeric.*

Dosages may vary, depending on the duration and severity of your symptoms. Follow package directions, or consult a qualified herbal practitioner.

What makes it worse?

• Taking too much *selenium* can cause your nails to become thin and brittle. Recommendation: If you are taking a vitamin and mineral supplement containing selenium, stop taking it for a period of at least 3 weeks, then resume with half your previous dose of selenium. If your nails improved off the supplement, but begin to become brittle after 3 or 4 weeks on even this reduced dose, further decrease your intake by half again.

• Excessive consumption of *citrus fruits, kale, and vinegar* can result in a protein and calcium imbalance that adversely affects nail health. Recommendation: Eat these foods in moderation.

————————— **Neuralgia** —————————

What is it?

When you feel pain along the course of a nerve, you suffer neuralgia. The causes of nerve pain vary from viral irritation of the nerve (as you would experience in shingles) to inflammation and irritation of nerves without discernible cause. An example of the latter category is the painful condition trigeminal neuralgia, also called *tic douloureux,* an excruciatingly painful disorder of one of the nerves that supplies sensation to your face. Although the causes of nerve pain are many, there are some similarities in the nutritional remedies that may help them. I invite you to read the discussion of Herpes Zoster (Shingles) for additional information about some of these nutrients, but let me augment that information with the following recommendations.

What helps it?

• *Thiamine* supplementation helps some people with trigeminal neuralgia. Recommendation: Take 25 to 50 mg thiamine per day, along with 50 mg B-complex.

• *Niacin* supplementation may help relieve the pain of trigeminal neuralgia in some people. Recommendation: Begin with 100 mg niacin, as niacinamide, along with 50 mg B-complex. Increase your dose of niacin to 250 mg, then finally to 500 mg per day if you do not experience flushing from the lower dose. Increase your B-complex dose to 100 mg per day with the higher doses of niacin. If after 4 to 6 weeks you have not seen any significant relief of symptoms, niacin probably will be of no benefit to you for this condition. Warning: Do not take niacin if you suffer from a liver disorder, gout, or high blood pressure.

• *Vitamin C with bioflavonoids* helps with your nerve impulse transmission. In addition, it has anti-inflammatory properties. Recommendation: Take 3000 to 6000 mg daily, in divided doses. That dynamic duo, *calcium* and *magnesium,* work together to maintain nerve impulse conduction. Recommendation: Supplement with a chelated form of calcium in a dosage of 2000 mg daily. Take 400 to 1000 mg of magnesium chloride daily.

Herbal remedies

• *Evening primrose* contains the amino acid tryptophan, which reduces pain and enhances one's pain threshold. Take the powdered form, as the oil extraction process causes much of the tryptophan to be lost.

• *Cayenne* contains capsaicin, which stimulates the release of endorphins, the body's natural painkillers. Increase the amount of cayenne and red pepper you use in your cooking.

Dosages may vary, depending on the duration and severity of your symptoms. Consult a qualified herbal practitioner, and let your physician know you've decided to try herbs. Some herbal remedies cannot be used in combination with conventional pharmaceuticals.

What makes it worse?
I know of no specific nutrients that worsen neuralgia.

─────────────── **Numbness and Tingling** ───────────────

What are they?
From time to time, we've all experienced that pins-and-needles sensation from sitting too long in one spot or from sleeping in an awkward position, or an electric shock sensation when we move the wrong way, but sometimes nutritional deficiencies can cause constant feelings or frequent episodes of numbness and tingling. Let's take a look at some possible causes.

What helps them?
• Deficiencies of *calcium* and *magnesium* can cause these sensations. Recommendation: Take a combination calcium and magnesium supplement (or separate tablets) providing 1000 mg of calcium and 500 mg of magnesium daily. If your symptoms have not responded within 2 to 4 weeks, deficiencies of these minerals probably were not the cause.

• Deficiency of *linoleic acid,* the raw material essential fatty acid from which your body makes the prostaglandin messengers (see the Yin and Yang of Human Health, pages 24–27), can cause numbness and tingling. Recommendation: Increase your intake of polyunsaturated and monounsaturated fats by using olive oil, canola oil, sunflower oil, dietary linseed oil, and safflower oil in cooking and dressings. And to further improve your response to essential fatty acids, begin with the proper macronutrient framework (see Section I, Macronutrients, page 23). To that nutritionally sound base add supplemental gamma-linoleic acid (GLA) and EPA fish oil in a ratio of 1:4 (GLA:EPA) 1 to 3 times daily. The EicoPro essential fatty acid product manufactured by Eicotec, Inc., of Marblehead, Massachusetts, contains ultrapure sources of linoleic acid and fish oils already combined in the proper ratio. If you cannot get that product, you can purchase linoleic acid in a product called evening primrose oil at most health and nutrition stores, and EPA fish oil as well. Because it is not as pure a form, the milligram dosing will be different. You can make a reasonable substitute by combining evening primrose oil capsules with fish oil capsules plus vitamin E. Take 500 mg of evening primrose oil (a source of linoleic acid in capsule form), plus 1000 mg EPA fish oil, plus 200 IU vitamin E 1 to 3 times a day. (Warning to diabetics: EPA fish oil can cause blood sugar fluctuations in some diabetics. Carefully monitor your blood sugar if you use this supplemental oil and discontinue its use if your blood sugar becomes difficult to control.)

• Deficiencies of the vitamins of the *B-complex* can cause numbness and tingling, since these vitamins all play important roles in normal nerve function. Recommendation: Take 100 mg B-complex daily. Plus, additional supplementation with the following B-group vitamins may also help:

• *Pantothenic acid* as calcium d-pantothenate 150 mg per day; 50 mg *vitamin* B_6 (pyridoxine) per day; 25 to 50 grams *thiamine* (vitamin B_1) per day; 100 mg *niacin* (vitamin B_3) per day; 2 to 5 mg *folic acid* per day; and 1000 *micro*grams *vitamin* B_{12} weekly to monthly.

Herbal remedies

• To supplement your calcium intake, use *pigweed,* the best plant source for this nutrient. Other plants that contain calcium include *stinging nettle, marjoram, red clover, thyme, basil, celery seed, dandelion, and purslane.*

• *Purslane* is also high in magnesium.

• Get your GLA from *black currant oil* or evening primrose oil.

Dosages may vary, depending on the duration and severity of your symptoms. Follow package directions, or consult a qualified herbal practitioner.

What makes them worse?

Mercury toxicity can cause numbness and tingling, and although you aren't likely to be supplementing your diet with mercury, the levels of mercury and other heavy metals have increased in some cold-water fish. Some fish oil supplements may contain unacceptable levels of mercury and other heavy metals, because their manufacturing process does not remove these toxic compounds from the oil. If you supplement with fish oil for this or other indications, I encourage you to purchase these oils from Eicotec, Inc., of Marblehead, Massachusetts. Their patented process ensures removal of heavy metals.

Obesity

What is it?

Although we often think of obesity in terms of weight, weight per se is not really a good measure to use. You can be overweight and not truly be obese, and on the other hand, you can be reasonably close to your "normal" weight and be overly fat. When we speak of obesity, we are talking about the excess storage of body fat.

Although there are a number of reasons why your body would take calories coming into it and store them away when you already have more than enough calories stored in the form of body fat, one of the most common reasons in Western society (and that includes you and me in the good old U.S.A.) centers around an inherited tendency to overproduce the hormone insulin when we eat certain kinds of food. We all produce insulin in response (primarily) to dietary starch and sugars. When we eat these things, our bodies absorb them, and our blood sugars rise, and that sends a signal to the pancreas to release insulin to bring the elevated blood sugar down by driving into our cells to be used or stored. Insulin does its work, falls back to normal, and that's the end of it until the next time we eat. At least, that's how it's supposed to happen.

Some people, however, inherit a tendency to produce too much insulin when they eat starchy or sugary foods, and although the insulin does its job in controlling the rise of blood sugar (sometimes too good a job, producing too low a blood sugar), the excess insulin doesn't fall quickly back down to normal. It's always hanging around, elevated long after the meal. The problem, in this instance, occurs because insulin does more than just regulate blood sugar. It also happens to be a very potent signal in the metabolism to store fat. When insulin levels are high, that should mean (if everything were working properly) you've just eaten a big meal and need to store some of it away for later. Let me illustrate why this should be.

Envision yourself dressed in animal skins, living 40,000 years ago on the savannahs of Ethiopia. Eating dinner doesn't mean run ning down to the local fast-food emporium, it means running down your food—on foot. When you were fortunate enough to have a big meal, having a metabolic means to store the extra calories (ones you couldn't use right away) would be a great help, since it might be a day or two or even three before you could eat a big meal again. Insulin filled a critical survival need for humankind then.

The problem, nowadays, is that it's more like three hours between meals instead of three days, and for those of us who readily produce too much insulin in response to a starchy meal, a few hours is hardly enough time for that insulin to have returned to zero. In these cases, insulin is always elevated to some degree. After a time, the sensors in the tissues that respond to the insulin and allow the blood sugar to go into the tissues become accustomed to the higher level of insulin they're always exposed to, and they quit responding to it. But your pancreas will respond to the challenge by making more insulin to meet the need and the levels of insulin climb higher. The sensors become accustomed to the higher level, the pancreas produces more, and so on, until even without food, your insulin may be 2, 3, 4, or even 8 or 10 times normal. (In some people the high insulin causes a cluster of problems, including high blood pressure, too little "good" cholesterol, and sugar intolerance, a condition called "Syndrome X.")

A high insulin level signals the fat cells to store, store, store! If all were working properly, it would only be high because lots of calories were coming in that needed to be stored. The irony is that in these cases the insulin level is high on no food at all and goes even higher when you eat. Is it any wonder, under these circumstances, that a body already overburdened with stored fat would continue to store? It's being told to by out-of-control insulin.

What can you do to reverse this process? Let's see.

What helps it?

• Obesity from insulin excess—which in my opinion is the commonest cause of obesity in the United States today—can only be controlled and never "cured." If you inherited a genetic tendency to overproduce insulin, all the weight loss in the world will not change that fact. But by taking control of the *composition of your diet,* you can make your insulin levels fall, and with that fall, the signal to store fat will fall silent. Keeping control of your insulin, through a lifetime of eating a properly constructed diet, will allow you to maintain your body fat at the correct percentage for good health. Recommendation: Begin by getting a good measure of your current body fat percentage and lean body weight. Refer to Macronutrients on page 23, where you will find several sources listed for methods to calculate lean body weight. (To estimate your fat percentage, subtract your lean body percentage from 100%.) Next, using the guidelines there, construct a diet for yourself that will contain about 45% of your day's total calories as lean protein (mostly chicken, fish, veal, and egg white), 35% nonstarchy carbohydrate (mainly from green vegetables and a *little* fruit), 20% monounsaturated fats—such as olive oil, canola oil, and 10% animal fat. Your diet should contain no sugar, corn syrup, high-fructose corn syrup, or products made with these substances, and no refined starches or meals, or products made with these. You should eat no fried foods. You should be certain to drink at least 64 ounces of water, unsweetened tea, or sugar-free fruit-flavored beverage each day. Remain on this diet until you approach your normal fat percentage.

• Because the storage and disposal of fat are nothing more than chemical reactions, each of which requires vitamin and mineral cofactors to operate efficiently, I recommend you take the recommended amounts of *vitamins and minerals* as described under Adult Supplementation along with supplemental *essential fatty acids,* gamma-linoleic acid (GLA) and fish oil (EPA), in a ratio of 1:4 (GLA:EPA) 1 to 3 times daily. The EicoPro essential fatty acid product manufactured by Eicotec, Inc., of Marblehead, Massachusetts, contains ultrapure sources of linoleic acid and fish oils already combined in the proper ratio. If you cannot get that product, you can purchase linoleic acid in a product called evening primrose oil at most health and nutrition stores, and EPA fish oil as well. Because it is not as pure a form, the milligram dosing will be different. You can make a reasonable substitute by combining evening primrose oil capsules with fish oil capsules plus vitamin E. Take 500 mg of evening primrose oil (a source of linoleic acid in capsule form), plus 1000 mg EPA fish oil, plus 200 IU vitamin E 1 to 3 times a day. (Warning to diabetics: EPA fish oil can cause blood sugar fluctuations in some diabetics. Carefully monitor your blood sugar if you use this supplemental oil and discontinue its use if your blood sugar becomes difficult to control.)

• *Lecithin* is a fat emulsifier and breaks down fat so the body can remove it. Recommendation: Take 1200 mg 3 times daily, before meals.

• *L-carnitine* breaks up fat deposits and aids in weight loss. Recommendation: Take 500 mg daily.

Herbal remedies

• *Aloe vera juice* improves digestion and cleanses the digestive tract.

• Make tea from these herbs and enjoy the diuretic benefits: *alfalfa, corn silk, dandelion, gravel root, horsetail, hydrangea, hyssop, juniper berries, parsley, thyme, white ash, and yarrow.*

• *Astragalus* increases energy and improves nutrient absorption. Caution: Do not take this herb if you have a fever.

• To improve digestion and aid in the metabolism of fat, use *butcher's broom, cardamom, cayenne, cinnamon, ginger, and green tea.* Caution: Use cinnamon sparingly if you are pregnant.

• *Fennel* is a natural appetite suppressant.

• *Fenugreek* dissolves fat within the liver.

• Suppress your appetite with *ephedra, guarana, and kola nut.* Caution: Do not use ephedra if you suffer from anxiety, glaucoma, heart disease, high blood pressure, or insomnia, or if you are taking an MAO (monoamine oxidase) inhibitor.

• The thyroid function is enhanced with *bladderwrack, borage seed, hawthorn berry, sarsaparilla, and licorice.* Caution: Excessive amounts or long-term use of licorice (over 6 weeks) can elevate blood pressure. Do not use this herb on a daily basis for more than 1 week, and avoid it completely if you have high blood pressure.

Dosage may vary, depending on the duration and severity of your symptoms. Consult a qualified herbal practitioner, and alert your physician to your decision to use herbs. Some herbal remedies cannot be used in conjunction with conventional pharmaceuticals.

What makes it worse?

• When you have a weight problem because of excess insulin—and unless you are known to have an adrenal or thyroid gland cause for your obesity, you probably do—*sugar* and all forms of *refined starches* are major culprits. They will keep your insulin elevated and keep you storing calories as body fat, make you retain fluid (see Hypertension), and keep you hungry as you try to diet.

• *Chewing gum* is not a good idea. It gets the digestive juices flowing and makes you feel hungry.

• The American Cancer Society has found that people who use *artificial sweeteners* actually gain, not lose, weight. These substances increase the appetite and slow down the digestive process.

Osteoporosis

What is it?

Thousands of fractured bones occur each year in America because of osteoporosis, or bone thinning. This most common metabolic bone disease in our country typically strikes women in their middle to later years, leading to such symptoms as severe backache, fracture of bones (especially the hip and ribs) with minimal injury, and collapse of vertebrae, the bones of the spine. Throughout our lives, our bones exist in a constant state of remodeling—laying down new bone, dissolving and removing old worn-out bone. In the middle to later years, especially as production of the reproductive hormones begins to wane, there tends to be more of the dissolving and removing than of the laying down. The bones become thinner, deficient in the minerals that keeps them strong and hard (calcium, magnesium, and phosphorus), and more susceptible to breaking. But waning levels of reproductive hormones are not the only cause of bone thinning. Steroid medications used regularly (as, for example, in rheumatoid arthritis, lupus erythematosus, or other inflammatory and autoimmune diseases) can cause bone thinning; excess thyroid hormone, whether produced naturally by your own thyroid gland or taken to excess in thyroid supplemental medications, causes it; excessive intake of vitamin D can thin your bones, too. There also seems to be an inherited tendency to develop osteoporosis with aging.

If you are a person at risk for bone thinning because of such a family history or because you fall into one of the other categories above, you will be keenly interested in what you can do to forestall bone loss. Let's see what nutrition can offer you.

What helps it?

• Deficiency in *calcium,* especially in women over age 35, may contribute to osteoporosis, although the problem seems to be more one of not absorbing it properly rather than extreme dietary deficiency. In earlier adult life, the reproductive hormones (especially in women) boost intestinal absorption of calcium to keep bones strong. With aging, calcium supplements will certainly help, but many women may also need prescription hormone replacement medications in order to absorb the calcium well. Recommendation: Take 1.5 grams (1500 mg) of calcium daily.

• Calcium works with its bone mineral partner, *magnesium,* a mineral necessary to activate the chemical reactions that form new bone. Recommendation: Take approximately 1 mg of magnesium for every 2 mg of calcium (a daily dose of 750 mg along with the recommended calcium dose of 1500 mg).

• Deficiency of *manganese,* another mineral important to normal bone formation, can weaken bone and make your bones less resistant to breaking. Recommendation: Take manganese aspartate (or other amino acid chelated manganese supplement) in a dose of 20 to 40 mg per day.

• Your body needs *folic acid* to properly build the fibrous collagen framework of bone onto which the mineral salts deposit. Without a strong framework, the bone will become weak and defective and more prone to breaking easily. Recommendation: Take 5 mg folic acid daily along with a 50 mg B-complex supplement, because the B vitamins work closely together. Warning: This dose of folic acid could mask a deficiency of B_{12}. Please read the discussion of both of these vitamins and ask your physician to regularly check your vitamin B_{12} status to detect deficiency.

• Like its B-vitamin cousin folic acid, your body needs *vitamin B_6* to properly build the fibrous framework that supports the bone minerals. Without a healthy framework, the bone is weakened. Recommendation: Take 50 mg vitamin B_6 once or twice daily along with 50 mg B-complex.

• A deficiency of *vitamin B_{12}* can prevent your body's bone-building cells from functioning properly. When these osteoblasts, as we call them, cannot do their work, but the bone-dissolving and removing cells (osteoclasts) work at a steady pace, the net result is more bone taken up than laid down and, therefore, weak, thin bones. Recommendation: Take 1000 *micro*grams daily.

• *Vitamin C with bioflavonoids* is important for collagen and connective tissue formation. Recommendation: Take 1000 mg daily.

• Your body must have plenty of *vitamin D* to effectively absorb calcium from the intestine. Recommendation: Because vitamin D is a stored vitamin, you must supplement it with great care. Begin by getting outside daily into fresh air and sunshine, where the action of sun on your skin can help your body produce vitamin D. Then to that add 400 IU to 800 IU (10 to 20 mg) of vitamin D to your diet in supplemental form. Please refer to the discussion of this vitamin to acquaint yourself with the symptoms of taking too much vitamin D. If you begin to develop any of the side effects of excess vitamin D, stop the supplementation for the moment and consult your physician.

• Deficiency of *vitamin K* may cause you to lose more calcium in your urine and consequently become somewhat deficient in calcium. With progressive calcium loss, your risk for bone (especially hip) fractures increases. Recommendation: Because intestinal bacteria usually produce sufficient vitamin K to meet our needs, it is unusual to become deficient except when prolonged or frequent courses of antibiotic medication have decimated the friendly bacteria of the colon. Because it is easy to take too much vitamin K, your best bet is to restore a normal complement of intestinal bacteria and let them do the producing of vitamin K for you. You may restore these friendly bacteria by eating cultured yogurt, drinking cultured buttermilk, or drinking sweet acidophilus milk daily. If you cannot tolerate milk products because of lactose intolerance, you can purchase acidophilus capsules at most health and nutrition stores. Take 2 or 3 of these capsules daily.

• Supplemental *boron* in your diet helps to prevent you from losing calcium and magnesium in your urine. Recommendation: Eat more foods rich in boron: nuts, beans, pears, grapes, peaches, and apples. In addition, take 3 mg boron per day for a minimum of 3 to 6 months to evaluate your response. You should be less troubled by symptoms such as backache, leg ache, and hip pain if you have responded to this remedy.

• *Zinc* enhances the action of vitamin D in helping your body absorb and use calcium to build stronger bones. Deficiency of zinc will lead to weakened bones that break easily. Because older people are often deficient in zinc, and because this is the age group most afflicted with osteoporosis and at higher risk for hip fractures, supplementation of zinc will help. Recommendation: Take a chelated form of zinc, such as zinc aspartate or zinc picolinate, in a dose of 20 to 50 mg per day. Warning: Supplementation of zinc in its ionic form can create deficiencies of other minerals, such as copper, by competing with them for absorption from the intestine. Chelation of the minerals (see discussion on pages 30–31, Section I) prevents this competition to get into the body, allowing you to fully absorb each of them.

Herbal remedies

• Boron raises estrogen levels, and estrogen preserves bones. *Dandelion* contains high levels of boron. It also contains a good deal of calcium and silicon.

• *Pigweed* contains an impressive amount of calcium, as do *marjoram, savory, red clover, purslane, and thyme.*

• Silicon has been studied for its effect on osteoporosis and has been found to prevent the disorder. *Horsetail* is one of the richest plant sources of the mineral. If you decide to use this herb, take it with a teaspoon of sugar. The sugar draws out the silicon. Make a tea and let it cool before drinking.

• *Parsley* contains a generous amount of boron. It also contains fluorine, another bone strengthener.

Dosage may vary, depending on the duration and severity of your symptoms. Consult a qualified herbal practitioner, and alert your physician to your decision to use herbs. Some herbal remedies cannot be used in conjunction with conventional pharmaceuticals.

What makes it worse?

• If your diet contains an excess of *phosphorus,* from too much animal protein or too many carbonated soft drinks, you may fail to absorb calcium from your food as well as lose more calcium from your urine. The ideal dietary ratio of calcium and phosphorus is 1:1, 1 mg of calcium for every 1 mg of phosphorus. Americans tend to eat more phosphorus than calcium, which looms large if you are at risk for bone thinning. Recommendation: Refer to Macronutrients in Section I, page 23, for dietary guidelines. Although you don't want to become deficient in protein, keep your intake to only that amount you need to provide for your lean tissues. Try to get most of your daily protein requirement from egg white and dairy sources, such as low-fat cottage cheese, yogurt, or milk, or soy products, such as tofu. Avoid carbonated soft drinks and yeast products.

• Drinking *alcohol* can also handicap your body's bone-forming cells, so that more bone is dissolved and removed than formed. The effect of alcohol is dose dependent, meaning that the more you drink, the worse the bone thinning becomes. Recommendation: Sharply restrict your alcohol intake if you are at risk for osteoporosis (see discussion of causes in "What is it?") to a level of no more than a single glass of wine, a single "lite" beer, or a single ounce of distilled liquor once or twice weekly. If you have osteoporosis, avoid alcohol on a regular basis entirely.

• *Caffeine* causes you to lose more calcium in your urine. One study* published in 1990 showed that women who drank over 2 cups of coffee per day were 53% more likely to fracture a hip; another study showed a threefold increase in hip fractures in women who drank over 4 cups per day compared to women who almost never drank coffee. (Research in this area primarily centers on women, since osteoporosis occurs much more commonly in women.) Since, for most Americans, a couple of cups of coffee per day constitutes average rather than heavy consumption, the information seems quite alarming. Other research has shown, however, that we can lessen the impact of this calcium-losing effect of coffee by making sure we get plenty of dietary calcium. Recommendation: If you are at risk for osteoporosis (as described in "What is it?" on page 446), reduce your intake of caffeine to less than 2 servings of coffee, tea, or caffeinated soft drinks per day. If you already have osteoporosis, you should totally eliminate caffeine from your diet. This includes regular coffee and tea, chocolate, and many soft drinks (although carbonated beverages will already be on your list of things to avoid, as just noted). If you currently drink more than a cup or two of coffee per day, you may experience caffeine-withdrawal headache and sleepiness as you decaffeinate your life. I have provided a schedule for decaffeinating yourself under Breast Disease, Benign, which you may follow to kick your caffeine habit without too much misery.

• A diet high in *sugar* also causes you to lose calcium in your urine, because it raises your insulin level (see Hypertension and Obesity for discussions of the harmful effects of high insulin on the human body). Recommendation: Sharply reduce or eliminate all sources of sugar from your diet: table sugar, corn syrup, high-fructose corn syrup, molasses, and all products made with these substances.

• A diet high in *fat* prevents you from absorbing calcium nor-

*D. Kiel, et al., "Caffeine and the Risk of Hip Fracture: The Framingham Study," *American Journal of Epidemiology* 132:675–84, October 1990.

mally from your intestine, because the fats bind with it, forming "soaps" in precisely the same way that frontier grannies cooked up batches of lye soap by mixing rendered fat (lard) with ashes. Your intestine cannot absorb these calcium soaps, which pass on through unchanged. Recommendation: Refer to discussion on page 23 to construct a diet for yourself that restricts fat to 30% of your day's calories.

• *Oxalic acid* is found in high amounts in foods such as almonds, asparagus, cashews, rhubarb, and spinach. Since oxalic acid inhibits calcium absorption, you would be wise to avoid or consume in moderation these foods.

——————— **Ovarian Cancer** ———————

What is it?

Thirty thousand cases of ovarian cancer are diagnosed annually, and 1 in every 65 women 85 years of age has cancer of the ovary. Preventive examinations, which discover cancer earlier, usually improve the chances for cure. Prevention is especially important for women at greatest risk: those who have had breast cancer and those who have a first-degree relative (mother, sister, or child) who has had ovarian cancer. Other causes include use of fertility drugs, delayed childbirth (past the age of 35), and having had few or no children.

Aside from early detection, what can you do nutritionally to reduce your risk of ovarian cancer? Let's see.

What helps it?

• *A nutritional regimen from the work of Dr. Linus Pauling improved survival of women with ovarian, breast, uterus, or cervical cancers from an average of 5.7 months to an average of 122 months:* 12 grams vitamin C per day; 1.5 to 3 grams niacinamide per day; 250 mg pyridoxine per day; B-complex (suggested dose 100 mg per day); 800 IU vitamin E per day; 30,000 IU beta-carotene per day; 2 to 500 *micro*grams selenium per day; plus at least the RDA for all other vitamins and minerals.

• A diet rich in fish, green vegetables, carrots, and whole grains helps to reduce your risk. The green vegetables and carrots probably boost immune function against cancer because they contain high amounts of *beta-carotene*. The fish, if they are cold-water varieties, also contain high amounts of *fish oil*, a substance that also helps control your body's production of the "good" eicosinoid messengers. Please refer to eicosinoids on pages 24–27 for more information about how these body chemicals keep you healthy. Refer also to Immune System Health in this section to learn more about how to maximize your immune defense system's ability to protect you from cancer.

• *Vitamin E* is an antioxidant that is important in the prevention of cancer. Foods high in vitamin E include vegetable oils, nuts, wheat germ, and whole grains. Recommendations: Be sure to eat more of the foods I mentioned. In addition, supplement with 1000 IU vitamin E daily. Use the emulsion form for easier assimilation and greater safety at high doses.

Herbal remedies
• See Breast Cancer.

What makes it worse?
• If you eat *fried* foods (even "healthy" foods, such as fish and green vegetables), you increase your risk of ovarian cancer. The high temperatures needed to fry foods cause alterations in the oils used to fry them. These changed oils can be cancer-causing. In a study of 16,000 Seventh-Day Adventists (a group chosen because, on the whole, they do not smoke or drink alcohol or coffee), women who ate fried eggs, fish, chicken, or potatoes increased their risk of fatal ovarian cancer. Recommendation: Try not to eat fried foods of any kind.

• A diet high in *animal fat,* from such sources as meat, eggs, and butter, may increase your risk for ovarian cancer. Again, in the Seventh-Day Adventist study mentioned above, women who ate eggs cooked in any fashion 3 or more times per week increased their risk of ovarian cancer by 3 times. One possible association among cancer, eggs, and meat may be that all these foods contain high amounts of arachidonic acid. This fatty substance is the forerunner of the "bad" group of prostaglandins (see eicosinoids, pages 24–27), which weaken your immune system. Eating large quantities of red meat and egg yolk provides your body with the raw material needed to produce large amounts of "bad" messengers. Recommendation: If you have a higher risk for developing ovarian cancer (as described on page 451), you should avoid red meat, eat only the whites of eggs, and use limited amounts of vegetable margarine in place of butter. If you carry no special risk for ovarian cancer but want to live prudently, you should limit consumption of red meat, egg yolk, and butter.

--- **Painful Periods** ---

(see Dysmenorrhea)

--- **Parkinson's Disease** ---

What is it?

Parkinson's disease affects 1.5 million Americans. This disease, of which approximately 50,000 new cases are diagnosed yearly, strikes all ethnic groups, and men approximately as often as women, usually beginning between the ages of 58 and 62. Ten percent of Parkinson's cases are found in patients less than age 40; 20% are found in patients between 40 and 50; 70% of the cases are found in patients 50 and older. This disorder of the nervous system occurs when something (and we usually don't know what) attacks a specific part of the brain responsible for producing a brain chemical called dopamine. The symptoms of dopamine deficiency gradually develop to include: slowness of motion, tremors of the hands at rest, loss of automatic motions such as swinging the arms when walking, walking with a shuffling gait of tiny steps, an expressionless face, scaly eczema of the face and scalp, and mild mental/intellectual deterioration. There are specific prescription medications that replace the lost dopamine and give some relief of symptoms. These medications should not be discontinued in favor of nutritional remedies, but along with medical therapy, some nutrients can help. Let's take a look.

What helps it?

• People with Parkinson's disease usually take a medication called L-dopa, which replaces their deficient dopamine. Taking this drug, however, can cause them to become deficient in *niacin,* a nutrient necessary for their brain to convert certain amino acid building blocks into natural L-dopa. Providing niacin in the diet can improve their symptoms by helping them to produce more of what they lack. Recommendation: Take 50 mg niacin 3 times per day. Warning: Taking supplementary niacin may alter the amount of prescription L-dopa needed. Be certain to advise your personal physician that you intend to take this vitamin before doing so, as he or she may need to reduce your medication. You may experience flushing;

this is normal. Do not take niacin if you have a liver disorder, gout, or high blood pressure.

• Deficiency of *folic acid* may contribute to the development or progression of symptoms in Parkinson's disease in some people. This theory—and it is merely a theory at this stage—suggests that some people develop nervous system degeneration of the type that leads to Parkinson's disease because they are born with an abnormality in the way their body metabolizes folic acid. The theory does not address whether supplementation of this nutrient would help to prevent the development of the disorder or alleviate symptoms. Recommendation: Because folic acid is a necessary vitamin for us all, my advice is that you endeavor not to become deficient in it, especially if Parkinson's disease runs in your family.

• Especially if taken early in the course of developing Parkinson's disease, *thiamine* may help to prevent the decline in dopamine that causes symptoms. Recommendation: Take thiamine in a daily dose of 50 to 100 mg per day along with 50 to 100 mg vitamin B-complex.

• In Parkinson's disease, the problem is not enough dopamine; we can only give the dopa form by mouth and must depend on the body's taking that medication and turning it into active dopamine. The chemical reaction that converts dopa to dopamine requires *vitamin B_6* to work effectively, and therefore, vitamin B_6 deficiency would hinder this conversion. Recommendation: Take 50 to 75 mg of vitamin B_6 3 times daily along with 50 to 100 mg of B-complex.

• *Vitamin C* may help to offset the unpleasant side effects of taking L-dopa, the medication most commonly used to treat Parkinson's disease. Although most people tolerate L-dopa well, some people who have been unable to tolerate taking their medication because of nausea or increased salivation can by taking vitamin C along with it reap the benefits of L-dopa without the misery. This vitamin is a powerful antioxidant that may slow the progression of the disease. Recommendation: Take 3000 to 6000 mg daily, in divided doses.

• *Selenium* is helpful as an antioxidant. Recommendation: Take 200 *micro*grams daily.

• People who eat foods high in *vitamin E* early in life have less likelihood of developing Parkinson's disease with aging. There is some suggestion in recent research that one of the contributing factors that damages and destroys the part of the brain responsible for producing dopamine (and thereby initiating Parkinson's disease) may be oxidative changes caused by free radicals. (Please refer to the in-depth discussions of oxidation and free radicals beginning on page 18 for more information about this process.) Because vitamin E acts as a potent antioxidant, a protector of tissues from damage by free radicals, it may help to prevent the disease. And it may also help to curb the progression of the disease once it has started. Recommendation: If you are a young person concerned about being at risk for developing Parkinson's disease (for example, because of family history, although no clearly inherited pattern is yet proposed), you may want to take vitamin E in doses of 800 IU per day as a means of protecting your tissues from oxidative damage. If you have (or know a person who has) Parkinson's disease, taking up to 3200 IU per day may help to slow the development of the disease and improve quality of life.

• Your body converts the amino acid *l-methionine* into an important brain chemical called S-adenosyl methionine, or SAMe. Taking prescription L-dopa can reduce the level of this brain chemical, and this deficiency can worsen muscle rigidity, mood, lack of strength, and poor attention span. Supplementing your diet with the raw material, l-methionine, from which SAMe is made may help to offset some of the deficiency. Recommendation: Take l-methionine in a dose of 1 gram per day for 1 week. Then, every week, increase the daily dose to 2, 3, 4, and finally 5 grams a day. Remain at this dose for 6 weeks to assess your response, which may include being in better spirits, moving more easily, sleeping better, improvement of concentration and attention span, feeling stronger, and having a stronger voice.

• *L-phenylalanine* alleviates symptoms. Recommendation: Take 100 to 500 mg daily. Warning: Do not take this supplement if you are pregnant or nursing, if you take an MAO (monoamine oxidase) inhibitor drug, or if you suffer from panic attacks, diabetes, high blood pressure, or PKU (phenylketonuria).

• Supplemental *essential fatty acids* providing increased amounts of linoleic acid seem to help reduce the resting hand tremors that trouble people with Parkinson's disease. These essential fatty acids occur in vegetable oils, but with aging and disease your body's ability to use these oils to make the "good" eicosinoid messengers from them declines. See the Yin and Yang of Human Health on pages 24–25 for more information on these "good" and "bad" messengers. Recommendation: To facilitate the best response from essential fatty

acids, begin with the proper macronutrient framework (see Section
I, Macronutrients, page 23). Then to that nutritionally sound base
add gamma-linoleic acid to EPA fish oil in a ratio of 1:4 (GLA:EPA)
1 to 3 times daily. The EicoPro essential fatty acid product manufactured by Eicotec, Inc., of Marblehead, Massachusetts, contains
ultrapure sources of linoleic acid and fish oils already combined in
the proper ratio. If you cannot get that product, you can purchase
linoleic acid in a product called evening primrose oil at most health
and nutrition stores, and EPA fish oil as well. Because it is not as
pure a form, the milligram dosing will be different. You can make a
reasonable substitute by combining evening primrose oil capsules
with fish oil capsules plus vitamin E. Take 500 mg of evening primrose oil (a source of linoleic acid in capsule form), plus 1000 mg
EPA fish oil, plus 200 IU vitamin E 1 to 3 times a day. (Warning to
diabetics: EPA fish oil can cause blood sugar fluctuations in some
diabetics. Carefully monitor your blood sugar if you use this supplemental oil and discontinue its use if your blood sugar becomes
difficult to control.)

Herbal remedies

• *Fava beans* contain L-dopa, the natural precursor of dopamine
in the brain. It is standard therapy for Parkinson's. As a pharmaceutical, it is incredibly expensive. But a can of beans costs around
$1.00. And Dr. James Duke, author of *The Green Pharmacy,* came
to the conclusion that it takes about one 16-ounce can of fava beans
to have a physiological effect on this disorder. Although it is always
important to let your physician know when you're trying natural
remedies, the point is absolutely critical in this case. Usually doctors
don't prescribe L-dopa until the disease is more advanced. Eating
fava beans at an early stage would be helpful. If you're already taking L-dopa, refrain from eating the beans until you've had a chance
to speak with your doctor. The fiber in fava beans helps prevent constipation, a common symptom of Parkinson's.

• *Evening primrose oil* reduces the tremors of Parkinson's, probably because it contains traces of tryptophan, an amino acid that
boosts the effectiveness of L-dopa. Try including ground seeds of
evening primrose in your baking.

• *Passionflower* contains two effective anti-Parkinson's compounds. I recommend taking a standardized tincture.

Dosages may vary, depending on the duration and severity of your symptoms. Consult a qualified herbal practitioner, and alert your physician to your decision to use herbs. Some herbal remedies cannot be used in conjunction with conventional pharmaceuticals.

What makes it worse?

• *Iron* can bind and render L-dopa and carbidopa (another similar drug used to treat Parkinson's disease) less effective. Recommendation: You should not take iron-containing vitamin and mineral supplements or iron supplements if you take these drugs, except at the direction of your personal physician.

• Excessive exposure to *manganese* dust (by breathing in the dust) such as might occur in an occupational or industrial setting can cause an illness resembling Parkinson's disease. There is no mention in the current literature that elaborates on whether you could develop problems from taking manganese supplements orally. Recommendation: Until more information comes to light about this nutrient, I would recommend that you not supplement the mineral over and above the amount needed to prevent deficiency (see listing for this nutrient).

• *Mercury* toxicity causes a nervous system disorder resembling Parkinson's disease, and people suffering from the disorder have been shown to have high mercury levels in their tissues. Recommendation: Mercury is not something you would ever supplement intentionally; however, because it may be helpful to supplement your diet with cold-water fish or with supplemental fish oil, be aware that these food sources can sometimes contain high levels of heavy metals, including mercury. (The Eicotec, Inc., essential fatty acid product recommended throughout this book uses fish oils cleansed of heavy metals by a patented process to ensure your safety.)

Peptic Ulcer Disease

(see also Heartburn)

What is it?

When your stomach or the first part of your intestine loses its mucous protective coating, the acid contents of your stomach can erode the lining, forming an ulcer. Typical ulcers can range in size from a millimeter or two in size (about as big as a large pinhead) to two centimeters (almost an inch). Symptoms of an ulcer include pain in the area around your stomach about an hour after you eat or pain in the stomach that wakes you in the wee hours of the morning, both of which food or antacids relieve. The symptoms may come and go.

Recent research has shown that a bacterial infection may be behind chronic ulcers that recur even following courses of medication to stop acid output (drugs such as Tagamet, Zantac, Pepcid, and Axid). Although healing your ulcer may require prescription medications, nutrition can play a crucial role. In Heartburn I have covered some of the nutrients that help this problem, but there are some differences. Let's take a look.

What helps it?

• See Heartburn.

• *Essential fatty acids* are the raw materials from which your body makes the prostaglandin messengers, both "good" and "bad." (Please refer to the Yin and Yang of Human Health, pages 24–27, for more information on these important body messengers.) The "good" group of messengers helps to protect you against ulcer disease by making your stomach and intestinal lining more resistant to damage and by speeding healing if damage does occur. Recommendation: To facilitate the best response from essential fatty acids, begin with the proper macronutrient framework (see Section I, Macronutrients, page 23). Then to that nutritionally sound base add gamma-linoleic acid (GLA) and EPA fish oil in a ratio of 1:4 (GLA:EPA) one to three times daily. The EicoPro essential fatty acid product manufactured by Eicotec, Inc., of Marblehead, Massachusetts, contains ultrapure sources of linoleic acid and fish oils already combined in this ratio. If you cannot get that product, you can purchase linoleic acid in a product called evening primrose oil at most health and nutrition stores, and EPA fish oil as well. Because it is not as pure a form, the milligram dosing will be different. You can make a reasonable substitute by combining evening primrose oil capsules with fish oil capsules plus vitamin E. Take 500 mg of evening primrose oil (a source of linoleic acid in capsule form), plus 1000 mg EPA fish oil, plus 200 IU vitamin E 1 to 3 times a day. (Warning to diabetics: EPA fish oil can cause blood sugar fluctuations in some diabetics. Carefully monitor your blood sugar if you use this supplemental oil and discontinue its use if your blood sugar becomes difficult to control.)

• *L-glutamine* is important in the healing of peptic ulcers. Recommendation: Take 500 mg of this amino acid on an empty stomach. Take with water or juice, but never with milk.

• Supplementation with *vitamin A* may help to prevent you from developing "stress" ulcers. When you have sustained a major physical or emotional trauma (a burn, major automobile accident, or internal injury from a fall or a blow), your body's natural response to the stress may cause an increase in the amount of stomach acid you produce as well as a reduced resistance to that acid on the part of your stomach lining. Recommendation: Under extreme physical stress, and under the supervision of your personal physician if possible, take 50,000 IU of vitamin A twice a day for no longer than 3 to 4 weeks. Please refer to the discussion of this vitamin in the A-to-Z Nutrient listings and acquaint yourself with the symptoms of taking too much vitamin A. Because your body can store this vitamin, toxic levels can build up. If you should develop any of the symptoms of vitamin A toxicity, you should promptly cease supplementation until levels can fall. Under less extreme stress, you may take the vitamin A forerunner, beta-carotene, instead of true vitamin A. Your body converts beta-carotene into vitamin A as it needs it. Take 25,000 to 50,000 IU beta-carotene per day.

• Deficiency of *vitamin B_6* may contribute to the development of stomach ulcers, and supplementation may promote healing of them. Recommendation: Take 50 to 100 mg of vitamin B_6 daily. You may increase to 150 mg if your symptoms warrant the increase; however, do not increase further. Permanent nerve damage has occurred at doses above 200 mg per day taken over a several-year period.

• Deficiency of *vitamin C* may increase your risk of peptic ulcer disease and bleeding from the ulcers, and supplementing this vitamin may speed your rate of healing. Recommendation: Take a minimum of 500 mg of time-release vitamin C 4 times a day. Refer to the discussion of this vitamin in the A-to-Z Nutrient listings for more information on its importance to health, as well as for instructions on how to take the vitamin in the crystalline or powdered form, which I prefer.

• Deficiency of *vitamin E* can cause stomach ulcers. Supplementation of this vitamin may help protect against stomach ulcers. This antioxidant also reduces stomach acid and relieves pain.

Recommendation: Take 400 to 800 IU of vitamin E, as d-alpha-tocopherol succinate, daily. Warning: Vitamin E can cause blood pressure elevation in some people. Please refer to the listing for this vitamin and follow the guidelines there for slowly and safely increasing your dose to the recommended level.

• *Vitamin K* is necessary for healing and to prevent bleeding. It also promotes nutrient absorption and has a neutralizing effect on the intestinal tract. A deficiency is common in those with digestive disorders. Recommendation: Take 100 *micro*grams daily. Increase your consumption of dark leafy green vegetables.

• For rapid relief of pain, drink a large glass of *water.* This dilutes stomach acid and flushes it out.

• *Bismuth,* the active ingredient in such stomach-soothing products as Pepto-Bismol, has proven in clinical testing to not only coat and soothe the inflamed stomach and intestinal lining but to actually kill *H. pylori,* the bacteria that seem to be responsible for keeping the ulcers going even with treatment. Physicians now routinely use "triple therapy" for chronic ulcers, which includes the acid-blocking drugs (Tagamet, Zantac, Axid, and Pepcid) plus an antibiotic medication (for example, tetracycline or metronidazole) and bismuth subsalicylate (Pepto-Bismol, Equate, and other similar products). Recommendation: Take 2 tablespoons bismuth subsalicylate 4 times per day. Note: Bismuth will darken your bowel movement to nearly black and can blacken the coating of your tongue. The changes are of no medical significance. Note also that these products contain an aspirin-like chemical; if you are on blood-thinning medication, medication for gout, or are aspirin allergic, you should not take them.

• Histamine (the same substance that causes allergic symptoms in your nose) stimulates the acid-producing cells in your stomach to release stomach acid. This stimulation is especially severe under stress and may be a major contributor to the development of stress ulcers. *Zinc,* because it prevents histamine release, may help to prevent stress ulcers. Recommendation: Take a chelated zinc supplement (such as zinc aspartate or zinc picolinate) in a dose of 20 to 50 mg twice a day. Warning: Supplementation of zinc in its ionic form can create deficiencies of other minerals, such as copper, by competing with them for absorption from the intestine. Chelation of the minerals (see discussion on pages 30–31, Section I) prevents this competition to get into the body, allowing you to fully absorb each of them.

Herbal remedies

• *Ginger* has anti-inflammatory activity, but it also contains more than 10 compounds that have anti-ulcer effects. The combination of honey and ginger is particularly effective. Honey has antibacterial action, and the two complement one another.

• *Licorice* contains a number of anti-ulcer compounds and is safe to use in moderate amounts. In larger amounts, or when used on a daily basis for longer than 6 weeks, it can produce headache, lethargy, loss of potassium, and high blood pressure. I suggest using licorice as a tea sweetener.

• Clinical trials suggest that *calendula* may be effective in treating ulcers. It has antibacterial, antiviral, and immune-boosting action. A tea can be made with about 5 teaspoons of fresh flowers. Lemon balm makes it even better.

• *Garlic* is an antibiotic. Cook with it, chop it up and mix it with other food, or just eat it plain, if you can.

• *Chamomile* is especially useful in treating ulcers. How's this for action: It's anti-inflammatory, antispasmodic, stomach-soothing, and antiseptic. Really, you can't go wrong with this herb.

• The anthocyanosides found in *bilberry and blueberry* offer protection against ulcers. They also stimulate production of mucus that protects the stomach lining.

Dosages may vary, depending on the duration and severity of your symptoms. Consult a qualified herbal practitioner, and alert your physician to your decision to use herbs. Some herbal remedies cannot be used in conjunction with conventional pharmaceuticals.

What makes it worse?

• See Heartburn.

• Although most medical research shows that *caffeine* doesn't cause stomach ulcers, it may worsen the symptoms from them. In most other conditions that caffeine makes worse, I would recommend you decaffeinate yourself and continue to enjoy your coffee; however, recent information suggests that *decaffeinated coffee* also stimulates the release of stomach acid. Recommendation: If you suffer with ulcers, your best bet is to slowly wean yourself off coffee (caffeinated or decaffeinated) over a period of 2 or 3 weeks and then remain off caffeine entirely. Becoming entirely caffeine-free means that you must also avoid caffeinated teas, chocolate (you may substitute with carob), and many soft drinks that contain caffeine.

• *Hot drinks* can trigger gastric discomfort. Allow teas and other hot beverages to cool before drinking them.

• Many experts believe that *food allergies* are a prime cause of ulcers. Carefully analyze your diet and remove from it any foods you suspect may cause you discomfort. If your symptoms improve, continue to avoid these foods permanently.

─────────── **Pregnancy** ───────────

What do you need?

• *Adequate protein and calories* from the first moment you recognize you're pregnant are absolutely necessary for a normal healthy baby and a normal healthy *you* afterward. Recommendation: Construct a diet for yourself that contains approximately 90 grams of lean protein from lean beef, chicken, fish, egg white, and dairy products. Add to that a wide selection of fresh fruits and vegetables, concentrating primarily on the dark green leafy vegetables, green vegetables, yellow-orange vegetables, richly pigmented fruits, and such starches as rice, whole grains, and oats. Don't avoid but try to limit your intake of concentrated starches such as potatoes and refined wheat starch. And keep your fat intake to about 30% of your total day's calories, with two-thirds of that fat coming from such oils as olive oil, canola oil, sunflower oil, and safflower oil. Only one-third of your fat intake should be from saturated animal sources, such as the fat in lean meats, chicken, and egg yolk. You should try to absolutely avoid refined flours and sugars of all types (see the listing for sugar on page 465).

• Your physician will likely prescribe a complete *prenatal multivitamin and mineral* containing at least the RDA for all nutrients. Be certain to take this vitamin every day. You may, with the approval of your obstetrician, take slightly higher amounts of some nutrients, such as:

• *Folic acid* has recently been shown to reduce the occurrence of birth defects involving the spinal canal. Recommendation: With the approval of your obstetrician, take 800 *micro*grams of folic acid per day during pregnancy. You will also want to ask your physician to check your level for vitamin B_{12} to be certain it is normal. If it is not, your physician may wish to provide you with supplemental B_{12} by injection.

• Supplemental *vitamin C* in a dose of 1 gram twice a day may help to relieve leg cramps, nausea, and vomiting associated with pregnancy. If you routinely take a dose of vitamin C higher than 2 grams per day, please see the following discussion under "What must you avoid?" concerning vitamin C. Larger doses (2000 to 4000 mg daily, in divided doses) taken before delivery may reduce labor pain.

• Deficiencies of *vitamin E* may increase the risk of complications of pregnancy such as pre-eclampsia (extreme fluid retention and high blood pressure in the last trimester). Studies have shown that vitamin E can be beneficial. Supplementation also decreases your chances for premature and low-birthweight infants. Recommendation: Take 400 IU per day of vitamin E as d-alpha-tocopherol succinate.

• Your *calcium* needs nearly double during pregnancy. If you did not take extra calcium prior to pregnancy, you should certainly begin to do so now to augment your dietary calcium intake. Recommendation: 1500 mg of calcium per day along with a dose of 750 mg of magnesium. (These two minerals work together to build bones and teeth—yours and your baby's.)

• Your *zinc* levels decline throughout pregnancy, falling on average by 30%, and a deficiency of zinc can increase your risk of miscarriage, premature delivery, complicated labor, low-birthweight babies, and toxemia (high blood pressure) of pregnancy. Recommendation: Take a chelated zinc supplement, such as zinc aspartate or zinc picolinate, in a dose of 20 mg per day. Warning: Supplementation of zinc in its ionic form can create deficiencies of other minerals, such as copper, by competing with them for absorption from the intestine. Chelation of the minerals (see discussion on pages 30–31, Section I) prevents this competition to get into the body, allowing you to fully absorb each of them.

• Especially those women who tend to retain fluid and have slightly elevated blood pressure during pregnancy can become deficient in *potassium*. Recommendation: By following the basic dietary guidelines just outlined, you will naturally eat more of the foods rich in potassium, such as broccoli, asparagus, tomatoes, citrus fruits, and bananas.

• During pregnancy, especially, your body requires a steady supply of the *essential fatty acid* raw materials needed for you to produce plenty of the "good" eicosinoid or prostaglandin messengers. The blood pressure–reducing effect of the "good" messengers is especially important for women who struggle with high blood pressure and fluid retention during pregnancy. Please refer to the Yin and Yang of Human Health, pages 24–27, for more information about the role of the messengers in good health. Recommendation: Begin by following the basic diet as outlined in this section. Then, with the approval of your personal obstetrician, add gamma-linoleic acid (GLA) and fish oil (EPA) in a ratio of 1:4 (GLA:EPA) once daily. The EicoPro essential fatty acid product manufactured by Eicotec, Inc., of Marblehead, Massachusetts, contains ultrapure sources of linoleic acid and fish oils already combined in the proper ratio. If you cannot get that product, you can purchase linoleic acid in a product called evening primrose oil at most health and nutrition stores, and EPA fish oil as well. Because it is not as pure a form, the milligram dosing will be different. You can make a reasonable substitute by combining evening primrose oil capsules with fish oil capsules plus vitamin E. Take 500 mg of evening primrose oil (a source of linoleic acid in capsule form), plus 1000 mg EPA fish oil, plus the 200 IU of vitamin E you will already be taking once a day. (Warning to diabetics: EPA fish oil can cause blood sugar fluctuations in some diabetics. Carefully monitor your blood sugar if you use this supplemental oil and discontinue its use if your blood sugar becomes difficult to control.)

Herbal remedies

• *Raspberry* is probably the most popular herb used during pregnancy. It relaxes the uterus. It helps women carry babies to term. It prevents many of the discomforts of pregnancy, including morning sickness. All this, and yet there's very little scientific proof that the herb accomplishes all that. However, pregnant women don't need scientific proof: If it works, it works!

• *Crampbark* soothes the uterus.

• *Blue cohosh* has been used by American Indians for centuries to induce labor. It contains a stimulator of uterine contractions. There have been stories that an overdose of this herb before term could cause you to lose your baby, so don't even go near this herb unless you discuss it with a qualified herbal practitioner. It is most often used to induce labor.

• *Jute* contains a great deal of folate, the B vitamin that prevents neural tube defects such as spina bifida.

• *St. John's wort* is soothing to the perineum during labor. After labor, its anti-inflammatory action eases the burning and swelling and speeds up healing of perineal tears.

• After birth, a dose of *shepherd's purse* can help stop bleeding.

One word of caution: Although these herbs have been used by women for centuries, every pregnancy is different. Please discuss with your doctor, midwife, or doula the use of any one or all of these herbs *before* using them.

What must you avoid?

• Babies born to mothers who drank *alcohol* during pregnancy have an increased risk for birth defects, learning and behavioral problems, hyperactivity, and shortened attention span. Recommendation: Do not drink alcohol during pregnancy. Mothers who consume more *caffeine* than that contained in about 2 cups of coffee risk causing stunted growth of their babies. Recommendation: Drink no more than 1 cup of coffee, caffeinated tea, or caffeine-containing soft drink per day. And remember, chocolate is loaded with caffeine, so you need to curb your chocolate consumption as well.

• Because *sugar* stimulates an increase in insulin, a high-sugar diet during pregnancy can stimulate massive weight gain, fluid retention, and blood pressure elevations that can prove difficult to correct (especially the excess weight) after delivery. I encourage you to read Obesity and Hypertension for more information about how dietary sugar can harm your health. Recommendation: Eliminate or sharply reduce your intake of sugar, corn syrup, high-fructose corn syrup, molasses, and all products made with these substances. I would also urge you to avoid keeping your sweet tooth fed by using artificial sweeteners during pregnancy. Try to enjoy the sweetness of whole fruits until delivery.

• Although deficiency of *vitamin A* during pregnancy can cause birth defects, too much vitamin A can as well. Recommendation: Take care not to exceed a daily intake of 8000 IU per day during pregnancy.

• During pregnancy you need adequate amounts of *vitamin B$_6$* for proper growth of your baby and to help curb nausea associated with the hormones of pregnancy. Recommendation: You should not take doses exceeding 20 mg per day, because higher doses may shut down breast milk production.

• During pregnancy, you should take no more than 2 grams of *vitamin C* per day, because infants born to mothers who take higher doses (5 grams or more) become dependent on the extra vitamin C and can develop signs of deficiency when the delivery abruptly separates them from their supplementation. Neither breast milk nor commercial infant formulas will supply the baby with the amount its body became used to in the womb. Recommendation: If you currently take more than 2 grams vitamin C per day, you may need to wean yourself down to this level during your pregnancy and then build back up to your previous level after delivery.

• Contrary to the old wives' tales about eating liver and needing iron to build you up during pregnancy, supplemental *iron* is probably not necessary unless your physician has documented by blood testing that you are deficient in iron. Taking extra iron can cause you to become deficient in other important minerals, such as zinc and copper. Recommendation: Except to correct deficiency, don't take extra iron supplements during pregnancy.

———— Premenstrual Syndrome (PMS) ————

What is it?

Menstrual cycling in women results from a complex interplay of reproductive hormones that surge and ebb at various points during the course of an approximately lunar month (28 days). Many women pass through cycle after cycle, blissfully unaware of the rising and falling of these hormones except during the specific several days of bleeding. As many as one-third of the women, however, suffer unpleasant symptoms that correlate with the hormonal fluctuations during especially the last 7 to 14 days of their monthly cycle. For perhaps 1 in 10 of these women, the symptoms—called premenstrual syndrome or PMS—trouble them nearly every month, while other women suffer only intermittently. What is the premenstrual syndrome?

The syndrome occurs in several distinct forms: emotional upheaval, including anxiety, irritability, insomnia, depression, forgetfulness, confusion, and lethargy; cravings for sweets, increased appetite, and intolerance to sugar (headache, heart palpitations, fatigue, and fainting); and fluid retention symptoms with weight gain puffiness of hands and feet, breast swelling and tenderness, and abdominal bloating and tenderness. Some women suffer with symptoms of all these forms, others only a few. If you suffer from premenstrual symptoms, can nutrition help? Let's see.

What helps it?

• *Proper dietary construction* will start you off on the road to better health and fewer symptoms. Recommendation: Please refer to Macronutrients on page 23, where you will find guidelines for constructing a diet for yourself that provides you with ½ gram of lean protein (lean beef, poultry, fish, and egg white) to support your muscle and organ tissues. The protein portion of your diet should constitute about 30% of your calories unless you are overweight (see Obesity). Another 40% of your day's calories should come from low-starch vegetables and fruits, and the final 30% of calories from fats and oils. By following these guidelines, you will stabilize your body fluid levels, prevent wild swings in blood sugar, and keep your cholesterol in line.

• The *essential fatty acids* in your diet are the raw materials from which your body makes a group of chemical messengers called prostaglandins. Please refer to the Yin and Yang of Human Health, pages 24–27, for more information about the critical role these messengers play in the symptoms that plague women with PMS: fluid retention, weight gain, headache, mood swings, and breast and abdominal tenderness. Recommendation: To facilitate the best response from essential fatty acids, begin with the proper macronutrient framework as outlined above. Then to that nutritionally sound base, add gamma-linoleic acid (GLA) and EPA fish oil in a ratio of 1:4 (GLA:EPA) 1 to 3 times daily. The EicoPro essential fatty acid product manufactured by Eicotec, Inc., of Marblehead, Massachusetts, contains ultrapure sources of linoleic acid and fish oils already combined in the proper ratio. If you cannot get that product, you can purchase linoleic acid in a product called evening primrose oil at most health and nutrition stores, and EPA fish oil as well. Because it is not as pure a form, the milligram dosing will be different. You can make a reasonable substitute by combining evening primrose oil capsules with fish oil capsules plus vitamin E. Take 500 mg of evening primrose oil (a source of linoleic acid in capsule form), plus 1000 mg EPA fish oil, plus 200 IU vitamin E 1 to 3 times a day. Warning to diabetics: EPA fish oil can cause blood sugar fluctuations in some diabetics. Carefully monitor your blood sugar if you use this supplemental oil and discontinue its use if your blood sugar becomes difficult to control.)

• Some research has shown that massive doses of *vitamin A* can help to relieve PMS symptoms. The downside of taking these very high levels of vitamin A (on the order of 300,000 IU per day) is that your body stores vitamin A, and at these levels toxic side effects occur readily. You can derive some of the benefit of increased vitamin A by taking the vitamin A forerunner, *beta-carotene,* which your body turns into active vitamin A as it needs it. Recommendation: Take 50,000 IU beta-carotene per day for 2 menstrual cycles to assess your response. If you see improvement of your symptoms, you may continue to supplement 25,000 IU to 50,000 IU per day. The only untoward side effect of beta-carotene is yellowing of your palms and soles. If this effect occurs, reduce your dose.

• Research testing has shown that women who suffer the emotional symptoms of PMS have fewer such problems if they take supplemental *vitamin B_6.* This vitamin also reduces water retention. Recommendation: Take vitamin B_6 in a dose of 50 to 100 mg per day. Warning: Do not increase your dose of B_6, since permanent nerve injury has occurred at doses of 200 mg taken daily over a period of several years.

• *Vitamin B_{12}* reduces stress and prevents anemia. Recommendation: take 200 *micro*grams daily.

• *Gamma-linoleic acid (GLA)* is vital to proper hormonal functioning. It improves cramps, cravings, muscle spasms, mood swings, depression, irritability, and breast tenderness. Borage oil is 24% GLA. Recommendation: Take one 1000 mg pill of borage oil daily.

• Women with PMS who have taken supplemental *vitamin E* report improvement of their symptoms of fluid retention, weight gain, breast tenderness, emotional upheaval, fatigue, and cravings for sweets. Recommendation: Take vitamin E, as d-alpha-tocopherol succinate, in a dose of 400 to 800 IU per day. Warning: Vitamin E can cause blood pressure elevation in some people. Please refer to the discussion of this vitamin and follow the guidelines there for slowly and safely increasing your dose to the recommended level.

• Deficiency of *magnesium* can cause the levels of certain brain chemicals to fall too low. This deficiency may contribute to the emotional symptoms you experience with PMS. Recommendation: Take 1000 mg magnesium chloride per day. (See listing for "dairy products or calcium" under "What makes it worse?" on page 470.)

• Deficiency of *zinc* during certain phases of the menstrual cycle can decrease your ability to produce and release progesterone, one of the major female reproductive hormones. Recommendation: Tak a chelated form of zinc, such as zinc aspartate or zinc picolinate, in a dose of 50 mg per day. Warning: Supplementation of zinc in its ionic form can create deficiencies of other minerals, such as copper, by competing with them for absorption from the intestine. Chelation of the minerals (see discussion on pages 30–31, Section I) prevents this competition to get into the body, allowing you to fully absorb each of them.

• *Isoflavones* are useful in alleviating mood swings associated with PMS. These phytoestrogens can be obtained from soybeans, peanuts, lentils, green peas, split peas, and beans. Recommendation: It is preferable to eat the organic form of isoflavones. Their equality to prescription hormonal supplements has been demonstrated, without the adverse side effects.

• *Exercise,* even in moderate amounts, is extremely helpful in alleviating PMS. Exercise increases oxygen levels in the blood, which improves nutrient absorption and toxin elimination. It also helps maintain hormone balance.

Herbal remedies

• *Chasteberry* relieves PMS because it balances hormones produced during women's monthly cycles. This increases other hormones, which leads to a shift in the estrogen-progesterone ratio. The result is less estrogen to cause or aggravate PMS. Caution: If you suffer from depression along with your PMS, do not use this herb. Some studies indicate that PMS with depression is caused by excess progesterone, a hormone whose level chasteberry raises.

• *Angelica* is used to treat PMS and cramps. Take 2 capsules between 400–500 mg twice daily to prevent PMS.

• Name the PMS complaint, and it can probably be helped with *evening primrose oil.* Some women take a capsule daily and increase that dosage to 3 to 4 once they feel the onset of PMS.

• *Valerian* promotes sleep and relieves the nervous tension of PMS.

• *Raspberry* has been touted for its ability to treat PMS. Make a tasty tea from this herb.

Dosages may vary, depending on the duration and severity of your symptoms. Follow package directions, or consult a qualified herbal practitioner.

What makes it worse?

• Avoid *simple carbohydrates and sugars* that will quickly raise your insulin levels. High insulin levels signal your kidneys to hold on to sodium, and therefore you retain more fluid. Insulin also stimulates your fat cells to store incoming calories as fat, promoting weight gain. And finally, insulin acts to make your body produce more of the "bad" prostaglandin messengers that will increase pain and inflammation, increase blood pressure, and increase uterine cramping and pelvic discomfort. Recommendation: If you suffer PMS regularly, eliminate or drastically reduce your intake of sugar, corn syrup, high-fructose corn syrup, molasses, and all products made with these substances. These restrictions are especially important during the last half of each menstrual cycle.

• Women who consume 4 to 15 caffeine-containing drinks per day (coffee, tea, soft drinks, or chocolate) suffer PMS at higher rates than women who drink little caffeine. Recommendation: Reduce your daily caffeine consumption to fewer than 4 caffeinated drinks per day. Reduce your intake of caffeine even more strictly (to no more than two caffeine-containing drinks) at least 3 days prior to the usual time of symptoms each month.

• Excessive consumption of *dairy products or calcium* supplements has been suggested as a cause of the emotional symptoms of PMS by creating a situation of dietary imbalance with calcium's fellow mineral, magnesium. Recommendation: If you take calcium supplements, be certain to also take half as much magnesium as calcium. Restrict your intake of dairy products in the week prior to your onset of symptoms and supplement with magnesium as recommended on page 468.

──────── Prostate Cancer ────────

What is it?

Cancer in the prostate gland is the most common form of male cancer, occurring in about 69 out of 100,000 men in the United States. As many as 70% of men in their 80s have at least microscopic evidence of cancer of the prostate; however, only about 6% of these men will have detected the cancer in their lifetimes. Men in their 50s rarely get prostate cancer. Ninety-five percent of all reported cases are in men between age 45 and 89. Although symptoms much like those from enlarged prostate—dribbling, frequency of urination, getting up many times in the night to urinate—occur with prostate cancer, many men have no symptoms at all, and for this reason, all men over 40 years of age should have a yearly examination by their personal physician to feel the prostate gland as well as to take a blood sample to determine their PSA (prostate-specific antigen, a body chemical produced by the prostate in bigger amounts in some situations, such as cancer). Nowadays, examination of the prostate gland is done by ultrasound. In this test, sound waves bounced off the gland generate patterns, not much different from sonar devices used by submarines to "see" the bottom or the depth finders fishermen use to track schools of fish and likely shapes of land below the water. The ultrasound test tells your physician about the size, shape, and consistency of your prostate gland better than even the standard rectal examination.

In addition to the early detection of cancers that regular examination by your physician can provide, what can you do nutritionally that might help? Let's take a look.

What helps it?

• A diet high in *fiber* helps to reduce your risk of prostate cancer by lowering your body's levels of reproductive hormones slightly. Men who eat the highest amounts of fiber have the fewest prostate cancers. Recommendation: Aim for a daily fiber intake of 40 to 50 grams, but don't try to reach that goal overnight or you will suffer abdominal bloating, gas, and cramping. Slowly increase your daily intake of high-fiber foods and add a bulk vegetable powder to that. I have outlined a slowly progressive fiber regimen under Colon, Spastic, that you may follow to gradually increase your intake to the recommended level. Deficiency of *vitamin A* increases the risk for prostate cancer. Taking supplemental vitamin A, however, can create problems itself, because your body can store this vitamin and its levels can build up to toxic amounts. You can still be sure your body has enough vitamin A by getting plenty of its forerunner, *beta-carotene*. Your body turns this vitamin relative into active vitamin A as it needs it. Recommendation: Increase your dietary intake of dark green leafy vegetables and yellow-orange vegetables, and add supplemental beta-carotene in a dose of 25,000 to 50,000 IU per day.

• Deficiency of certain of the B vitamins may increase your risk of prostate cancer. These are: *riboflavin, thiamine, and vitamin B_6.* Recommendation: Take 50 mg of riboflavin, 100 mg of thiamine, and 100 mg of vitamin B_6 along with a single 100 mg tablet of full

B-complex daily. The B vitamin family works best when all its members are present.

• Deficiency of *zinc* may increase risk of cancer because zinc nourishes the prostate gland and is vital for proper immune function. Take 50 to 100 mg of zinc gluconate lozenges daily. Do not exceed this amount. Additionally, increase your consumption of foods high in zinc, such as mushrooms, pumpkin seeds, seafood, spinach, sunflower seeds, and whole grains.

• Research shows that *soybeans* and *soy products* such as tofu, soy flour, and soy milk have cancer-fighting properties due to the presence of a protein called genistein. This protein retards tumor growth by preventing the growth of new blood vessels to feed the tumor.

Herbal remedies
• See Prostate Enlargement.

What makes it worse?
• A diet high in *saturated fat* may increase your risk of cancer of the prostate, according to some studies. Although the reason for this effect is not clear, it may be that a high fat intake weakens the killing power of certain immune fighters, leaving you more vulnerable to cancer development. Cancers occur when a cell is damaged and it ceases to function normally or to obey your body's normal controls. You depend upon your immune system to vigilantly protect you from this everyday process. Recommendation: Eat a diet that is reduced in fat content. Try to eat no more than 30% of your total day's calories as fat, with only 10% of your day's total as saturated (animal) fat.

• Avoid *red meat.* According to the *Journal of the National Cancer Institute,* men who eat red meat 5 times or more weekly have a risk of prostate cancer that is almost 3 times higher than that for men who eat red meat less than once weekly.

———— Prostate Enlargement ————

What is it?
The prostate gland, responsible for producing the seminal fluids in which the sperm "swim," sits under the bladder and surrounds the tube leading from the bladder to the outside. With aging, the prostate gland enlarges in size and, because of its location, can prevent normal urine flow. Most men, if they live long enough, will develop a

least some degree of prostate gland enlargement, and by age 80, as many as 40% of them in the United States will have had surgery to remove a part of their enlarged gland.

Symptoms of prostate enlargement include a weak urine stream, dribbling of urine, difficulty getting your urine stream started and stopped, and incomplete emptying of your bladder. When urine remains sitting in your bladder, it can more easily become infected. The obstruction to urine flow caused by the enlarged gland can become so severe that you cannot pass urine at all. This complication is a true emergency for which you must seek immediate medical attention.

Do vitamins and minerals play a role in reducing the risk for enlargement? It appears that they might. Let's see how.

What helps it?

• There is some evidence in the laboratory—and so far only experimental—that certain minerals can cause the prostate cells to grow in size and number. In these laboratory tests, *selenium* was able to counteract this growth stimulation. What that may mean to prostate gland enlargement in people is at this point uncertain. Recommendation: As of this writing, I have no hard science to suggest that selenium will help to prevent prostate enlargement; however, the mineral is beneficial to your health in other ways. I would recommend a daily dose of 100 *micrograms* of selenium for general health purposes, and it may help your prostate as well. The jury is still out.

• *Zinc* has been shown to reduce the size and symptoms of the enlarged prostate gland in a number of medical studies. Recommendation: Take a chelated form of zinc, such as zinc aspartate or zinc picolinate, in a dose of 80 mg daily. Do not exceed this amount, as large dosages (over 100 mg) have been shown to depress immune function. Warning: Supplementation of zinc in its ionic form can create deficiencies of other minerals, such as copper, by competing with them for absorption from the intestine. Chelation of the minerals (see discussion on pages 30–31, Section I) prevents this competition to get into the body, allowing you to fully absorb each of them.

• Researchers originally isolated the prostaglandin messengers (see eicosinoids, pages 24–27) from the prostate gland, which is quite rich in them. Your body takes *essential fatty acids* in your diet as the raw material to make the prostaglandins; however, some of the steps in this process slow down with age. Some research suggests that the slowing down of prostaglandin production may in part contribute to the enlargement of the prostate gland. Supplementation of already activated fatty acids bypasses the body's sluggish conversion and may help to reduce the size of the gland. Recommendation: To facilitate the best response from essential fatty acids, begin with the proper macronutrient framework as outlined on page 467. Then to that nutritionally sound base add gamma-linoleic acid (GLA) and EPA fish oil in a ratio of 1:4 (GLA:EPA) 1 to 3 times daily. The EicoPro essential fatty acid product manufactured by Eicotec, Inc., of Marblehead, Massachusetts, contains ultrapure sources of linoleic acid and fish oils already combined in the proper ratio. If you cannot get that product, you can purchase linoleic acid in a product called evening primrose oil at most health and nutrition stores, and EPA fish oil as well. Because it is not as pure a form, the milligram dosing will be different. You can make a reasonable substitute by combining evening primrose oil capsules with fish oil capsules plus vitamin E. Take 500 mg of evening primrose oil (a source of linoleic acid in capsule form), plus 1000 mg EPA fish oil, plus 200 IU vitamin E 1 to 3 times a day. (Warning to diabetics: EPA fish oil can cause blood sugar fluctuations in some diabetics. Carefully monitor your blood sugar if you use this supplemental oil and discontinue its use if your blood sugar becomes difficult to control.)

• To protect the skin tissue, you need a healthy supply of *beta-carotene*. Recommendation: Supplement with 25,000 IU daily. Warning: Do not use this supplement if you have diabetes.

Herbal remedies

• Zinc has been shown to reduce the size of the prostate, and *pumpkin seeds* are high in zinc. These seeds also prevent testosterone from being transformed into dihydrotestosterone. And finally, pumpkin seeds contain certain amino acids that, when researched, have been shown to relieve symptoms of enlarged prostate.

• *Saw palmetto* gives comfort and relief because it contains a compound that inhibits the action of the enzyme that turns testosterone into dihydrotestosterone. Studies show the effectiveness of this herb.

• *Stinging nettle* also inhibits the effect on the conversion of testosterone. German herbalists recommend 2 to 3 teaspoons of extract daily.

Dosages may vary, depending on the duration and severity of your symptoms. Consult a qualified herbal practitioner, and alert your physician to your decision to use herbs. Some herbal remedies cannot be used in conjunction with conventional pharmaceuticals.

What makes it worse?

I know of no specific nutrients that contribute to prostate enlargement.

Psoriasis

What is it?

In psoriasis the skin erupts in patches of raised, red, flat-topped plateaus covered with silvery scaling skin. The patches most commonly occur on the elbows, knees, and scalp, but can also erupt in folds of skin, in the ear canals, and even on the external genital organs. Although the disease usually confines itself to your skin and scalp, it can also attack your joints, causing symptoms of pain, swelling, and redness.

You inherit a tendency to develop psoriasis, but a case of mistaken identity triggers its onset. I refer you to Autoimmune Disorders for more information on how your body's immune defenders mistakenly turn on your own tissues, as is the case in psoriasis and other such diseases. Physical and emotional stress seem to worsen the rashing of psoriasis, and the rash may erupt in areas where you cut or scrape your skin.

There are a number of excellent medical treatments that help to reduce the inflammation and scaling rash in psoriasis, but nutrition can be a helpful remedy in addition to medical therapy. Let's examine what nutrients seem to help in psoriasis.

What helps it?

• Proper dietary construction can reduce your tendency for psoriatic eruption. But how do you properly construct a basic diet to meet your needs? Begin by being certain to eat a diet that provides the proper macronutrient framework, as described on page 23. Your basic dietary needs will consist of sufficient high-quality lean protein to provide a minimum of ½ gram of protein for every pound of your lean body mass. High-quality protein should make up about 30% of your day's calorie needs. Another 40% should be carbohydrate, coming mostly from high-fiber, low-starch fruits and vegetables, and the final 30% should come from fats and oils (20%

monounsaturated and polyunsaturated oils such as olive oil, canola oil, safflower and sunflower oil, and 10% saturated fats of animal origin).

• Your body needs a steady supply of *essential fatty acids* that it can use as raw materials to produce prostaglandin messengers. (See the Yin and Yang of Human Health, pages 24–27, for a more in-depth discussion of these chemicals as mediators of pain, inflammation, and immune system health.) Recommendation: To a nutritionally sound basic diet, add gamma-linoleic acid (GLA) and EPA fish oil in a ratio of 1:4 (GLA:EPA) 1 to 3 times daily. The EicoPro essential fatty acid product manufactured by Eicotec, Inc., of Marblehead, Massachusetts, contains ultrapure sources of linoleic acid and fish oils already combined in the proper ratio. If you cannot get that product, you can purchase linoleic acid in a product called evening primrose oil at most health and nutrition stores, and EPA fish oil as well. Because it is not as pure a form, the milligram dosing will be different. You can make a reasonable substitute by combining evening primrose oil capsules with fish oil capsules plus vitamin E. Take 500 mg of evening primrose oil (a source of linoleic acid in capsule form), plus 1000 mg EPA fish oil, plus 200 IU vitamin E 1 to 3 times a day. (Warning to diabetics: EPA fish oil can cause blood sugar fluctuations in some diabetics. Carefully monitor your blood sugar if you use this supplemental oil and discontinue its use if your blood sugar becomes difficult to control.)

• *Application of essential fatty acids to your skin* can also help to reduce scaling and inflammation. Although you can break open capsules of evening primrose oil and apply the contents to your skin, the oil is somewhat sticky. A product called Eicoderm, manufactured by Eicotec, Inc., of Marblehead, Massachusetts, is the only product of which I am aware that provides gamma-linoleic acid (GLA) in a form that absorbs readily into your skin. Recommendation: Apply Eicoderm to the psoriatic rash 2 to 4 times daily.

• People with psoriasis often have mild deficiency of *vitamin A,* which may contribute to their skin problems by a means not entirely clear. Because your body can store vitamin A and a buildup of the vitamin can cause toxic symptoms, you should not supplement with excess vitamin A. Your body can produce active vitamin A from its nontoxic relative, *beta-carotene,* however, and this gives you a means to prevent deficiency safely. Recommendation: Take 25,000 IU of beta-carotene daily. If you have diabetes, do not use this supplement.

• Exposure to *sunlight* (or to the ultraviolet B irradiation in sunlight) has long been known to clear the rash in psoriasis. Dermatologists frequently prescribe ultraviolet light (sunbed) therapy for their patients with severe psoriasis. Recent research suggests that the sunlight helps because it stimulates your skin to produce vitamin D, and that it is actually an increase in vitamin D which alleviates the rash. Recommendation: In mild cases of psoriasis, I would recommend you get outdoors for a minimum of 30 minutes to 1 hour each day in sunny weather. Do not burn your skin, just spend a little time outdoors each day in the sunlight.

• Your body must have *selenium* to make its own natural antioxidant, glutathione peroxidase. This potent antioxidant helps to curb your body's production of some of the inflammatory eicosinoid messengers that worsen your rash. (See eicosinoids, pages 24–27.) Recommendation: Take selenium aspartate in a dose of 100 to 200 *micro*grams per day.

• Early research into the nutritional factors that might help people suffering with psoriasis showed *lecithin* gave some relief. Recommendation: Take soy lecithin granules in a dose of 3 grams per day.

• *Vitamin E* neutralizes free radicals that damage the skin. Recommendation: 400 to 1200 IU daily. Use an emulsion form for easier assimilation.

• Although further research needs to be done, studies show that *shark cartilage* is effective in treating psoriasis, without the toxicity of standard drugs. It seems to inhibit the growth of blood vessels to stop the spread of the disorder. Itching and scaling clear first, then redness gradually fades. Recommendation: Talk to your doctor first, but should you decide to try this technique, take 1 gram per 15 pounds of body weight daily, divided into 3 doses. Allow 2 to 3 months to see results.

• *Carrot juice* combined with a small amount of green vegetable juice contains an abundance of valuable nutrients. Recommendation: Drink 8 to 16 ounces of this combination daily.

Herbal remedies
• Ancient Egyptians and Indians rubbed what historians presume was psoriasis with plants containing psoralens and then sat in the sun. *Bishop's weed* contains an abundance of one of these psoralens. These compounds inhibit cell division, slowing down the skin cells

that cause psoriasis. Caution: High doses of psoralens can be carcinogenic. If this herb irritates your skin, discontinue use.

• *Angelica* also contains psoralens. Ingest the herb and then spend some time in the sun. But beware: Discontinue use if any irritation develops. And remember that high dosages of psoralens can be carcinogenic.

• Europeans use *chamomile* to treat this disorder. Apply a chamomile cream directly to the affected areas. Caution: If your itching becomes worse, discontinue use.

• Many naturopaths consider *licorice* to be more effective than hydrocortisone when treating psoriasis. Apply an extract directly to the affected area using a clean cloth.

• *Lavender oil* is praised by aromatherapists for its healing powers. Apply the essential oil directly to the skin; do not ingest.

• *Milk thistle* contains 8 anti-inflammatory compounds that act on the skin. Take as a tea or tincture, or in capsules.

Dosages may vary, depending on the duration and severity of your symptoms. Follow package directions, or consult a qualified herbal practitioner.

What makes it worse?

• Some recent research has shown that people who develop psoriasis tend to drink more *alcohol* than those who don't. Whether alcohol acts as a triggering stimulus is not clear. Recommendation: If you have a family history for psoriasis, you would be well advised not to drink alcohol. If you have psoriasis, drink alcohol only sparingly or not at all.

• A diet high in *red meat and egg yolk* may promote inflammation and eruption of your psoriatic rash because of the high amounts of arachidonic acid that these two foods contain. Arachidonic acid is the forerunner from which your body makes the "bad" line of prostaglandins that promote inflammation. Recommendation: Limit your intake of these foods to 1 serving per week or less.

• People with psoriasis who have been placed on very restricted diets (rice diets and liquid fasting programs) often experience clearing of their rashes. This benefit may occur because their usual diet contains one or more foods to which they are sensitized or allergic. *Food sensitivities* may be a contributing cause to the waxing and waning of your psoriatic rashes. Recommendation: You may want to consult an allergy specialist to do some blood and skin testing for food allergies to help narrow your search for foods that cause you trouble. Armed with the information you gain from these tests, you must undertake a systematic elimination trial of each food individually to determine if it indeed is a culprit in your disease. Please refer to Food Allergy for information about how to conduct an elimination trial.

Psoriatic Arthritis

What is it?

Arthritic disorders come in a variety of forms, with the most common ones being rheumatoid arthritis, osteoarthritis, systemic lupus erythematosus, and a group that we refer collectively to as the spondylopathies or spinal arthritic diseases. This last group includes ankylosing spondylitis, a disorder called Reiter's syndrome, and psoriatic arthritis, which is the combined inflammatory condition that involves the skin (see Psoriasis) and the joints. What these last three arthritic conditions share is a tendency to attack the joints of the spine and lower back and the same immune system marker. For a more detailed discussion of all these forms of arthritis, I refer you to my previous book entitled *If It Runs in Your Family: Arthritis* (Bantam, 1992). You will also find information pertinent to psoriatic arthritis in this listing under Arthritis and Immune System Health.

Arthritis occurs in about 15 to 20% of people with psoriasis, frequently striking the low back and pelvic girdle joints, the finger joints closest to the nails, and often one or more of the major joints: a hip, knee, shoulder, ankle, or elbow. Usually—in fact, about 80% of the time—the onset of the skin condition precedes the development of joint problems, and the more severe the psoriasis, the more likely the chance for arthritis.

What helps it?
- See Arthritis, Immune System Health, Psoriasis.

Herbal remedies
- See Arthritis, Immune System Health, Psoriasis.

What makes it worse?
- See Arthritis, Immune System Health, Psoriasis.

———————— **Raynaud's Syndrome** ————————

What is it?

The condition we call Raynaud's syndrome or Raynaud's phenomenon, a disorder common to young women, causes episodes of abrupt spasm of the arteries supplying blood to the hands. The attack usually begins with loss of color (white hands) as the blood supply suddenly diminishes, followed by purplish tingeing (blue hands) as the length of time without adequate blood flow increases, and finally by fiery color, throbbing pain, and tingling as the blood vessel spasm relaxes and blood returns (red hands). These paroxysmal blood vessel spasms can occur because of cold temperature (an exaggerated form of the blood vessel constriction that normally occurs in all people's hands in cold weather) or because of emotional upset. If these episodes continue for longer than 3 years (with no other medical explanation for them), we call the condition Raynaud's syndrome. From time to time, the frequency and duration of attacks deprives the skin of the fingertips of blood long enough to cause skin damage, forming ulcers that repeatedly must scab over and heal.

Medical treatment usually consists of keeping the hands protected from cold (wearing warm gloves) or injury, and stopping smoking (components in tobacco smoke cause spasm of the blood vessels, too). Sometimes physicians prescribe medications to prevent the blood vessel spasm (such as nifedipine, Procardia). And occasionally, some people may require surgery to cut the nerves that supply the blood vessel wall, so that they can no longer send signals to constrict. But in addition to any medical treatment that might be necessary, what can nutrition offer? Let's look.

What helps it?

• A number of medical studies have shown that people with Raynaud's phenomenon developed fewer attacks and that the duration of the attacks was shorter when they took supplemental *niacin*. This is probably because niacin dilates small arteries, thereby improving circulation. Recommendation: Take niacin, as inositol nicotinate, 500 to 1000 mg 4 times per day. The inositol combination slows the release of the niacin. You could also try time-release niacin in a dose of 250 mg 3 times daily. Warning: Niacin can cause flushing (redness and warmth of your face, neck, and sometimes entire body) in bigger doses. Reduce your dose if you experience flushing or elevation of blood pressure.

• *Vitamin E* has been shown to decrease the spasm and speed healing of skin ulcers. It also improves circulation and dissolves clots in the legs, heart, and lungs. Recommendation: Take vitamin E, either as d-alpha-tocopherol succinate or as alpha-tocopherol nicotinate, in a dose of 200 IU each day and gradually work up to 1000 IU daily. You can also pierce the capsules of vitamin E and rub the oil onto the healing ulcerated areas (but not on new ulcers). Warning: Vitamin E can cause elevation of blood pressure in some people. Please refer to the discussion of this vitamin for information on how to increase your dose slowly and safely.

• Women who suffer from Raynaud's phenomenon become deficient in *magnesium* upon exposure to cold temperatures. One theory suggests that the low magnesium may contribute to the tendency for the blood vessels to spasm. Recommendation: Take magnesium aspartate in a dose of 750 mg daily during cold weather. Since magnesium works with calcium, it is important to take a calcium supplement as well. Take 1500 mg calcium daily. This combination also protects the arteries from stress caused by sudden changes in blood pressure.

• *Coenzyme Q_{10}* improves tissue oxygenation. Recommendation: Take 100 to 200 mg daily.

• The *bioflavonoids* seem to improve blood flow through tiny blood vessels by reducing the "stickiness" of red blood cells. Some people with Raynaud's phenomenon from various causes have shown improvement—fewer and milder attacks, healing of ulcers, and relief of pain—from taking these compounds. Recommendation: Take 1000 mg bioflavonoid complex (containing rutin) twice daily for 4 weeks to assess your response. If your symptoms improve, continue this regimen in cold weather.

• *Essential fatty acids* are the raw materials your body uses to produce a group of powerful body chemicals called the eicosinoids, some of them "good," some of them "bad." (See the Yin and Yang of Human Health, pages 24–27, for more information about these messengers.) The "good" members of this family of chemicals help to dilate and relax blood vessels, reduce inflammation, and speed healing—in short, they do everything that a person suffering from Raynaud's phenomenon could hope for. Recommendation: To facilitate the best response from essential fatty acids, begin with a proper macronutrient framework. Then to that nutritionally sound base add gamma-linoleic acid (GLA) and EPA fish oil in a ratio of 1:4 (GLA:EPA) 1 to 3 times daily. The EicoPro essential fatty acid product manufactured by Eicotec, Inc., of Marblehead, Massachusetts, contains ultrapure sources of linoleic acid and fish oils already combined in the proper ratio. If you cannot get that product, you can purchase linoleic acid in a product called evening primrose oil at most health and nutrition stores, and EPA fish oil as well. Because it is not as pure a form, the milligram dosing will be different. You can make a reasonable substitute by combining evening primrose oil capsules with fish oil capsules plus vitamin E. Take 500 mg of evening primrose oil (a source of linoleic acid in capsule form), plus 1000 mg EPA fish oil, plus 200 IU vitamin E 1 to 3 times a day. (Warning to diabetics: EPA fish oil can cause blood sugar fluctuations in some diabetics. Carefully monitor your blood sugar if you use this supplemental oil and discontinue its use if your blood sugar becomes difficult to control.)

Herbal remedies

• The oil made from *evening primrose* contains a generous amount of GLA, a substance believed to relieve symptoms of this disorder.

• *Garlic* improves circulation. Studies indicate it is useful in treating Raynaud's. Add more garlic to your diet, or take in capsule form.

• *Ginkgo* also enhances blood circulation. This herb is widely used in Europe to treat Raynaud's. Don't take any more than 240 mg daily or you may experience diarrhea, irritability, and restlessness.

• Mix some *red pepper* with vegetable oil and rub on your fingers.

Dosages may vary, depending on the duration and rate of your symptoms. Consult a qualified herbal practitioner, and let your physician know of your desire to use herbs. Some herbal remedies cannot be used safely along with conventional pharmaceuticals.

What makes it worse?

• Sometimes allergic reactions to food or *food sensitivities* can trigger Raynaud's phenomenon. Discovering what of the many foods or food additives could be responsible takes time. You may want to enlist the aid of an allergy specialist to perform some blood or skin testing to help narrow down the field. Once you're armed with a list of probable suspects, your job begins in earnest. You must systematically eliminate each food or substance individually. I have described this process, called an elimination trial, in detail under Food Allergy. Refer to that discussion for further information.

——————— **Restless Leg Syndrome** ———————

What is it?

If you sometimes lie down to rest at night or for an afternoon nap, and you can rest but your legs can't, you may suffer from a disorder called restless leg syndrome or "jumpy legs." The problem may occur not only with "rest" but in such situations as sitting to watch a movie or a play. The symptoms in your legs (and occasionally arms) include pain, numbness, lightning stabs, crawling, tingling, burning, and occasionally muscle cramping when you are resting or still, but disappear or improve with movement. The restlessness of your legs, then, is an attempt to relieve the strange or unpleasant sensations you feel. The more severe the problem with restless legs, the more disrupted your rest in general becomes, and you may experience insomnia and even depression over not being able to rest properly. Can vitamins, minerals, and nutrients make a difference? Yes. Let me tell you how.

What helps it?

• Eating a *properly constructed diet* may result in quite dramatic and prompt relief of symptoms. Recommendation: Refer to Macronutrients on page 23 and follow the guidelines contained there to construct a diet for yourself that provides plenty of high-quality lean protein to make up about 30 to 35% of your daily caloric intake. Another 35 to 40% should come from fresh, whole fruits and a wide selection of low-starch vegetables, such as dark green leafy vegetables, green vegetables, and yellow-orange vegetables, and starches coming primarily from rice and oats. The final 30% of your day's calories should come from fats and oils.

• Sometimes restless legs occur with a deficiency of *folic acid*. Your physician can determine deficiency by checking the amount of folate in your blood. Recommendation: If you are deficient in folic acid, you should take 5 mg of folic acid daily until your blood values return to normal. Warning: High doses of folic acid can hide a deficiency in vitamin B_{12}. Your physician must also periodically check your blood for deficiency of this vitamin and supplement it if necessary. Refer to the discussion of these vitamins for more information.

• Deficiency of *vitamin E* can also cause restless legs in some people. Recommendation: Take vitamin E, as d-alpha-tocopherol succinate, in a dose of 400 IU per day for at least 4 to 6 weeks to assess your response. Warning: Vitamin E can cause elevation of blood pressure in some people. Please refer to the listing for this vitamin for information on how to slowly and safely increase your dose to the recommended level.

• In cases of true deficiency of *iron,* some people develop restless legs. Because you shouldn't take excess iron when you don't have a deficiency of this mineral, you should ask your physician to check the level of iron in your blood. Recommendation: If you are mildly iron deficient, take a chelated iron supplement, such as iron glycinate, in a dose of 10 to 20 mg per day. If you cannot find a chelated form of iron, you may take 90 mg ferrous sulfate 2 to 3 times daily, along with 500 mg of vitamin C at each dose. The vitamin C helps you absorb the iron better by chelating it. Refer to chelation on pages 30–31 for more information on why this is important.

• Before the FDA removed all the *tryptophan* supplements from the shelves across America, many people with restless legs and insomnia benefited from taking this amino acid. Although it's now quite clear that the tryptophan itself wasn't the problem, but a contaminant in the processing of a single manufacturer, there's still no tryptophan on the market. Recommendation: If the FDA ever decides that it will allow this amino acid back onto the market, you may try taking 1 gram (1000 mg) of tryptophan once or twice daily. You can still derive benefits from tryptophan by consuming foods high in the amino acid. These include turkey, bananas, figs, dates, yogurt, milk, tuna, and whole grain crackers. Warning: Because you can't know if an old bottle of tryptophan contains the contaminant that caused severe and fatal muscle damage in those who took it, absolutely *do not* use any old, leftover tryptophan supplement you may have around.

What makes it worse?

• There is some suggestion in the literature that some people may develop restless legs because of wildly swinging blood sugar. In some clinical settings, people suffering restless legs noted dramatic and significant improvement in their symptoms from eliminating *sugar* from their diets. Recommendation: Eliminate or sharply reduce your intake of sugars, including: table sugar, corn syrup, high-fructose corn syrup, molasses, and all products made with these substances.

• In one study, all 62 patients who eliminated *caffeine* and other related compounds found in tea and chocolate noted improvement of their symptoms. Recommendation: Eliminate or sharply curtail your intake of caffeine from all sources, including coffee, tea, chocolate, and soft drinks. If you currently consume fairly high amounts of caffeine-containing foods and beverages, undertake your decaffeination slowly. I have described a regimen of gradual caffeine withdrawal under Breast Disease, Benign, that should help you decaffeinate yourself without the headache and sleepy stuporous feeling that may occur with abrupt caffeine withdrawal.

Rheumatoid Arthritis

What is it?

Rheumatoid arthritis (RA) is a severe and potentially crippling form of arthritis that occurs when your immune defense system mistakenly turns its destructive power on its own body's tissues. In this case, the immune system defends you from your own joints and the tissues surrounding them, causing pain, redness, swelling, decreased movement, and, if untreated, deformity and crippling caused by destruction of the cartilage surfaces covering the ends of the bones. I have described how this process occurs in more detail under Autoimmune Disorders, and you may wish to read that discussion for more information. Rheumatoid arthritis should always demand the regular attention of a physician expert in treating this condition, because prompt and vigorous treatment can spare you from deformity and crippling. Nutrition and nutritional remedies can help, but you should not substitute them for medications or physical remedies your personal physician may prescribe.

One of my previous books concerned how to reduce your risk for various forms of arthritis including rheumatoid arthritis—*If It Runs in Your Family: Arthritis* (Bantam, 1992), and I had significantly more space to devote to this disease than I will have here. I encourage you to read that book if you want more information about the nutritional and environmental factors that influence this disease. But in the space allotted here, let's take a look at what nutrients may help.

What helps it?

• Malnutrition may contribute to the development of RA. Eating a properly constructed diet that provides sufficient complete lean protein to support your muscles and organs is of paramount importance. Recommendation: Refer to the discussion of Macronutrients that you will find on page 23, and from those general guidelines construct a diet for yourself that provides ½ gram of complete lean protein (poultry, fish, seafood, egg white, and occasional lean beef) for every pound of your lean tissue (instructions on how to calculate lean tissue weight are provided in the discussion). You should aim for the dietary percentages given there: 30% of your day's total number of calories from protein; 40% from low-starch vegetables, whole fresh fruits, rice and oats; and 30% from fats and oils. Avoid or sharply reduce your intake of nutritionally blank foods, such as refined sugars: table sugar, corn syrup, high-fructose corn syrup, molasses, and products made with these substances. Make your nutrition count.

• In a number of medical studies, people with RA who took *pantothenic acid* noted improvement of their symptoms of morning stiffness, pain, and ability to perform their daily activities. Recommendation: Take pantothenic acid, as calcium d-pantothenate, in a dose of 250 to 500 mg 3 to 4 times daily for a period of 4 weeks to assess your response. If your symptoms improve, you may continue to take 250 mg daily.

• People with RA develop very fragile capillaries, especially in their forearms and lower legs, and consequently always have a crop of dark red/purple bruises from minor trauma. Many of the medications RA sufferers must take worsen this problem. *Vitamin C* helps to reduce this tendency to bruise. Recommendation: Take a minimum of 500 mg time-release vitamin C 2 to 4 times daily. You may want to refer to the discussion of this important vitamin for more information on its many health benefits.

• Deficiency of *vitamin E* may contribute to the inflammation and pain in RA and other forms of severe arthritis of the spine. In some studies, the relief of pain and improvement in mobility of arthritic joints from supplemental vitamin E equaled that of prescription strength anti-inflammatory medications. Recommendation: Take vitamin E, as d-alpha-tocopherol succinate, in a dose of 400 to 800 IU per day. Warning: Vitamin E can cause elevation of blood pressure in some people. Please refer to the listing for this vitamin for information on how to slowly and safely increase your dose to the recommended level.

• Your body uses dietary *essential fatty acids* as the raw materials to produce a family of powerful body chemicals called the eicosinoids. Some of these chemical messengers are "good" for you, reducing inflammation, pain, and swelling, and others are "bad." (Please refer to the Yin and Yang of Human Health, pages 24–27, for more information about these substances.) Because RA is an inflammatory disease—inflammation caused by your immune defense system's misguided attack produces the pain, redness, swelling, and damage to the joints—having more of the "good" messengers can only help. Recommendation: To the nutritionally sound basic diet just recommended, add gamma-linoleic acid (GLA) and EPA fish oil in a ratio of 1:4 (GLA:EPA) 1 to 3 times daily. The EicoPro essential fatty acid product manufactured by Eicotec, Inc., of Marblehead, Massachusetts, contains ultrapure sources of linoleic acid and fish oils already combined in the proper ratio. If you cannot get that product, you can purchase linoleic acid in a product called evening primrose oil at most health and nutrition stores, and EPA fish oil as well. Because it is not as pure a form, the milligram dosing will be different. You can make a reasonable substitute by combining evening primrose oil capsules with fish oil capsules plus vitamin E. Take 500 mg of evening primrose oil (a source of linoleic acid in capsule form), plus 1000 mg EPA fish oil, plus 200 IU vitamin E 1 to 3 times a day. (Warning to diabetics: EPA fish oil can cause blood sugar fluctuations in some diabetics. Carefully monitor your blood sugar if you use this supplemental oil and discontinue its use if your blood sugar becomes difficult to control.)

• From old wives' tales to mountain folklore, *copper* has figured in as a remedy for arthritis. And medical research supports the belief that copper deficiency may indeed play a role in activity of RA. Studies comparing copper bracelets to identical-appearing aluminum bracelets showed that when the 240 people participating wore copper, their symptoms improved, and when they wore the look-alike aluminum, their symptoms worsened. Exactly how copper on the skin exerts this beneficial effect is unclear, but you can't argue with the results. Other studies have shown that taking brief courses of copper supplementation may also help. Recommendation: If you would like to wear a copper bracelet, I don't see why you shouldn't. You may also take copper salicylate in a dose of 64 mg daily with meals for no longer than 10 days at a time, and not more often than every 3 to 4 months.

• The battle that rages in arthritic joints between your misguided immune defenders and your innocent joint tissues produces high concentrations of toxic free radicals at the scene. Refer to oxidation and free radicals beginning on page 18 for more information. Your body requires *selenium* to produce its own powerful free radical scavenger, glutathione peroxidase, to combat these toxic compounds released by the immune defenders. Recommendation: Take selenium aspartate in a dose of 100 to 200 *micro*grams per day.

• As RA progresses, your body's level of *zinc* falls significantly. As the zinc falls, inflammation becomes worse. It's a vicious cycle. Recommendation: Take zinc in a chelated form, such as zinc aspartate or zinc picolinate, in a dose of 20 mg twice per day. Warning: Supplementation of zinc in its ionic form can create deficiencies of other minerals, such as copper, by competing with them for absorption from the intestine. Chelation of the minerals (see pages 30–31, Section I) prevents this competition to get into the body, allowing you to fully absorb each of them.

• Some research has shown benefit in reducing inflammation can occur with injections into arthritic joints of a special anti-inflammatory chemical called *superoxide dismutase* or SOD. You may see this substance sold as tablets or capsules; however, these forms will be of no value to you. Stomach acid destroys the enzyme before you can absorb it. Recommendation: Don't waste your money purchasing SOD to take by mouth.

• *Boron* is a trace mineral required for healthy bones. Recommendation: 3 mg daily.

• *Sea cucumber* is a rich source of lubricating compounds found in all connective tissues, especially joints and joint fluid. Check out your local health food store for sea cucumber; if they don't carry it, you can always request that it be ordered. Allow 3 to 6 weeks to note improvement.

Herbal remedies
    See Arthritis.

What makes it worse?

• Many people who suffer from RA will see dramatic improvement of their symptoms when they avoid certain kinds of food. *Food sensitivities,* although they may not cause the disease, can certainly contribute to flare-ups of pain, swelling, and stiffness. Because any food, beverage, or food additive could be a culprit, you may want to consult an allergy specialist to perform some skin and blood testing to help narrow your list of suspects. Armed with that information, you will have to systematically eliminate each suspect individually. I have provided the details of how to conduct this systematic search, called an elimination trial, under Food Allergy.

• A diet high in *red meat and egg yolks* may worsen inflammation and pain in RA, because of the high amounts of arachidonic acid these foods contain. Arachidonic acid is the forerunner of the "bad" group of eicosinoid messengers (see discussion of essential fatty acids on page 487) that promote inflammation and increase pain and swelling. Recommendation: Sharply reduce your intake of these foods, eating them no more often than once a month or so.

Ringing in the Ears

(see Hearing Loss)

Scaly Skin and Scalp

(see Dermatitis)

Scleroderma

What is it?

Scleroderma means "hard skin." In this disorder—which probably occurs because the body's immune defenses mistakenly turn on its own tissues—the body lays down layers of fibrous tissue (the same kind of tissue as the scar tissue used to repair wounds) in the skin and sometimes in the internal organs. Most of the time (roughly 80%), the scarring affects only the skin. Another 20% of people, however, may develop problems from scarring in the intestinal tract, the kidney, and the heart. The disorder affects about two to three times more women than men and usually begins in the 30s and 40s. Symptoms include thickening and puffiness of the skin, difficulty swallowing, coughing, and shortness of breath. Scarring in and around the smaller blood vessels causes Raynaud's syndrome (see its listing) in about 90% of people with scleroderma. This same blood vessel scarring can cause kidney and heart problems. If you have scleroderma, you should regularly consult with the physician caring for you, but in addition to the medications your physician may prescribe, nutrition may offer some help.

What helps it?

• Supplemental *vitamin E* seems to improve symptoms in people with scleroderma (both limited to the skin and involving the internal organs). Recommendation: Take 600 IU of vitamin E, as d-alpha-tocopherol succinate, 3 times daily 15 minutes before meals for 4 to 6 weeks to assess your response. If your symptoms improve, maintain your intake at a dose of 800 IU taken once per day. Warning: Vitamin E can cause elevation of blood pressure in some people. Please refer to the listing for this vitamin for information on how to slowly and safely increase your dose to the recommended level.

• Your body uses dietary *essential fatty acids* as the raw materials to produce a family of powerful body chemicals called the eicosinoids. Some of these chemical messengers are "good" for you, reducing inflammation, pain, and swelling, and others are "bad." (Please refer to the Yin and Yang of Human Health, pages 24–27, for more information about these substances.) These messengers, the "good" ones at least, help to reduce inflammation and may even help to reduce the scarring, so encouraging your body to make more of the "good" messengers can only help. Recommendation: To a nutritionally sound basic diet (see discussion of Macronutrients, page 23), add gamma-linoleic acid (GLA) and EPA fish oil in a ratio of 1:4 (GLA:EPA) 1 to 3 times daily. The EicoPro essential fatty acid product manufactured by Eicotec, Inc., of Marblehead, Massachusetts, contains ultrapure sources of linoleic acid and fish oils already combined in the proper ratio. If you cannot get that product, you can purchase linoleic acid in a product called evening primrose oil at most health and nutrition stores, and EPA fish oil as well. Because it is not as pure a form, the milligram dosing will be different. You can make a reasonable substitute by combining evening primrose oil capsules with fish oil capsules plus vitamin E. Take 500 mg of evening primrose oil (a source of linoleic acid in capsule form), plus 1000 mg EPA fish oil, plus 200 IU vitamin E 1 to 3 times a day. (Warning to diabetics: EPA fish oil can cause blood sugar fluctuations in some diabetics. Carefully monitor your blood sugar if you use this supplemental oil and discontinue its use if your blood sugar becomes difficult to control.)

Herbal remedies

• *Aloe* is effective in treating a number of various skin disorders. Apply the gel right from the plant directly to the area, or apply a commercial cream.

• Ointment made from *calendula* works on skin problems because it is antibacterial, antifungal, anti-inflammatory, and antiviral.

• *Gotu kola* is an Indian herb that stimulates the regeneration of skin cells and the underlying connective tissue. Use in tincture form.

Dosages may vary, depending on the duration and severity of your symptoms. Follow directions on the package, or consult a qualified herbal practitioner.

What makes it worse?

• I could find no mention in the medical literature of any specific nutrient that has been documented to make scleroderma worse. Since the disorder is one of too much fibrous tissue being laid down in tissues and fibrous tissue means basically collagen, the chief protein component of fibrous tissue, and since vitamin C is required for the proper manufacture of collagen, it would seem to make medical sense that you wouldn't want to take in more vitamin C than absolutely that amount essential to prevent deficiency. That should mean an intake in the neighborhood of 60 mg per day. I have no hard science to support this thinking; it is just an intriguing theory.

—————— Seborrheic Dermatitis ——————

What is it?

Dry scaling patches of skin can occur for a variety of reasons. When the patches involve the scalp, eyebrows, skin behind the ears, the face, especially the creases beside the nose, the navel, skin over the breastbone, and the eyelids, the cause is usually seborrheic dermatitis (also called seborrhea). This kind of chronic dermatitis seems to run in families, but nutrition, hormones, infection, and physical or emotional stress may cause flare-ups of activity. Seborrhea is primarily an inflammatory problem, although the irritated skin occasionally becomes infected, too. One theory exists, however, that suggests that the root cause of this kind of dermatitis might be an allergic reaction to the common scalp yeast fungus *Pityrosporum ovale* and, therefore, that antifungal medications might help. Indeed the drug ketoconazole does seem to stop the scaling in some seborrhea sufferers, but not all. Since inflammation and infection still play important roles in this skin disorder, nutritional therapies that decrease inflammation or that improve your resistance to infection should help.

What helps it?

See listings for Autoimmune Disorders, Dermatitis, and Immune System Health.

Herbal remedies

See listings for Autoimmune Disorders, Dermatitis, and Immune System Health.

What makes it worse?

See listings for Autoimmune Disorders, Dermatitis, and Immune System Health.

Shingles
(see Herpes Zoster)

Sinus Infection

What is it?

Some people seem to be always afflicted with infections in their sinuses, hardly whipping one infection down before the next one begins, bouncing from one antibiotic to another. If this picture describes you, here's my advice. Ask your personal physician or an ear, nose, and throat specialist to thoroughly evaluate your sinuses, including sinus X-ray studies. Be certain that you don't keep getting infected because of some structural abnormality in the sinus cavities, such as polyps or cysts. Also consult with an allergy specialist to be certain that it's not untreated allergies to pollen, weeds, trees, dust, pets, or foods that keep things stirred up. An inflamed sinus tract will more easily infect. As far as what nutrition can do to help, I have already described the nutrients that help related conditions and frequent infections almost wherever they occur.

What helps it?

• See Allergies, Common Cold, and Immune System Health.

Herbal remedies

• See Allergies, Common Cold, and Immune System Health.

What makes it worse?

• See Allergies, Common Cold, and Immune System Health.

——————— Skin Cancer ———————

What is it?

Cancerous growths of the skin occur, as cancers do in all tissues, when something damages the DNA (the genetic material in the nucleus, or "command and control" center) of a cell. Once the damage occurs, the cell goes haywire and ceases to function normally or to obey the body's normal controls. These "rogue" cells then begin to rapidly divide and invade the normal tissue around them. You depend upon a vigilant and ever-ready immune defense system to spot these cells gone bad, to attack them, and to destroy them. Most of the time, that happens without a hitch. Sometimes, however, one such cell slips through and forms a small cancer. In your skin, the damaging stimulus is usually ultraviolet irradiation from sun exposure, which sets the stage for development of one of the three basic types of skin cancer: basal cell carcinoma, squamous cell carcinoma, and malignant melanoma. It is believed that 20% of Americans who live to age 65 will develop skin cancer. Eight hundred thousand cases are diagnosed yearly. An even more disturbing statistic is the one that shows a steady 4% rise in melanoma yearly since 1973.

Basal cell cancers usually arise in sun-exposed areas of skin, such as the face, nose, ears, chest, and arms, but occasionally in other areas. They are slow growing, pearly in appearance, often with tiny capillary blood vessels attached to them. They originate, as the name implies, from rogue cells deep at the base of the skin.

Squamous cell cancers arise from damage to cells closer to the surface. They are very common on the faces, lips, noses, ears, arms, and upper chest of fair-skinned people who spend too much time in the sun—farmers, lifeguards, construction workers, sun worshipers. These cancers also grow fairly slowly and can be removed by simple office surgery procedures when caught early.

Malignant melanoma, as its name implies, is the bad actor of skin cancers. These cancers develop when pigment-producing cells go haywire. They tend not to look like much at first, but can rapidly spread to sites in the body far distant from their origins. It is these kinds of skin cancer that make it so important that you notice any change in a mole. If it grows, changes color, changes shape, or becomes painful or itchy, you should immediately consult your personal physician, a dermatologist, or a surgeon adept at skin cancer removal, for an examination. If the mole is suspicious to the physician, he or she should refer you to an expert in melanoma removal (unless he or she so qualifies) to minimize the chance of spread of the bad cells to other areas by improper removal.

In addition to surgical treatments—and let me stress that especially in the case of melanoma I said *in addition* to and *not instead of* them—what can nutrition offer? Let's see.

What helps it?

• The risk of malignant melanoma appears to be higher in people with the lowest intakes of *vitamin E*. Because vitamin E is a powerful antioxidant, this effect may be because it softens the damage that ultraviolet irradiation causes to the skin cells. Recommendation: Take vitamin E in a dose of 400 to 800 IU per day. Good food sources include asparagus, green leafy vegetables, raw nuts, wheat germ, and cold-pressed vegetable oils. Warning: Vitamin E can cause elevation of blood pressure in some people. Please refer to the listing for this vitamin for information about how to slowly and safely increase your intake to the recommended level.

• In laboratory animals, supplemental *beta-carotene* along with vitamin E caused epidermoid cancers (the same general type of cell as those of the skin) to shrink in size. Again, what this may mean to human skin cancers is at this point uncertain. Recommendation: While I cannot cite any hard science to give a specific recommendation for beta-carotene, I would encourage you to not let yourself become deficient in this forerunner of vitamin A by eating a diet containing plenty of the foods rich in it, such as dark green leafy vegetables and yellow-orange vegetables. You may even want to supplement your intake with 25,000 IU (15 mg) of beta-carotene in capsule form.

• Deficiencies of *selenium,* because it is necessary for your body to manufacture its own potent free radical scavenger (see oxidation and free radicals, beginning on page 18), may increase the risk for several types of cancer, including skin cancer. Selenium has also been shown to protect against UV damage. Recommendation: Take selenium aspartate in a dose of 100 to 200 *micro*grams daily.

• *Vitamin C* is a powerful anticancer agent that boosts immunity. Recommendation: 5000 to 20,000 mg daily, in divided doses.

• *Vitamin A* contains potent antioxidants that destroy free radicals. Recommendation: 50,000 to 100,000 IU daily for 10 days. Use emulsion form for better assimilation and greater safety at high doses. Warning: If you are pregnant, do not exceed 8,000 IU daily.

• A *diet high in antioxidants* is important in preventing cancer. Eat carrots, sweet potatoes, squash, spinach, broccoli, cabbage, turnips, and citrus fruits.

• In addition, because a healthy immune system offers you the best protection against the development of cancers in the first place, you may want to also read the information provided under Immune System Health.

Herbal remedies
• See Breast Cancer.

What makes it worse?
• Certainly, you must avoid *sun exposure* by wearing blocking preparations on your skin, including lips and ears, and wearing protective clothing and a wide-brimmed hat when outdoors. And when at all possible, stay in the shade.

• A diet high in *polyunsaturated fats* may increase your risk for malignant melanoma. No explanation has yet emerged for why these fats should increase risk, only that they may. Just because a fat or oil is not from an animal source or saturated doesn't make it good for you. Recommendation: Limit your intake of total fat and oil to 30% of your day's calories; 20% of these calories should be polyunsaturated fats and 10% saturated.

• Certain *medications* increase your risk for skin cancer because they make the skin more susceptible to sun damage. These include antibiotics, antidepressants, diuretics, antihistamines, sedatives, estrogen, and acne medications such as retinoic acid. Recommendation: Talk to your health care provider or pharmacist if you suspect any medication you are taking may increase your risk for skin cancer.

• See also Immune System Health, which contains information about nutrients that may hamper the ability of your immune defense system to guard you well.

Skin Health

What to take

Follow the guidelines suggested under Adult Supplementation, General, paying particular attention to the vitamins and minerals listed below:

- essential fatty acids
- zinc
- beta-carotene
- vitamin E
- vitamin C

Solar Keratosis
(see Age Spots)

Sore Throat

What is it?

Sore throats need no introduction. We've all had them at one time or another. They occur most commonly from infection with viruses, bacteria, and fungi (yeast), but chronic drainage from allergies can make your throat sore as well. Sometimes sore throats occur when stomach acid backs up (refluxes) into the esophagus and back of the throat.

Any sore throat that lasts more than a few days that you cannot gargle away with warm salt water, or has fever or a rash associated with it, demands the attention of your physician. But once you have a good idea—from among the many possibilities—of what's causing your throat to be sore, nutrition can help.

What helps it?

See Allergies, Common Cold, Heartburn, Immune System Health, Yeast Infections.

Herbal remedies

• See Allergies, Common Cold, Heartburn, Immune System Health, Yeast Infections.

• *Eucalyptus* helps ease sore throats in two ways: It has a cooling effect on inflamed tissue, and it has astringent action as well. Crush the leaves and make a tea.

What makes it worse?

See Allergies, Common Cold, Heartburn, Immune System Health, Yeast Infections.

Sprue

(see Celiac Sprue)

Stomach Cancer

What is it?

Cancers of the stomach occur most commonly in men over age 40, representing the eighth most frequently occurring male cancer. Early symptoms of stomach cancer very often mimic indigestion or heartburn: vague fullness in the stomach, nausea, belching, and loss of appetite, especially for meat symptoms that often don't prompt a visit to the doctor. Stomach cancers occur more commonly in people who have chronic stomach ulcers, severe stomach irritation and damage from vitamin B_{12} deficiency, and abuse alcohol.

If you suffer from more than a week or two of these kinds of symptoms—especially if you are a man over 40—you must be certain to have your personal physician check the symptoms. Don't ignore these seemingly innocuous symptoms, treating them yourself, hoping they will go away. In stomach cancer—as in most cancers—the name of the game is prevention: leading a lifestyle that reduces your risk. There are a number of nutritional dos and don'ts that may help. Let's look.

What helps it?

• Deficiency of *vitamin A* may increase your risk for stomach cancer. Recommendation: Because your body can store vitamin A, building up levels that could become toxic to you, I recommend that you increase your intake of *beta-carotene,* the vitamin A relative that your body converts to active vitamin A as it needs it. Eat more foods containing beta-carotene, such as dark green leafy vegetables and yellow-orange vegetables. And you can supplement your food intake with 25,000 IU beta-carotene per day.

• Deficiency of *vitamin B₁₂* can cause damage to the stomach (called atrophic gastritis) that increases your risk for stomach cancer. Recommendation: Take 500 *micro*grams vitamin B_{12}, in sublingual form once a week. Because the B vitamins work best together, you should also take 50 to 100 mg of B-complex each day.

• Your best defense against cancer is a *healthy diet.* In addition to antioxidant vitamins and minerals, there are naturally occurring substances in foods that have powerful anti-cancer properties. These include beta-carotene, quercetin, indoles and thiocyanates (in cruciferous vegetables), and omega-3 fatty acids. Recommendation: Eat an abundance of carrots, cantaloupe, squash, broccoli, cauliflower, onions, and tuna.

• *Phytochemicals* are naturally occurring substances in plants that protect the body against cancer. Cancer formation is a multistep process, and phytochemicals block one or more of those steps. Almost every grain, legume, fruit, and vegetable has been found to contain these substances. Recommendation: Base your meals around fruits, vegetables, and grains. These can be eaten raw or cooked; the healthy properties of phytochemicals are not affected by cooking.

• People with high intakes of *vitamin C* are less likely to develop stomach cancer. Some researchers believe that one of the major causes of stomach cancer involves the damaging effect of a certain class of chemicals, called nitroso compounds, on the stomach. Among these, the nitrosamines that are produced when meat is fried or burned on the grill have already gained national news attention as potential cancer-causing substances. Because vitamin C is a powerful antioxidant, it helps to protect the stomach from the damage these caustic chemicals cause. (For more information, refer to oxidation and free radicals, beginning on page 18.) Vitamin C may also improve the killing power of certain immune defenders, further helping to protect you. Recommendation: Take a minimum of 1000 mg of time-release vitamin C 5 to 7 times a day. If you suffer indigestion from taking vitamin C in tablet form, you may tolerate taking the crystalline powder better. Please refer to the discussion of this vitamin for more information and how to use the powder.

• Deficiency of *vitamin E* may also increase your risk of stom ach cancer. Again, most likely because vitamin E is a potent antioxidant, it helps to protect the lining of the stomach from damage by cancer-causing chemicals in the foods we eat. Recommendation: Take vitamin E, as d-alpha-tocopherol succinate, in a dose of 400 to 600 IU per day. Warning: Vitamin E can cause elevated blood pressure in some people. Please refer to the discussion of this vitamin for information about how to slowly and safely increase your dose to the recommended level.

• Because *selenium* works with vitamin E when your body produces its own potent free radical scavenger, glutathione peroxidase, a deficiency of selenium may make you unable to make this important natural antioxidant. Recommendation: Take selenium aspartate in a dose of 100 to 200 *micro*grams per day.

• Your body uses dietary *essential fatty acids* as the raw materials to produce a family of powerful body chemicals called the eicosinoids. Some of these chemical messengers are "good" for you, reducing inflammation, pain, and swelling, and others are "bad." (Please refer to the Yin and Yang of Human Health, pages 24–27, for more information about these substances.) Some research suggests that these messengers, the "good" ones at least, may inhibit the growth of cancer cells, so encouraging your body to make more of the "good" messengers can only help. Recommendation: To a nutritionally sound basic diet (see Macronutrients on page 23), add gamma-linoleic acid (GLA) and EPA fish oil in a ratio of 1:4 (GLA:EPA) 1 to 3 times daily. The EicoPro essential fatty acid product manufactured by Eicotec, Inc., of Marblehead, Massachusetts, contains ultrapure sources of linoleic acid and fish oils already combined in the proper ratio. If you cannot get that product, you can purchase linoleic acid in a product called evening primrose oil at most health and nutrition stores, and EPA fish oil as well. Because it is not as pure a form, the milligram dosing will be different. You can make a reasonable substitute by combining evening primrose oil capsules with fish oil capsules plus vitamin E. Take 500 mg of evening primrose oil (a source of linoleic acid in capsule form), plus 1000 mg EPA fish oil, plus 200 IU vitamin E 1 to 3 times a day. (Warning to diabetics: EPA fish oil can cause blood sugar fluctuations in some diabetics. Carefully monitor your blood sugar if you use this supplemental oil and discontinue its use if your blood sugar becomes difficult to control.)

• *Vitamin B_3* (niacin) has been discovered to play a major role in preventing and treating cancer, probably because B vitamins improve circulation and build red blood cells. Recommendation: Take 100 mg daily. Warning: Do not take niacin if you have a liver disorder, gout, or high blood pressure.

Herbal remedies
• See Breast Cancer.

What makes it worse?
• Foods containing *nitrate,* a food additive. Recommendation: Eliminate from your diet bacon, luncheon meats, hot dogs, and smoked or cured meats.

• Limit your intake of *soybean products.* They contain enzyme inhibitors.

• Avoid refined *sugars.* A significant correlation turned up in a 1985 study of 50,000 German households between the intake of refined sugars and stomach cancer in both men and women. Sugar has a strongly irritative and damaging effect on the intestinal lining, not to mention its role in depressing your immune defenses. Recommendation: Eliminate all refined sugars from your diet: table sugar, corn syrup, high-fructose corn syrup, molasses, and all products made with these substances.

• Although several studies have reported that people who develop stomach cancer drink more *milk* than people who do not, I do not feel that this finding implicates milk or even the saturated fat in the milk as a cancer-causing agent. The association may be as straight-forward as this: People who have stomach cancer typically develop symptoms of indigestion, sometimes for years before being diagnosed. Since milk is the hands-down favorite old wives' remedy for indigestion, perhaps these people drink more milk because they have more indigestion. Recommendation: I remain unconvinced that in the case of milk and stomach cancer there is a cause and effect at work.

Stress

What is it?
You've heard of it, probably suffered from it, but do you understand what it is? Let's look. In medicine, we say that stress occurs when events of life overwhelm our capacity to deal with them. The

stressful event can be a good one (a promotion, a new job, a move to a new home, a marriage) or a bad one (loss of a job, loss of a loved one, divorce, a threat to financial security or health), but either kind of event can require emotional adjustments that may overwhelm us. Throughout our lives, each of us will face one or more of these emotional challenges; some we may handle with unruffled aplomb and others may stagger us beneath their weight. Our reaction to stress does not necessarily equate with the magnitude of the event, but rather with our own perception of its importance—that is, for a small child, the loss of a favorite toy will elicit sorrowful wails or a teenager may rage and rail over hair that won't cooperate but may accept the death of a loved one with outward calm. Typical reactions to stress include: anxiety, depression, escape (running away, withdrawing into ourselves, drinking alcohol, engaging in extramarital affairs), rage, and fear. Under stress, we may become restless, irritable, tired, or tense. We may want to sleep all the time or be unable to sleep much at all. We may eat voraciously and gain weight or find food unappealing and lose pounds. And we may even develop physical complaints, such as headache, joint and muscle aches, vision problems, skin rashes, gastritis, ulcers, or other gastrointestinal disturbances.

Whether the stress is good or bad, emotional, physical, or both, the toll it exacts on your body is much the same. One critical area that especially takes a beating under stress is your immune system. In the dozen or so years of my general practice, I can think back to more than one bride with strep throat on the eve of her wedding, countless patients falling ill before a big trip, singers and actors developing bad colds under the hectic schedule of a performance. I even had a patient who developed a bladder infection every time her mother-in-law came to town. People under stress fall victim more easily to infections because the body's production of immune fighters falls off measurably during periods of physical or emotional stress. Although you may not be able to change the stressful event (and if it's a good one, may not even want to), you *can* withstand the stress better with good nutrition. The role of vitamins, minerals, and other nutrients in helping you combat stress rests primarily on bolstering your immune system and replacing those nutrients that your body uses in greater amounts during stress. Let's take a look at what nutrition can offer.

What helps it?

• *Proper dietary construction* forms the base of your nutritional fortress against stress. Under stress your body's requirement for complete protein increases from a base level of about 0.5 gram of protein per pound of lean body tissue (see Macronutrients, page 23, for more information) to a need of at least 0.6 grams for each pound of lean body mass. This increased need occurs because under stress your body uses amino acids (the building blocks of protein) to produce more "stress hormones." Recommendation: Using the information in the eicosinoid discussion, calculate your body's lean tissue weight (lean body mass), then feed it a minimum of 0.6 grams of high-quality complete protein per day. By that rule, if you calculated a 100-pound lean tissue weight, you would need to eat 100×0.6 or 60 grams of protein per day. A good rule of thumb is that 1 ounce of lean meat, fish, poultry, or seafood provides about 7 grams of protein, 1 ounce of fluid milk provides about 1 gram of protein, and 1 egg white provides about 6 grams of protein. So a daily 60 gram protein need could come from 8 to 9 ounces of lean animal protein, or from some combination of the protein choices above.

You should design a diet for yourself under stress that provides about 35% of your day's calories as high-quality protein (with enough to feed your lean tissues as a bare minimum amount), another 35% as low-starch fruits and vegetables, and another 30% as fat (20% monounsaturated or polyunsaturated oils and 10% animal fats).

• It is common for people suffering from stress to be deficient in *magnesium*. This deficiency can result in anxiety, fear, and, in some extreme cases, hallucinations. Recommendation: Supplement with 1000 mg daily. To balance the magnesium, take a 2000 mg supplement of calcium as well.

• *Pantothenic acid* (vitamin B_5) is an antistress vitamin needed by the thymus gland. Recommendation: Take 500 mg daily.

• *Vitamin B_{12}* is involved in the production of myelin, which covers and protects our nerves. The association of a deficiency of this vitamin and impaired nervous system function is well established. Recommendation: Take 100 to 500 *micro*grams daily.

• The *B vitamins* are necessary for proper functioning of the nervous system. Recommendation: If possible, have your physician administer intramuscular injections of 1 cc B-complex weekly. Injections work more quickly. If you must use a tablet, take 100 mg daily

• Your need for *vitamin C* (ascorbic acid) increases dramatically under stress. Recommendation: If you do not currently take vitamin C in supplemental form, begin by taking a single 500 mg time-release capsule of vitamin C daily. After several days, increase your dose to twice daily, then three times daily, then four times per day. Please read the discussion of vitamin C beginning on page 50 for information on how to increase your daily intake of vitamin C to your level of tolerance. Bear in mind that it is not uncommon for an adult to tolerate 4 to 15 grams of vitamin C per day under physical or emotional stress. Your bowel will tell you when you've gone over your limit.

• *Zinc* protects the cells from free radical damage. Recommendation: Take 50 mg daily in zinc gluconate form.

• Stress reduces your *potassium* supply. Recommendation: Take 99 mg daily.

• *Amino acids* supply protein, which the body uses rapidly during times of stress. Recommendation: Visit your local natural foods store and purchase a free-form amino complex. Take according to the label.

• See also Immune System Health.

Herbal remedies

• *Bilberry* prevents destruction of cells throughout the body.

• *Catnip* is an antistress herb that also promotes sleep.

• To relax the nerves, use *chamomile*. It is a pleasant-tasting sleep aid.

• *Hops* eases nervousness and stress.

• To achieve a total mind-body relaxation, use *kava kava*.

• *Skullcap* is good for nervous disorders. It also promotes sleep.

• When taken at bedtime, *valerian* is a powerful sleep aid. Taken anytime, it calms the nerves.

Dosages may vary, depending on the duration and severity of your symptoms. Consult a qualified herbal practitioner, and let your physician know of your desire to use herbs. Some herbal remedies should not be used in combination with conventional pharmaceuticals.

What makes it worse?

• *Sugar* and other *refined starches* create an even bigger drain on your body's levels of vitamin C and the B vitamins.

Recommendation: Eliminate or sharply restrict your intake of these food substances, especially under stressful circumstances.

• *Processed foods* create stress on the system. Recommendation: Avoid or sharply curtail your consumption of processed foods and others that create a stressful internal environment: carbonated soft drinks, chocolate, eggs, fried foods, pork, red meat, white flour products, heavy spices, junk/snack foods.

• See also Immune System Health.

Substance Abuse

What is it?

Addiction exists when the body becomes so accustomed to the presence of a foreign substance that it can no longer function properly if the substance is withheld. This is why a person who is addicted to a drug experiences withdrawal symptoms if suddenly deprived of the drug. Signs of drug addiction include a decreased desire to work or socialize, extreme drowsiness, inattentiveness, frequent mood swings, restlessness, personality changes, and a loss of appetite. Other symptoms include slow, slurred speech and a change in the eye pupils.

The following recommended dosages are for adults. For a child under the age of 17, use half to three-quarters of the recommended dosage.

• The *B vitamins* are needed to rebuild the liver when a person is under stress. Injections work best because they are assimilated quickly. Recommendation: Under a physician's supervision, take 2 cc daily of vitamin B-complex along with 1 cc *vitamin B_{12}*.

• *Calcium* and *magnesium* nourish the central nervous system and help control tremors. Recommendation: Take 1500 mg calcium and 1000 mg magnesium at bedtime. Use chelate forms.

• *L-glutamine* promotes healthy mental functioning and has a calming effect. Recommendation: Take 500 mg 3 times daily on an empty stomach.

• *L-tyrosine* and the herb valerian root taken every 4 hours have given good results for cocaine withdrawal. Recommendation: Take 500 mg L-tyrosine twice daily on an empty stomach. Take with 2 tablets valerian root with water or juice, but not milk. Warning: Do not take tyrosine if you take an MAO (monoamine oxidose) inhibitor drug.

• *Glutathione* detoxifies drugs to reduce their harmful effect while it reduces the desire for drugs and alcohol. Recommendation: Take 1000 mg daily.

• *L-phenylalanine* is fuel for the brain and has been found to be useful in treating withdrawal symptoms. Recommendation: Take 1500 mg upon arising. Warning: Do not take if you are pregnant or nursing, or suffer from panic attacks, diabetes, high blood pressure, or PKU (phenylketonuria).

• *Pantothenic acid* is essential for the adrenal glands and for reducing stress. Recommendation: Take 500 mg 3 times daily.

• *Vitamin C* detoxifies the system and lessens the craving for drugs. Recommendation: Increase your consumption of citrus fruits, berries, leafy green vegetables, tomatoes, cantaloupe, cauliflower, potatoes, and peppers. Take 2000 mg vitamin C every 3 hours. Use a buffered form for safety at high dosages and easier assimilation.

• *Niacinamide* is important for brain function. Recommendation: Take 500 mg 3 times daily. Do NOT take niacin in place of niacinamide. High doses of niacin can be toxic.

• Minimize withdrawal symptoms by *withdrawing slowly.* The dosage should be decreased gradually over a period of 4 weeks or longer. And don't try to do it alone; seek help and counseling at a hospital or from a professionally trained expert.

Herbal remedies

• Calm your nerves using *valerian root.* To promote sleep, take this herb within an hour before bedtime.

• *Siberian ginseng* helps ease the symptoms of cocaine withdrawal. Caution: Do not take this herb if you have hypoglycemia, high blood pressure, or a heart disorder.

• Replenish your supply of minerals with *alfalfa.*

• *Burdock root and red clover* cleanse the bloodstream.

Dosages may vary, depending on the duration and severity of your symptoms. Consult a qualified herbal practitioner, and talk to your doctor before beginning herbal remedies. Some remedies cannot be used in combination with conventional pharmaceuticals.

What makes it worse?

• Most addicts suffer from malnutrition. Nutrient supplementation at high doses is essential. Emphasize raw, fresh foods in the diet to obtain their maximum nutrient content.

──────────── **Swimmer's Ear** ────────────

What is it?

Swimmer's ear—or external otitis as we call it in medicine—occurs when bacteria or fungi set up an infection in the skin of the outer ear canal. The tendency to infection increases with swimming because the ear canal remains wet much of the time, softening the skin and making it easier for the infecting agents to set up housekeeping. But swimming is only one of the factors that can make an ear canal vulnerable. Hot humid weather can trap perspiration in the canal, too frequent cleaning with cotton-tipped applicators or cleaning solutions such as alcohol can damage the skin, and conversely, impacted ear wax can trap water behind the plug and soften the skin of the canal.

Once an infection begins, however, you should consult with your physician because some infections will require antibiotic or antifungal ear drops or tablets to kill the infection. Making yourself a more resistant host, however, will help to reduce your chances of developing an infection in the first place, and nutrition definitely plays a key role in that regard.

What helps it?

• You can reduce the chance of infection of the canal by carefully drying the ear canal after swimming. Recommendation: Drain each ear canal by laying your head, ear down, on a dry towel for several minutes or by using a blow-dryer for hair drying on its lowest setting to gently dry the canal. Follow either of these maneuvers by dropping 2 or 3 drops of a mixture of ½ white vinegar and ½ rubbing alcohol into each canal.

• See also the listings for Frequent Infections and Immune System Health.

Herbal remedies

• See Chronic Ear Infection.

What makes it worse?

• See also the listing for Immune System Health.

──────────── **Tinnitus** ────────────

(see Hearing Loss)

Tiredness
(see Fatigue)

Ulcerative Colitis
(see Colon, Spastic)

Urinary Tract Infections

What are they?

Although urinary tract infections occur in both sexes, women suffer far more of them, primarily because of simple anatomical differences. The urethra (the tube leading from the bladder to the outside) in men is usually four or five inches in length and opens freely to the outside. In women, however, the tube is only about an inch or so in length, and the opening to the outside lies within the skin folds of the external genitalia, a short hop from the vaginal tract opening and only a few inches from the rectal opening. Although the urine usually remains sterile (totally free of bacteria), the same cannot be said for the vaginal or rectal tracts, both of which teem with bacteria. Women, then, are designed in a way that makes it easier for bacteria from these two adjacent areas to scuttle up that tube and into the bladder. To prevent that, nature has endowed women with a good immune defense system that constantly patrols the urethral tube on the lookout for bacteria trying to make their way in. As long as that system works well, a woman can fend off bladder and kidney infections. But let stress, illness, physical injury, or nutritional deficiency enter the picture, and the slight dip that may occur in immune defenses can leave the door open to the bacteria that are always trying to gain entry. In addition to the general nutritional recommendations you will find under Immune System Health, let me offer a few other specifics.

What helps them?

• *Water* can be your best ally. Recommendation: Drink a minimum of 64 ounces of fluid a day. A solid fluid intake will keep your bladder filling and that will encourage you to empty it often.

• Research shows that *cranberry juice* acidifies the urine, destroys bacteria buildup, and promotes healing. Recommendation: Drink at least 8 ounces of pure, unsweetened cranberry juice daily. If you cannot find pure cranberry juice, cranberry capsules can be substituted.

• *Vitamin C* helps to provide an acid environment in your urine hostile to most bacteria. Recommendation: Take a minimum of 1000 mg of vitamin C 3 to 4 times daily.

• See Immune System Health.

Herbal remedies
• See Immune System Health.

What makes them worse?
• A diet high in *sugar* increases your risk for urinary tract infections. Recommendation: If you suffer frequent bladder or kidney infections, eliminate or drastically curtail your intake of sugars, including table sugar, corn syrup, high-fructose corn syrup, molasses, and all products made with these substances.

——————— Urticaria ———————
(Hives)

What is it?
You probably know this disorder by its more common name: hives. This allergic skin rash erupts in irregularly shaped, raised, red, flat-topped itching patches that appear suddenly and then wax and wane. When you develop urticaria, it is usually because you've been around something, eaten or drunk something, taken medication, been bitten by something, or breathed in something you are allergic to. But this same kind of skin rashing can come from sun exposure, from temperature extremes (such as a very hot shower), and occasionally from stress. The cause behind the development of the hives is the release of the histamine into the skin. Refer to Allergies for more information about histamine and its role in allergic symptoms.

Because urticaria may precede more serious allergic problems, such as swelling in your breathing passages and severe low blood pressure, you should always consult with your physician about the appearance of this kind of rash. Although there are specific medications that your physician may prescribe to help combat an outbreak of hives, nutrition can also help. Let's take a look at what you can do.

What helps it?
• Hives that occur when you get out in the sun may improve by taking *beta-carotene*. Recommendation: Increase your consumption

of dark green leafy vegetables and yellow-orange vegetables rich in this vitamin A relative. You can also take 25,000 IU of supplemental beta-carotene per day.

• *Acidophilus* reduces allergic reactions. Recommendation: Take 2 capsules 3 times daily with meals.

• *Vitamin B$_{12}$* prevents nerve damage and promotes normal skin growth. Recommendation: Take 2000 *micro*grams daily. Use an under-the-tongue form.

• *Niacin* helps to prevent the release of histamine from immune defenders controlling your allergic response. Recommendation: Take niacin, as niacinamide, in a dose of 100 to 250 mg per day. Warning: Niacin can cause flushing sensations (redness and warmth of the skin) in some people. If you develop flushing, reduce your dose or discontinue the vitamin.

• *Vitamin C* along with the *bioflavonoids* helps to decrease the leakiness of capillaries that allows allergic swelling to develop in the urticarial patches, as well as around the lips and eyes and the hands. Recommendation: Take a minimum of 500 mg of vitamin C plus bioflavonoid complex 2 to 4 times daily. Increase your dose by 500 to 1000 mg in the face of an outbreak of hives. If you already take vitamin C, you can add a 500 to 1000 mg dose of bioflavonoid complex to your daily intake of C.

• To reduce outbreaks, take *vitamin D*. Recommendation: Supplement with 400 IU daily.

• *Vitamin E* is a powerful antioxidant that improves circulation to the skin tissue. Recommendation: Take 600 IU daily.

• Deficiency of *magnesium* may promote urticaria. Recommendation: Take magnesium aspartate in a dose of 250 to 500 mg per day.

• *Zinc* heals skin tissue and is necessary for maintaining proper levels of vitamin E in the blood. Recommendation: Take 50 mg daily in the form of zinc gluconate.

Herbal remedies

• Apply *aloe vera gel* directly to the hives.

• *Alfalfa, cat's claw, chamomile, echinacea, ginseng, licorice, nettle, sarsaparalla, and yellow dock* can relieve the discomfort of hives. Caution: Do not use chamomile on an ongoing basis, and avoid it completely if you are allergic to ragweed. Do not use ginseng or licorice if you have high blood pressure.

Dosages may vary, depending on the duration and severity of your symptoms. Follow package directions, or consult a qualified herbal practitioner.

What makes it worse?

• Continued exposure to any substance you are *allergic* to will, of course, keep the urticaria going. It is sometimes quite difficult to figure out what's causing the hives, and so you might want to consult an allergy specialist to perform some skin and blood testing to help you narrow your list of suspects. Once you know what to avoid, your course is simple.

——— Vegetarian Supplementation ———

What to take:

There are a variety of diets that are considered "vegetarian." A lacto-vegetarian includes plant foods and dairy products in the diet. A lacto-ovo-vegetarian consumes both dairy and eggs. These two types of vegetarian diets can easily meet the DRI for all nutrients. If you are a strict vegetarian (vegan) who eats no animal protein (no egg, milk, or fish), you need to plan more carefully to ensure adequate amounts of iron, riboflavin, calcium, zinc, and vitamin B_{12}. The American Dietetic Association supports appropriately planned vegetarian diets, and recognizes them as "healthful, nutritionally adequate, and providing health benefits in the prevention and treatment of certain diseases." These diseases include coronary artery disease, hypertension, lung and colorectal cancer, and renal disease.

• Vegetable sources of proteins, such as beans, peas, and grains, were once believed to be deficient in one or more essential amino acids. But it increasingly appears that Western vegetarians rarely show protein or amino acid deficiencies. Research has shown that vegetarians need not be concerned with combining proteins, and scientists almost universally reject this outdated concept. Part of the reason that balancing amino acids is unnecessary is because the body's requirement for essential amino acids seems to be much less important than researchers once believed. Good sources of protein include legumes, lentils, nuts, soy products, tempeh, tofu, and whole grains.

• If you are a vegan, I suggest taking the following supplement just to be sure you're getting enough of these vital nutrients:

Riboflavin, 50 mg per day.

Iron should be supplemented only if you are deficient. Iron deficiency affects about 10% of America's population. Consume iron-rich foods such as dried beans, dark green leafy vegetables, blackstrap molasses, and cooked lentils. You can boost your iron absorption by eating foods rich in vitamin C at each meal. Vitamin C assists with iron uptake. Broccoli, cauliflower, dark leafy greens, tomatoes, cantaloupe, oranges, strawberries, and honeydew are high in vitamin C.

Eliminating caffeine with meals is another way to boost iron absorption. Coffee has been shown to decrease iron absorption by 39%, tea by 64%. This probably happens due to tannins and other substances that bind with the iron and make assimilation more difficult.

If you believe you are deficient in iron, seek the advice of your physician or nutritionist. The daily recommended dosage is 18 mg.

• *Vitamin B_{12}* is found naturally only in animal products. Nutritional yeast, fortified soy milk, and enriched cereals are also possible sources. The most reliable source, however, is a supplement in sublingual (under the tongue) form in a dose of 300 *micro*grams daily. Take a single 50 mg B-complex supplement along with your B_{12}.

• *Calcium* requirements for vegans may be somewhat lower than those for meat-eaters because vegans tend to consume less protein. High levels of protein intake increase the amount of calcium lost from the body. But calcium is an important nutrient, and it is vital that adequate amounts are absorbed. Foods high in calcium include dark leafy green vegetables, broccoli, legumes, fortified soy milk, and blackstrap molasses. Note that these are some of the same foods high in iron content.

The recommended daily dosage of calcium is 1000 mg daily for adults aged 19 through 50, and 1200 mg daily for adults 51 years and older. Again, supplement only if you suspect a deficiency and have discussed it with your physician.

• Studies show *zinc* intake to be lower or comparable in vegetarians compared to nonvegetarians. Although most studies show that zinc levels in hair, serum, and saliva are in the normal range in vegetarians, there is a low bioavailability of zinc from plant foods. And since we don't completely understand the effects of marginal zinc levels, it is important to meet the daily dosage of 50 mg. Foods high in zinc include whole grains, tofu, miso, nuts, wheat germ, and legumes. Supplement only after consultation with your physician.

─────────────── **Vertigo** ───────────────

(see Inner Ear Dysfunction)

─────────────── **Wound Healing** ───────────────

What is it?

When you cut, burn, or otherwise damage your skin, healing forces immediately spring into action. In the first 48 hours, your body's repair cells begin to quickly lay down new fibers of connective tissue to bridge the gap or patch the damaged area. Over the next couple of weeks, this first wave of repair completes the initial job of scarring the wound closed. Over a period of the next 2 years, slower-working artisans of repair move into the area to remodel the quick initial work, improving the appearance and strength of the scar. Nutrition plays an important role in healing wounds. Let me show you how.

What helps it?

• *Proper basic nutrition,* providing all the building materials your repair machinery needs to do the job, is an absolute requirement for speedy wound healing. Malnourishment, such as often occurs in third world countries or among our own country's frail older people, hinders the body's ability to heal wounds. Recommendation: Refer to Macronutrients on page 23 to construct a diet meeting all essential requirements for protein, carbohydrate, and fat. You will find instructions there about how to determine the amount of protein your body needs to flourish, grow, and repair itself.

• Your body uses dietary *essential fatty acids* as the raw materials to produce a family of powerful body chemicals called the eicosinoids, which are important in wound healing and the formation of the best possible scar. (Please refer to the Yin and Yang of Human Health, pages 24–27, for more information about these substances.) Recommendation: To a nutritionally sound basic diet (see Macronutrients on page 23), add gamma-linoleic acid (GLA) and EPA fish oil in a ratio of 1:4 (GLA:EPA) 1 to 3 times daily. The EicoPro essential fatty acid product manufactured by Eicotec, Inc.

of Marblehead, Massachusetts, contains ultrapure sources of linoleic acid and fish oils already combined in the proper ratio. If you cannot get that product, you can purchase linoleic acid in a product called evening primrose oil at most health and nutrition stores, and EPA fish oil as well. Because it is not as pure a form, the milligram dosing will be different. You can make a reasonable substitute by combining evening primrose oil capsules with fish oil capsules plus vitamin E. Take 500 mg of evening primrose oil (a source of linoleic acid in capsule form), plus 1000 mg EPA fish oil, plus 200 IU vitamin E 1 to 3 times a day. (Warning to diabetics: EPA fish oil can cause blood sugar fluctuations in some diabetics. Carefully monitor your blood sugar if you use this supplemental oil and discontinue its use if your blood sugar becomes difficult to control.)

• You can also apply *essential fatty acid oils* to the healing scar to improve its appearance. The Eicotec, Inc., manufacturer of Marblehead, Massachusetts, makes a product called Eicoderm, which to my knowledge is the only commercially available essential fatty acid preparation specifically designed to absorb easily into the skin. Recommendation: Apply Eicoderm oil twice daily to your skin. If you cannot find this product, you may apply the contents of an evening primrose oil capsule to the healing scar twice daily, but the oil doesn't penetrate as readily and tends to be sticky.

• Supplementation of *pantothenic acid,* one of the B vitamins, may help to speed the normal healing process. Recommendation: Take 250 mg of pantothenic acid twice a day along with a 50 to 100 mg dose of B-complex.

• Deficiency of *thiamine* may hinder the laying down of collagen (the chief protein of fibrous tissue used to repair damaged skin). Recommendation: Take 100 mg thiamine daily along with 50 mg of B-complex.

• Deficiency of *vitamin A* can lead to the laying down of a weaker scar. Recommendation: Because your body stores vitamin A, potentially toxic levels of the vitamin can build up over time. With an injury, however, I would recommend that you take vitamin A in a dose of 10,000 IU per day for approximately 1 week, then switch to beta-carotene in a daily dose of 25,000 IU.

• Your body must have *vitamin C* to hook the subunits of collagen, the chief protein of fibrous repair tissue, tightly together. Deficiency of vitamin C leads to weak collagen that more easily tears and breaks down. Refer to the discussion of this important vitamin in the A-to-Z Nutrient listings as well as to Scurvy, its deficiency disease, for more information about vitamin C's role in building strong tissues. Recommendation: Take a minimum of 2,000 mg of vitamin C 2 to 3 times daily following injury.

• *Vitamin E* helps to reduce the scarring of wounds both when taken by mouth and when applied to the skin. Recommendation: Following injury, take vitamin E, as d-alpha-tocopherol succinate, in a dose of 600 to 800 IU per day. Once the wound is sealed (no raw, open, or weeping areas are visible), begin to massage the contents of a single vitamin E capsule into the developing scar twice a day.

• The minerals *copper, zinc, and manganese* all are needed to form strong collagen for repairing wounds. Their main function is to increase absorption of other necessary nutrients, such as vitamin C. Recommendation: If you eat fresh leafy greens, organ meats, or whole grain products on a daily basis, it is highly unlikely that you need to supplement copper. However, copper is essential for the utilization of vitamin C, so take 2 mg daily if you suspect a deficiency. Take 20 mg of zinc and 20 mg of manganese. You should always take minerals in chelated form (see pages 30–31, Section I) to ensure that you don't become deficient in one mineral from taking increased amounts of another one.

Herbal remedies

• *Tea tree oil* makes an excellent wound healer due to its antiseptic action, which fights bacteria and fungi. If you have sensitive skin, pure oil may irritate it. If this is the case, dilute by putting several drops in a couple teaspoons of vegetable oil.

• Commission E advises using *calendula* to reduce inflammation and heal wounds. It is probably most effective in cream form for this purpose.

• *Comfrey* contains allantoin, which heals wounds. Apply it directly to the wound, either by rubbing fresh leaves on the area, or by using commercial creams.

• *Arnica* disinfects cuts and other wounds. Commission E recommends that you apply arnica flowers directly to wounds. For a compress, use 1 to 2 teaspoons per cup of boiling water. Steep until cool, soak a clean cloth in it, and apply.

• *Garlic* is a natural antibiotic. Cut a clove and apply it directly to the wound.

Dosages may vary, depending on the duration and severity of your symptoms. Follow package directions, or consult a qualified herbal practitioner.

What makes it worse?

• I know of no specific nutrients that of themselves impede wound healing.

Yeast Infections

What is it?

When we speak of a "yeast" infection, what we usually mean is infection with a specific fungus, *Candida albicans*. Virtually all of us have "colonies" of this usually harmless yeast fungus living peacefully in our intestinal tract (and vaginal tract in women). *Candida* behaves in an opportunistic fashion, by which I mean it lives peacefully, minding its own business, keeping quiet, knowing its place, if you will, until something provides an opportunity for it to rise up in revolt. That something might be a course of antibiotics that wipes out all the competing bacteria in the area, or a severe infection that occupies your immune system on other fronts, or diabetes, or diseases such as AIDS that cripple the immune system. Whatever the cause, given the opportunity, the yeast fungi begin to grow unrestricted and causes infection. In the mouth, overgrowth of yeast causes a disorder known as thrush, in which white patches form on the inner surface of the cheeks, lips, and throat. In babies, the yeast makes its move when wet or dirty diapers remain too long against tender skin, causing a diaper rash. In women, courses of antibiotics may kill off the friendly bacteria in the vaginal tract, paving the way for yeast to grow, causing the typical itchy white discharge called a yeast infection.

What can you do nutritionally to help curb the opportunities for yeast overgrowth? Let's see.

What helps it?

• *Proper dietary construction* is the place to begin, because it will not only eliminate some of the foods and substances you will need to avoid, but it will provide you with everything you need to nurture a healthy immune system to keep the yeast in check. Refer to Macronutrients on page 23, and from the guidelines there, construct a basic diet for yourself that first provides you with sufficient dietary protein to preserve and maintain your lean tissues (about $\frac{1}{2}$ gram of complete protein for every pound of your lean body weight). You'll find methods to determine how much you need there, too. Lean protein should constitute about 30% of your day's total calories. Another 40% should come from low-starch vegetables and fruits. Restrict your intake of the higher-starch vegetables, such as corn, potatoes, and wheat, including cornmeal and flour. When you are inclined to develop yeast infections, you want to eliminate yeast-containing foods and mold-containing foods, which mean breads, rolls, beer, and aged cheeses. The final 30% of your diet should come from cold-pressed oils (about 20%) and saturated fats (about 10%).

• *Biotin* is essential in healing this disorder, as it inhibits yeast. Recommendation: 300 *micro*grams 3 times daily.

• To restore normal vaginal bacteria, use *Acidophilus*. Recommendation: Take 2 capsules 3 times daily, with food. Some people who tend to develop yeast infections may be deficient in *folic acid*. Recommendation: Take folic acid 2 mg per day along with a 50 mg B-complex supplement. The B vitamins work best together.

• A true *deficiency of iron* can increase your chances of developing recurring yeast infections. And in the case of true deficiency, supplementing iron will help. Because overloading yourself with iron can be detrimental when you aren't deficient, you should ask your physician to test your blood to determine whether you need to take extra iron. Recommendation: If deficient, you should take 10 to 20 mg per day of iron glycinate (a chelated iron supplement). If you cannot find such a chelated iron supplement, you may take 90 mg ferrous sulfate twice daily along with 500 mg time-release vitamin C, which will help you absorb the iron.

• *Vitamin A* is a potent free radical scavenger that aids in vaginal healing. Recommendation: Take 50,000 IU daily. Warning: Do not exceed 8000 IU daily if you are pregnant.

• Yeast infection can lead to *vitamin B* deficiency. Recommendation: Take 100 mg of a yeast-free formula daily.

• When your body is fighting infection, you need extra amounts of *vitamin D, calcium, and magnesium*. Recommedation: Take 400 IU vitamin D, 1500 mg calcium, and 750 mg magnesium.

• Deficiency of *selenium* may increase your tendency to develop yeast infections, although we don't understand exactly why. Recommendation: Take 100 *micro*grams selenium aspartate per day.

• Deficiency of *zinc* may increase your tendency to develop yeast infections, because among other reasons, it reduces the killing power of certain immune fighters against the yeast. Recommendation: Take a chelated form of zinc, such as zinc aspartate or zinc picolinate, in a dose of 20 mg per day. Warning: Supplementation of zinc in its ionic form can create deficiencies of other minerals, such as copper, by competing with them for absorption from the intestine. Chelation of the minerals (see pages 30–31, Section I) prevents this competition to get into the body, allowing you to fully absorb each of them.

• Normalizing your intake of *essential fatty acids* may improve your resistance to yeast infections, but we don't understand exactly why. Certainly, the "good" prostaglandin messengers seem to boost immune function, but at this point, there is no hard science to verify this theory. Recommendation: To a nutritionally sound basic diet (see discussion on page 515), add gamma-linoleic acid (GLA) and EPA fish oil in a ratio of 1:4 (GLA:EPA) 1 to 3 times daily. The EicoPro essential fatty acid product manufactured by Eicotec, Inc., of Marblehead, Massachusetts, contains ultrapure sources of linoleic acid and fish oils already combined in the proper ratio. If you cannot get that product, you can purchase linoleic acid in a product called evening primrose oil at most health and nutrition stores, and EPA fish oil as well. Because it is not as pure a form, the milligram dosing will be different. You can make a reasonable substitute by combining evening primrose oil capsules with fish oil capsules plus vitamin E. Take 500 mg of evening primrose oil (a source of linoleic acid in capsule form), plus 1000 mg EPA fish oil, plus 200 IU vitamin E 1 to 3 times a day. (Warning to diabetics: EPA fish oil can cause blood sugar fluctuations in some diabetics. Carefully monitor your blood sugar if you use this supplemental oil and discontinue its use if your blood sugar becomes difficult to control.)

Herbal remedies

• Because it stimulates white blood cells to soak up yeast, *echinacea* is especially effective in treating this disorder.

• *Garlic* is used to treat yeast infections because it is an antibiotic.

• *Goldenrod* contains compounds that battle *Candida* organisms. Make an astringent tea and drink it, or use it as a douche.

• *Sage* contains a number of *anti-Candida* compounds.

• *Cranberry* helps treat candida infections. Drink pure, unsweetened cranberry juice, at least 2 or 3 glasses daily.

• *Tea tree oil* is a powerful antiyeast herb.

• American researchers found that an extract of *spicebush bark* had powerful action against yeast infections.

Dosages may vary, depending on the duration and severity of your symptoms. Follow package directions, or consult a qualified herbal practitioner.

What makes it worse?

A diet high in *sugar* promotes yeast growth in the intestinal tract. Recommendation: Eliminate or sharply reduce your intake of refined sugars of all types, including table sugar, corn syrup, high-fructose corn syrup, molasses, honey, and all products made with them.

BIBLIOGRAPHY

"Aim for the Target." *Natural Health.* (May 1999), pp. 96–97.

Angier, Natalie. "Chemists Learn Why Vegetables Are Good for You." *New York Times,* April 13, 1993.

Atkins, Robert C. *Dr. Atkins' Nutrition Breakthrough.* New York: Bantam Books, 1986.

Balch, James F., M.D., and Phyllis A. Balch, C.N.C. *Prescription for Nutritional Healing.* New York: Avery Publishing Group, 1997.

Braverman, Eric R. "Sports and Exercise: Nutritional Augmentation and Health Benefits." *Journal of Orthomolecular Medicine* 6, nos. 3 & 4 (1991), pp. 191–201.

Cathcart, R. F. "The Third Face of Vitamin C." *Journal of Orthomolecular Medicine* 7, no. 4 (1992), pp. 197–200.

Challem, Jack. "How to Use Nutritional Supplements." *Natural Health.* (March/April 1993) pp. 88–105.

Challem, Jack and Renate Lewis. "What's Missing from the RDAs?" *Natural Health* (January/February 1993), pp. 57–59.

Cheraskin, E. "Vitamin C . . . Who Needs It?" Excerpted in *Health and Nutrition Update* 7, no. 4 (Winter, 1992), pp. 4–16.

Commission on Life Sciences, National Research Council. Food and Nutrition Board. *Recommended Dietary Allowances.* 10th ed. Washington, D.C.: National Academy Press, 1989.

Committee on Diet and Health, Food and Nurtition Board. *Diet and Health: Implications for Reducing Chronic Disease Risk.* Washington, D.C.: National Academy Press, 1989.

Duke, James, Ph.D. *The Green Pharmacy.* Pennsylvania: Rodale Press, 1997.

Eades, Michael R. *Thin So Fast.* New York: Warner Books, Inc., 1989.

Fariss, M. "Oxygen Toxicity: Unique Cytoprotective Properties of Vitamin E Succinate in Hepatocytes." *Free Radical Biology and Medicine* 9 (1990).

Goldberg, Burton. *Alternative Medicine: The Definitive Guide.* Tiburon, CA: Future Medicine Publishing. 1997.

Gorner, Peter. "Scientists Try to Tame Molecular 'Sharks.' " *Chicago Tribune,* December 11, 1991, Section 1, p. 1.

Kissir, Susan. "Treat Alcoholism with Nutrition." *Natural Health* (January/February 1993), pp. 48–53.

Lieberman, Shari. *The Real Vitamin and Mineral Book, Second edition.* New York: Avery Publishing Group, 1997.

Long, Patricia. "C of Vitamin." *Hippocrates* (February 1993).

Matz, Robert. "Magnesium: Deficiencies and Therapeutic Uses." *Hospital Practice* (April 30, 1993), pp. 79–92.

McKeown, L.A. "Vitamin E May Cut LDL Oxidation." *Medical Tribune,* April 29, 1993, p. 5.

Mindell, Earl. *Vitamin Bible for the 21st Century.* New York: Warner Books, 1999.

Mindell, Earl and Virginia Hopkins. *Prescription Alternatives.* New York: Keats Publishing, 1998.

Newbold, Herbert L. *Mega-Nutrients: A Prescription for Total Health.* Los Angeles: The Body Press, 1987.

Null, Gary, Ph.D. *The Complete Encyclopedia of Natural Healing.* New York: Kensington Publishing Corporation, 1998.

Olson, Robert E., ed. *Present Knowledge in Nutrition.* 5th ed. Washington, D.C.: The Nutrition Foundation, Inc., 1984.

Pauling, Linus. *Vitamin C and the Common Cold.* New York: Bantam Books, 1971.

Pauling, Linus. *How to Live Longer and Feel Better.* New York: Avon Books, 1986.

Peirce, Andrea. *The American Pharmaceutical Association Practical Guide to Natural Medicines* New York: William Morrow and Co, Inc., 1999.

Priestly, Joan C. "Highly Beneficial Results in the Treatment of AIDS." *Journal of Orthomolecular Medicine* 6, nos. 3 & 4 (1991), pp. 174–180.

Remmington, Dennis, Garth Fisher and Edward Parent. *How to Lower Your Fat Thermostat.* Provo, Utah: Vitality House International, Inc. 1987.

Shils, Maurice and Vernon Young. *Modern Nutrition in Health and Disease.* 7th ed. Philadelphia: Lea & Febiger, 1988.

Skerrett, P.J. "Mighty Vitamins." *Medical World News* (January 1993), pp. 24–32.

Skerrett, P.J. "Fat May Cut Gallstone Risk in Dieters." *Medical Tribune,* March 11, 1993.

Skerrett, P.J. "Low Selenium Linked to Precancerous Colon Polyps." *Medical World News* 34, no. 34 (April 1993).

Theodosakis, Jason, Barry Fox and B. Adderly. *The Arthritis Cure.* New York: St. Martin's Press, 1997.

Tierney, Lawrence M., Jr., M.D., et al., eds. *Current Medical Diagnosis and Treatment.* Norwalk, Connecticut: Appleton & Lange, 1993.

Vinson, J.A. and P. Bose. "Comparative Bioavailability to Humans of Ascorbic Acid Alone or in a Citrus Extract." *American Journal of Clinical Nutrition* 48 (1988).

Voet, Donald and Judith. *Biochemistry.* New York: John Wiley and Sons, 1990.

Werbach, Melvyn R. *Nutritional Influences on Mental Illness: A Sourcebook of Clinical Research.* Tarzana, California: Third Line Press, Inc., 1991.

Werbach, Melvyn R. *Nutritional Influences on Mental Illness: A Sourcebook of Clinical Research.* 2nd ed. Tarzana, California: Third Line Press, Inc., 1993.

Williams, Eleanor R. *Nutritional Principles, Issues, and Applications.* New York: McGraw-Hill, Inc., 1984.

Yudkin, John. *The Penguin Encyclopedia of Nutrition.* Middlesex, England: Penguin Books, 1986.

Web sites:
www.accessexcellence.org
www.all-natural.com
www.bewell.com
www.eatright.org
www.healthy.net
www.mayohealth.org
www.mothernature.com

www.nap.edu
www.newcenturynutrition.com
www.niaid.nih.gov
www.nutritionsciencenews.com
www.planetrx.com
www.realtime.net
www.sciencedaily.com
www.vrg.org
http://lef.org/prod_hpabstracts/php-ab120.html

INDEX